Clinical Embryology for Medical Students

D1340623

Little, Brown's Paperback Book Series

Basic Medical Sciences

Boyd & Hoerl	Basic Medical Microbiology
Colton	Statistics in Medicine
Daube et al.	Medical Neurosciences
Friedman	Biochemistry
Kent	General Pathology: A Programmed Text
Levine	Pharmacology
Miller	Peery & Miller's Pathology
Reich	Hematology
Richardson	Basic Circulatory Physiology
Roland et al.	Atlas of Cell Biology
Selkurt	Physiology
Sidman & Sidman	Neuroanatomy: A Programmed Text
Siegel, Albers, et al.	Basic Neurochemistry
Snell	Clinical Anatomy for Medical Students
Snell	Clinical Embryology for Medical Students
Streilein & Hughes	Immunology: A Programmed Text
Valtin	Renal Dysfunction
Valtin	Renal Function
Watson	Basic Human Neuroanatomy

Clinical Medical Sciences

Clark & MacMahon	Preventive Medicine
Eckert	Emergency-Room Care
Grabb & Smith	Plastic Surgery
Green	Gynecology
Gregory & Smeltzer	Psychiatry
Judge & Zuidema	Methods of Clinical Examination
Nardi & Zuidema	Surgery
Niswander	Obstetrics
Thompson	Primer of Clinical Radiology
Wilkins & Levinsky	Medicine
Ziai	Pediatrics

Manuals and Handbooks

Alpert & Francis	Manual of Coronary Care
Arndt	Manual of Dermatologic Therapeutics
Berk et al.	Handbook of Critical Care
Bochner et al.	Handbook of Clinical Pharmacology
Children's Hospital Medical Center, Boston	Manual of Pediatric Therapeutics
Condon & Nyhus	Manual of Surgical Therapeutics
Friedman & Papper	Problem-Oriented Medical Diagnosis
Gardner & Provine	Manual of Acute Bacterial Infections
Iversen & Clawson	Manual of Orthopaedic Therapeutics
Klippel & Anderson	Manual on Techniques of Emergency and Outpatient Surgery
Massachusetts General Hospital	Clinical Anesthesia Procedures
Massachusetts General Hospital	Diet Manual
Massachusetts General Hospital	Manual of Nursing Procedures
Neelon & Ellis	A Syllabus of Problem-Oriented Patient Care
Papper	Manual of Medical Care of the Surgical Patient
Samuels	Manual of Neurologic Therapeutics
Shader	Manual of Psychiatric Therapeutics
Snow	Manual of Anesthesia
Spivak & Barnes	Manual of Clinical Problems in Internal Medicine: Annotated with Key References
Wallach	Interpretation of Diagnostic Tests
Washington University Department of Medicine	Manual of Medical Therapeutics
Zimmerman	Techniques of Patient Care

Little, Brown and Company
34 Beacon Street
Boston, Massachusetts 02106

By the same author

Clinical Anatomy for Medical Students

Clinical Embryology for Medical Students

Second Edition

Richard S. Snell, M.D., Ph.D.

Professor and Chairman, Department of Anatomy
The George Washington University School of Medicine and Health Sciences
Washington, D.C.

Little, Brown and Company, Boston

To My Students—Past, Present, and Future

Preface

Embryology provides a basis for understanding gross anatomy and an explanation of many of the congenital anomalies that are seen in clinical medicine. The purpose of this book is to give the student a concise account of the development of the human body. At the end of all pertinent chapters there is a description of the more common congenital anomalies that a practicing physician is likely to encounter. References to embryological literature are included so that students can acquire a deeper knowledge of specific areas of interest, should they so desire.

In this second edition, the simple illustrations have been retained and photographs of clinical cases have been added. Clinical problems requiring embryological knowledge for their solution are also presented at the end of each chapter.

This book has not been written with the idea of replacing the larger reference textbooks of embryology. From extensive teaching experience in medical schools in the United States and in Great Britain, and from conversations with senior medical students and faculty colleagues, I have become aware of the need for a concise, simplified account of human development from the clinical point of view. This need has become particularly important in recent years because of the extensive curriculum revisions taking place in many medical schools.

I thank the many students, colleagues, and friends who have consciously or unconsciously stimulated me to write this book. I am most grateful to the following clinical colleagues at The George Washington University Medical Center who have provided me with photographic examples of congenital anomalies: Dr. John P. Adams, Professor and Chairman of Orthopaedic Surgery; Dr. Gordon Avery, Professor of Child Health and Development; Dr. Mervyn Elgart, Associate Professor of Dermatology and of Child Health and Development; Dr. David S. Friendly, Assistant Professor of Ophthalmology and of Child Health and Development; Dr. Pandit Klug, Assistant Professor of Medicine; Dr. Lawrence S. Lessin, Associate Professor of Medicine and of Pathology (Hematology); Dr. Harry Miller, Professor and Chairman, Department of Urology; Dr. Ronald J. Neviaser, Associate Professor of Orthopaedic Surgery; Dr. Mark M. Platt, Associate Professor of Neurology and of Child Health and Development; Dr. Judson G. Randolph, Professor and Director of Pediatric Surgery; Dr. Lewis W. Thompson, Associate Professor and Director of Plastic Surgery.

I am also greatly indebted to Dr. Robert Chase, Emile Holman Professor of Surgery and Chairman, Department of Surgery, Stanford University School of Medicine, Stanford, California, for additional photographs of clinical cases. I wish to extend my sincere thanks to my artists, Mrs. Terry Dolan, Mrs. Virginia Childs, and Mr. Kenneth Finan, for their careful interpretation of my rough sketches for the illustrations, and for their patience in executing the final artwork, and to the librarians of The George Washington University School of Medicine for their help in procuring for me much-needed reference material. I am greatly indebted to Miss Sonia Malitsky for her skill in typing the manuscript.

R. S. S.

Washington, D.C.

Contents

Clinical Embryology for Medical Students

SPERMATOGENESIS

The term *spermatogenesis* is applied to the sequence of events by which spermatogonia are transformed into spermatozoa within the testes.

The Testes and Their Ducts

The testes are paired ovoid organs situated in the scrotum (Fig. 1-1). The descent of the testes from the abdominal cavity into the scrotum (Chap. 16) is important, since it has been found that spermatogenesis will only take place normally if the testes are at a lower temperature than that of the abdominal cavity. Each testis has a thick fibrous capsule, the *tunica albuginea* (Fig. 1-2), which is thickened posteriorly to form the *mediastinum testis*. Extending from the inner surface of the capsule to the mediastinum is a series of fibrous septa which divide the interior of the organ into about 250 lobules. Lying within each lobule are one to three coiled *seminiferous tubules*. Each tubule is in the form of a loop, the ends of which are continuous with a *straight tubule*. The straight tubules open into a network of channels within the mediastinum testis called the *rete testis*. Situated within each lobule between the seminiferous tubules are delicate connective tissue and groups of rounded *interstitial cells* that produce the male sex hormone *testosterone*.

The rete testis is drained by *efferent ductules* into the long much-coiled duct, the *epididymis* (Figs. 1-1 & 1-2), which is situated on the posterior surface of the testis. The duct of the epididymis becomes continuous with the thick-walled *vas deferens*. This emerges from the lower end or *tail* of the epididymis and passes up through the inguinal canal into the abdomen. On reaching the posterior surface of the bladder, it joins the duct of the *seminal vesicle* to form the *ejaculatory duct,* and this in turn opens into the prostatic part of the *urethra*.

Seminiferous Tubule

The wall of the seminiferous tubule (Fig. 1-2) has a basement membrane lined by an epithelium consisting of a number of layers of cells. The basal layer of cells is of two types: the scattered, tall, pyramid-shaped *Sertoli cells,* which extend from the basement membrane to the lumen of the tubule, and, lying between these cells, the numerous germinal cells, the *spermatogonia*. The spermatogonia are of two types, A and B. Type A spermatogonia are the stem cells, which undergo mitotic division to form additional

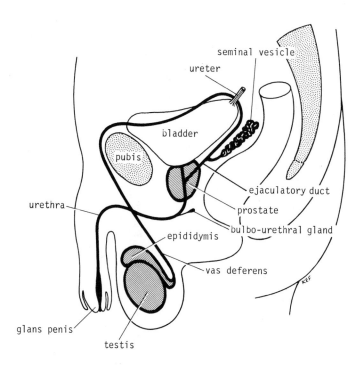

Fig. 1-1. Male reproductive system as seen in sagittal section.

type A spermatogonia and a more differentiated type B spermatogonia. After this division, type B spermatogonia now divide by mitosis into *primary spermatocytes.* The latter cells migrate toward the middle zone of the seminiferous epithelium and then undergo meiotic division into smaller *secondary spermatocytes,* each containing half the number of chromosomes of the primary cell. The secondary spermatocytes soon divide to form the smallest cells, the *spermatids,* which become embedded in the cytoplasm of the free ends of Sertoli cells. The spermatids now undergo a series of morphological changes with the ultimate formation of *spermatozoa.* The nucleus of the spermatid condenses and becomes slightly flattened and elongated in shape. It forms most of the sperm head. Granules within the vacuoles of the Golgi apparatus coalesce to form the *acrosomic granule.* This granule then spreads out over the surface of the nucleus as a thin membrane called the *acrosomal cap.* The centrioles move to the side of the nucleus opposite the acrosomal cap. There, one of the centrioles gives rise to an *axial filament* that grows out and penetrates the cell surface. At the same time the mitochondria migrate toward the axial filament and become arranged around it in the form of a sheath or collar. At the distal end of the mitochondrial collar is a ring-like structure, the *terminal ring.* The collar and terminal ring lie within the *middle piece* or *body* of the spermatozoon. The remainder of the cytoplasm is cast off from the developing spermatozoon and degenerates. The fully formed spermatozoon now leaves the Sertoli cell and becomes free within the lumen of the seminiferous tubule. It has been estimated that the total duration of spermatogenesis is 64 days. The spermatozoon moves successively through the straight tubules, rete testis, and efferent ductules to the epididymis. It is believed that contractile elements in the

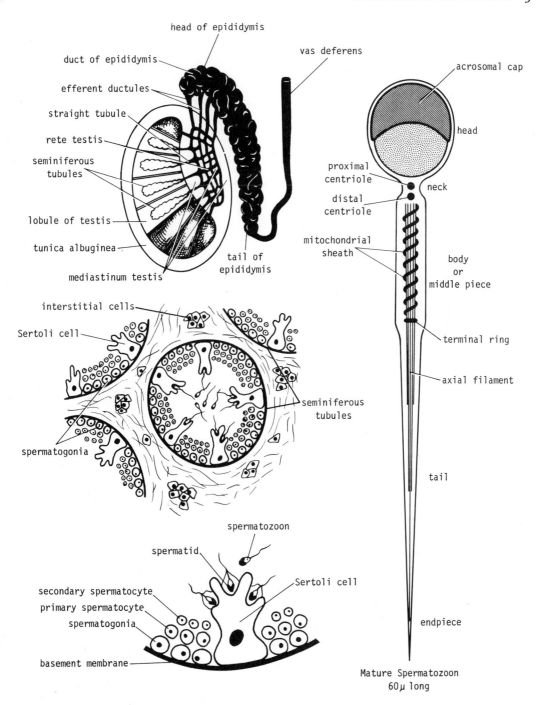

Fig. 1-2. Spermatogenesis.

walls of these tubes are responsible for this movement. The spermatozoon, while lying within the epididymis, undergoes further maturation as seen by the increase in motility and fertilizing power.

Spermatogenesis begins at about 14 years of age, but it does not start at that time unless the testes are in the scrotum. Not all seminiferous tubules are actively producing spermatozoa at the same time. Moreover, areas of germinal epithelium in a single tubule may be active while other areas may be temporarily dormant. Spermatogenesis continues into advanced old age, but after middle age, increasing numbers of atrophic tubules are found.

Mature Spermatozoon

The mature spermatozoon measures about 60 μ in length. The structure of a mature spermatozoon is seen in Figure 1-2. It consists of a *head, neck, body,* and *tail.* The head is formed largely by the condensed nucleus and is covered by the cell membrane. Covering the anterior half of the nucleus under the membrane is the acrosomal cap. Behind the head is the neck containing the two centrioles. The axial filament arises from the distal centriole, and in the body consists of a pair of central fibrils surrounded by two concentric rings of nine fibrils. Outside the concentric rings, a further ring of coarse fibrils is present. Mitochondria are arranged spirally around the axial filament within the middle piece or body. The spiral collar of mitochondria ends distally at a terminal ring. The tail contains the pair of central fibrils surrounded by the two concentric rings of nine fibrils. The outer coarse fibrils are present only at the proximal end of the tail. The fibrils of the tail are enclosed in a sheath of transversely oriented fibrils. Near the end of the tail the sheath is absent. The spermatozoon is covered by a thin layer of cytoplasm and a cell membrane. It is thus seen that the head of the spermatozoon contains the structures responsible for the transmission of genetic information and the remainder of the spermatozoon is concerned with locomotion.

OOGENESIS

The term *oogenesis* is applied to the sequence of events by which oogonia are transformed into ova within the ovaries.

Ovary

The mature ovaries are paired ovoid organs situated within the pelvis (Fig. 1-3). Each is suspended from the posterior surface of the *broad ligament* of the uterus by a short mesentery, the *mesovarium* (Fig. 1-4). The ovaries are surrounded by a thin fibrous capsule, the *tunica albuginea.* This is covered externally by a single layer of cuboid cells called the germinal epithelium. The term *germinal epithelium* is a misnomer, since it does not give rise to ova (for further details see p. 224). The germinal epithelium is a modified area of peritoneum and is continuous with the squamous mesothelial cells of the general peritoneum at the hilum of the ovary where the mesovarium is attached. The ovary has an outer *cortex* and an inner *medulla,* but the division between the two is ill defined. Embedded in the connective tissue of the cortex are the *ovarian follicles* in different stages of development. The medulla consists of very vascular connective tissue.

Ovarian Follicles

During early fetal development primordial germ cells migrate from the yolk sac into the developing ovaries. These cells then differentiate into *oogonia.* By the third prenatal month, the oogonia start to undergo a number of mitotic divisions within the cortex of the ovary to form the *primary oocytes.* The oocytes now enter the prophase of their first meiotic division, and by the time of birth they are in a late stage of prophase of their

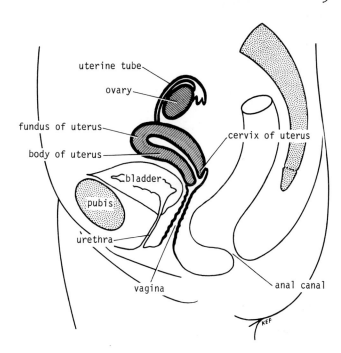

uterine tube

ovary

fundus of uterus

body of uterus

cervix of uterus

bladder

pubis

urethra

vagina

anal canal

KEF

Fig. 1-3. Female reproductive system
as seen in sagittal section.

meiotic division. The primary oocytes become surrounded by a single layer of flattened cells and are known as *primordial
follicles.* The surrounding cells are termed
granulosa cells. Many oogonia and primary
oocytes degenerate during the fifth and sixth
months of fetal life (for details see Chap. 16).
The surviving primordial follicles mainly
occupy the periphery of the cortex. The nucleus of the oocyte is large, pale, and centrally
placed. Little chromatin is seen, but the nu-
cleolus is prominent. The cytoplasm is pale,
and yolk granules are evenly dispersed
throughout it. At birth there may be over
700,000 follicles present in the two ovaries.
The number diminishes with age so that
about 40,000 survive to puberty.

At puberty, as a result of hormonal stimulation from the pituitary, the ovarian cycles
begin. With each cycle, many follicles in both
ovaries start to enlarge, but gradually one
follicle only gains ascendancy and reaches
maturity, while the remainder degenerate
and become *atretic follicles.* As a result, one
ovum normally ovulates during each ovarian

cycle. It has been estimated that only from
300 to 400 follicles come to full maturity and
liberate ova from the ovaries during the reproductive life of a woman.

The primordial follicles increase in size
after puberty in response to the *follicle-
stimulating hormone* (FSH) of the pituitary.
The granulosa cells become cuboid in shape
and begin to divide so that the oocyte is surrounded by a number of layers of granulosa
cells. These cells now secrete around the
oocyte a hyaline material consisting of glyco-
proteins. This material forms the *zona pellucida.* As the oocyte increases in size, irregular spaces filled with clear fluid, the *liquor
folliculi,* appear among the granulosa cells.
These spaces later coalesce to form a single
cavity, the *follicular antrum.* The granulosa
cells, which line the cavity, make up the
membrana granulosa. The oocyte, still surrounded by granulosa cells, the *cumulus
oophorus,* projects into the antrum from one
side. At this stage of development the follicle
is known as a *graafian follicle.* While the follicle has been increasing in size, the sur-

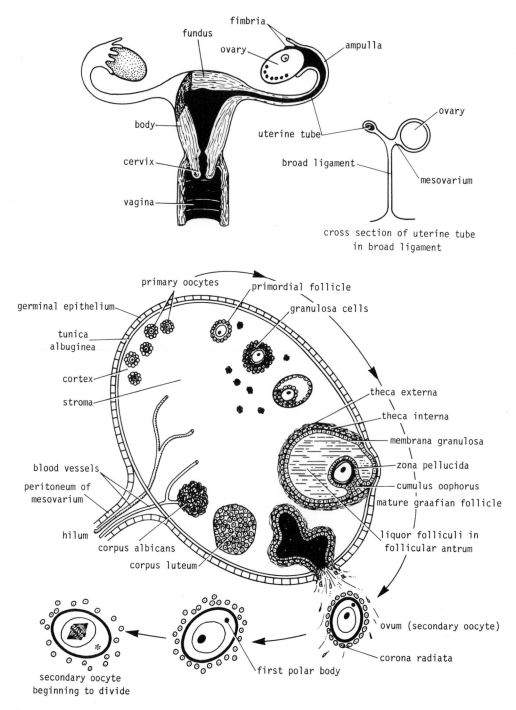

Fig. 1-4. Maturation of an ovarian follicle.

rounding stroma has been differentiating into an inner vascular layer of secretory cells, the *theca interna,* and an outer connective tissue layer, the *theca externa.* After 10 to 14 days of growth, the follicle measures about 10 mm in diameter and bulges slightly from the free surface of the ovary.

As the ovarian follicles mature under the influence of the FSH of the pituitary, the ovary begins to elaborate *estrogens.* The exact site of origin of these hormones is not known, but the cells of the theca interna and the granulosa cells are probably responsible for their genesis.

Ovulation

The meiotic division of the primary oocyte which began during the third month of fetal development is finally completed a few hours before ovulation occurs, and the *secondary oocyte* and the *first polar body* are formed. The first polar body, which receives only a little cytoplasm, lies between the zona pellucida and the cell membrane of the secondary oocyte (Fig. 1-4). As a result of the continued accumulation of liquor folliculi, the tense graafian follicle now ruptures, and the secondary oocyte, the zona pellucida, and the cumulus oophorus, now known as the *corona radiata,* escape into the peritoneal cavity. Immediately after ovulation the secondary oocyte undergoes the second meiotic division to form the *mature ovum* and the *second polar body;* however, this division is not completed until after fertilizaton has taken place. When the second polar body is formed, the first and second polar bodies undergo rapid breakdown and disappear. The mature ovum has a diameter of about 120 μ.

Following ovulation, the walls of the follicle collapse and the cells of the membrana granulosa are thrown into folds. Blood from the ruptured capillaries of the theca interna fills the remains of the antrum and clots. The cells of the membrana granulosa and the theca interna are stimulated by the *luteinizing hormone* (LH) of the pituitary. They enlarge and their cytoplasm accumulates lipid. Later a yellow pigment appears in the cytoplasm. These modified cells are known as *luteal cells,* and together they form the *corpus luteum.* The luteinized theca interna cells continue to produce estrogens, and the luteinized granulosa cells start to produce progesterone. As the result of continued hormonal stimulation from the pituitary, the corpus luteum enlarges for about 10 days after ovulation, reaching a diameter of about 2 cm, when it may be seen on the surface of the ovary as a yellowish projection surrounded by an area of hyperemia. If fertilization does not occur, the LH of the pituitary decreases in amount and the corpus luteum begins to involute. The secretion of progesterone diminishes, and the corpus luteum is finally converted into a fibrous scar, the *corpus albicans.*

Recently, it has been shown that the administration of progesterone will inhibit the process of ovulation. This finding has led to the preparation of contraceptive compounds that may be taken orally and that completely arrest the process of maturation of the follicles. It is of clinical interest to note that the ovaries may be artificially stimulated to ovulate by the administration of the pituitary FSH followed by the chorionic gonadotropic hormone or by treatment with the synthetic nonsteroid *clomiphene.* This may be of value in cases of sterility resulting from anovulation.

CHROMOSOMAL CHANGES DURING SPERMATOGENESIS AND OOGENESIS

In the human somatic cell there are 46 chromosomes, consisting of 22 pairs of *autosomes* and one pair of *sex chromosomes* (XY or XX). The different pairs of autosomes vary in size, but the two members of any given pair of autosomes are identical. The sex chromosomes in the female (XX) are also identical, but in the male there is one X and a much shorter Y chromosome. The spermatogonia and oogonia possess 46 chromosomes. When mitotic division of these cells occurs with the formation of the primary spermatocytes and oocytes, respectively, each chromosome splits longitudinally so that each daughter cell receives the identical number of chromosomes as the mother cell. When the primary spermatocytes and oocytes divide meiotically, the secondary spermatocytes and oocytes receive only half (haploid) the number of chromosomes, i.e., 23. In the male 22 + X chromosomes go to one secondary spermatocyte and 22 + Y chromosomes pass to the other. In the female 22 + X chromosomes pass to the secondary oocyte and 22 + X chromosomes go to the first polar body. The term *first polar body* is given to the very much smaller of the two daughter cells which receives very little cytoplasm from the mother cell.

In the male, the second meiotic division of the secondary spermatocytes to form spermatids takes place so that two spermatids are produced with 22 + X chromosomes and two with 22 + Y chromosomes. In the female, the secondary oocytes divide in a similar manner so that one ovum is formed with 22 + X chromosomes and a *second polar body* is formed (resulting from unequal distribution of cytoplasm from the mother cell) with 22 + X chromosomes. At the same time, the first polar body may divide to form two additional secondary polar bodies. By this means, in the male one spermatogonium with 44 autosomes and one pair of XY chromosomes eventually give rise to 8 spermatozoa. Four of the spermatozoa have 22 autosomes and one X sex chromosome and four have 22 autosomes and one Y sex chromosome. In the female, one oogonium with 44 autosomes and one pair of XX chromosomes eventually give rise to two ova with 22 autosomes and one X sex chromosome.

If fertilization should occur and a spermatozoon with 22 + Y chromosomes enters an ovum with 22 + X chromosomes, a male child will result. If, on the other hand, a spermatozoon with 22 + X chromosomes enters an ovum, a female child will result. The above chromosomal changes are depicted in Figure 1-5.

MALFORMATION OF SPERMATOZOA AND OVA

Abnormal spermatozoa are frequently found in the *semen* (see page 13). Spermatozoa may have abnormally small heads or abnormally large heads. They may have tapering or narrow heads. Spermatozoa with two or more tails or with one tail and two heads may be present. Although having a normal morphological appearance, spermatozoa may lack normal motility. Normal spermatozoa move rapidly and progress in a straight line, while abnormal forms are sluggish and tend to move in a circle or move in an irregular pattern. It is difficult to estimate accurately what percentage of spermatozoa may be abnormal without loss of fertility. It is believed that as many as 10 percent may be abnormal without loss of fertility.

The formation of abnormal ova is believed to be an extremely rare condition. More than one oocyte may be seen in a developing follicle, but these usually degenerate before ovulation takes place.

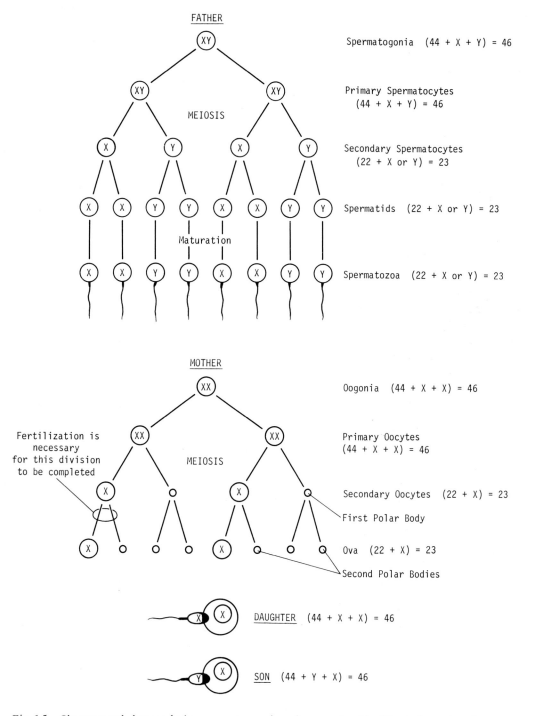

FATHER

Spermatogonia (44 + X + Y) = 46

Primary Spermatocytes
(44 + X + Y) = 46

MEIOSIS

Secondary Spermatocytes
(22 + X or Y) = 23

Spermatids (22 + X or Y) = 23

Maturation

Spermatozoa (22 + X or Y) = 23

MOTHER

Oogonia (44 + X + X) = 46

Fertilization is
necessary
for this division
to be completed

Primary Oocytes
(44 + X + X) = 46

MEIOSIS

Secondary Oocytes (22 + X) = 23

First Polar Body

Ova (22 + X) = 23

Second Polar Bodies

DAUGHTER (44 + X + X) = 46

SON (44 + Y + X) = 46

Fig. 1-5. Chromosomal changes during spermatogenesis and oogenesis with ultimate formation of zygote.

Clinical Problems
Answers on page 427

1. A 75-year-old man visited his physician and asked his advice about marrying a 28-year-old woman. He said that they were very fond of one another and wanted to have children. He was concerned that his advanced age might interfere with his ability to have intercourse and produce viable spermatozoa. Using your knowledge of anatomy and physiology, what advice would you give this patient?

2. A concerned mother consulted a pediatrician about her 14-year-old son. He was starting to date girls and return home late after school dances. When he was a 2-year-old, she had noticed that when he was being bathed he often fondled his penis and displayed erections. She thought he might be "oversexed" and might get a "nice girl into trouble." Using your knowledge of anatomy and physiology, what advice would you give this mother?

3. A 26-year-old male intern at a children's hospital was surprised to see on looking in the shaving mirror that his right parotid and right submandibular regions were swollen. He was also experiencing a slight headache and malaise and noted some discomfort in the parotid region on opening and closing his mouth. The diagnosis of mumps was made, and he was sent home to bed. One week later he developed severe pain in the left testicle. On examination, the right testis was seen to be normal, but the left one was tense, acutely tender, and slightly swollen. The intern had a pyrexia of 101° F. A diagnosis of left-sided orchitis was made secondary to the mumps infection. Using your knowledge of anatomy and physiology, do you think that sterility will follow this infection?

4. An 18-year-old man was medically examined prior to entering the army. On physical examination he was found to have bilaterally undescended testes (cryptorchidism). Based on your knowledge of anatomy and physiology, what advice would you give this patient?

5. A mother asked her physician to explain what is meant by the terms *puberty*, *menarche*, *adolescence*, and *menopause*. She also asked if her daughter could become pregnant once she had started to menstruate. What would you tell this mother?

6. An 18-year-old woman visited her physician for a premarital examination and to discuss conception control. Can you explain the action of contraceptive drugs?

7. A fourth-year medical student was asked in an examination what therapeutic methods exist for the treatment of anovulation associated with secondary amenorrhea. He was also asked if there were any complications associated with the treatment. How would you have answered these questions?

REFERENCES

Baker, G. T. A Quantitative and Cytological Study of Germ Cells in Human Ovaries. *Proc. Roy. Soc.* [*Biol.*] 158:417, 1963.

Bawa, S. R. The Fine Structure of the Sertoli Cell of the Human Testis. *J. Ultrastruct. Res.* 9:459, 1963.

Bishop, D. Sperm Motility. *Physiol. Rev.* 42:1, 1962.

Blandau, R. H., and Rumery, R. E. Fertilizing Capacity of Rat Spermatozoa Recovered from Various Segments of the Epididymis. *Anat. Rec.* 139:209, 1961.

Blandau, R. H., White, B. J., and Rumery, R. E. Observations on the Movements of the Living Primordial Germ Cells in the Mouse. *Fertil. Steril.* 14:482, 1963.

Block, E. A. Quantitative Morphological Investigation of the Follicular System in Newborn Female Infants. *Acta Anat.* 17:201, 1953.

Chiquoine, A. D. The Development of the Zona Pellucida of the Mammalian Ovum. *Amer. J. Anat.* 106:149, 1960.

Clermont, Y., and Huckins, C. Microscopic Anatomy of the Sex Glands and Seminiferous Tubules in Growing and Adult Male Albino Rats. *Amer. J. Anat.* 108:79, 1961.

Clermont, Y., and Leblond, C. P. Renewal of Spermatogonia in the Rat. *Amer. J. Anat.* 93:475, 1953.

Clermont, Y., and Leblond, C. P. Spermiogenesis of Man, Monkey, Ram and Other Mammals as Shown by Periodic Acid–Schiff Technique. *Amer. J. Anat.* 96:229, 1955.

Clermont, Y., and Leblond, C. P. Differentiation and Renewal of Spermatogonia in the Monkey. *Amer. J. Anat.* 104:237, 1959.

Clermont, Y., and Perey, B. Quantitative Study of the Cell Population of the Seminiferous Tubules in Immature Rats. *Amer. J. Anat.* 100:241, 1957.

Denver Conference. A Proposed Standard System of Nomenclature of Human Mitotic Chromosomes. *Lancet* 1:1063, 1960.

Fawcett, D. W. The Structure of Mammalian Spermatozoon. *Int. Rev. Cytol.* 7:195, 1958.

Fawcett, D. W. Sperm Tail Structure in Relation to the Mechanism of Movement. In *Spermatozoon Motility,* edited by D. W. Bishop. American Association for the Advancement of Science, Washington, D.C. Publication No. 72, p. 147.

Fawcett, D. W., and Burgos, M. H. The Fine Structure of Sertoli Cells in Human Testis. *Anat. Rec.* 124:401, 1956.

Ford, C. E., and Hamerton, J. L. The Chromosomes in Man. *Nature* (London) 178:1020, 1956.

Franchi, L. L., Mandl, A. M., and Zuckerman, S. The Development of the Ovary and the Process of Oogenesis. In *The Ovary,* edited by S. Zuckerman, A. M. Mandl, and P. Eckstein. Academic, New York, 1962.

Hamilton, W. J. Phases of Maturation and Fertilization in Human Ova. *J. Anat.* 78:1, 1944.

Mancini, R. E., Narbaitz, R., and Lavieri, J. S. Origin and Development of the Germinative Epithelium and Sertoli Cells in the Human Testis: Cytological, Cytochemical and Quantitative Study. *Anat. Rec.* 136:477, 1960.

Manotaya, T., and Potter, E. L. Oocytes in Prophase of Meiosis from Squash Preparations of Human Fetal Ovaries. *Fertil. Steril.* 14:378, 1963.

Mazia, D. Mitosis and the Physiology of Cell Division. In *The Cell,* edited by J. Brachet and A. E. Mirsky. Academic, New York, 1961. Vol. 3, p. 80.

McCary, J. L. Physiological and Psychological Factors of Sexual Behavior. In *Human Sexuality,* edited by J. L. McCary. Van Nostrand, Princeton, 1967.

McKay, D. G., Hertig, A. T., Adams, E. C., and Danziger, S. Histochemical Observations on the Germ Cells of Human Embryos. *Anat. Rec.* 117:201, 1953.

Ohno, S., Klinger, H. P., and Atkin, N. B. Human Oogenesis. *Cytogenetics* (Basel) 1:42, 1962.

Parkes, A. S. The Reproductive Life Cycle. *Sci. J.* 6:26, 1970.

Pinkerton, H. M., McKay, D. G., Adams, E. C., and Hertig, A. T. Development of the Human Ovary: A Study Using Histochemical Techniques. *Obstet. Gynec.* 18:152, 1961.

Tijo, J. H., and Levan, A. A Chromosome Number in Man. *Hereditas* (Lund) 42:1, 1956.

Witschi, E. Migration of the Germ Cells of the Human Embryos from the Yolk Sac to the Primitive Gonadal Folds. *Contrib. Embryol.* 32:67, 1948.

Zuckerman, S. Origin and Development of Oocytes in Foetal and Mature Mammals. In *Sex Differentiation and Development,* edited by C. R. Austin (*Mem. Soc. Endocrinol.,* No. 7, pp. 63–70). Cambridge University Press, London, 1960.

STORAGE AND TRANSPORT OF SPERMATOZOA

At the conclusion of spermatogenesis, the spermatozoa become detached from the Sertoli cells and lie free in the fluid of the seminiferous tubules. At this stage of their development they are nonmotile and are passively transported in groups into the efferent ductules of the testis and the duct of the epididymis by the contraction of smooth muscle in the walls of these passages and by the action of the ciliated epithelium. The spermatozoa accumulate in the epididymis and are nourished with the secretion of the lining epithelium. About 20 days are required for the spermatozoa to traverse the 4- to 6-meter length of the tortuous duct of the epididymis. During this period they become motile and attain their full physiological state, which they retain for a limited period. If ejaculation does not occur, they degenerate and die.

The introduction of spermatozoa into the vagina involves erection of the penis and ejaculation of the seminal fluid. Friction between the glans penis and the vaginal mucosa, reinforced by other afferent nervous impulses and psychological factors, results in a reflex discharge along the sympathetic nerve fibers to the smooth muscle of the duct of the epididymis and the vas deferens on each side, the seminal vesicles, and the prostate. The smooth muscle contracts and the spermatozoa, together with the secretions of the seminal vesicles and prostate, are discharged into the prostatic urethra. The fluid is now joined by the secretions of the bulbo-urethral glands and penile urethral glands and is then ejected from the penile urethra as a result of the rhythmic contractions of the bulbospongiosus muscle, which compress the urethra. Meanwhile, the sphincter of the bladder contracts and prevents a reflux of the spermatozoa into the bladder. The spermatozoa and the secretions of the several accessory glands constitute the *seminal fluid* or *semen.*

SEMEN

The average volume of the ejaculate is about 3.5 ml. The spermatozoa are suspended in the secretions of the accessory glands termed the *seminal plasma.* The average concentration of spermatozoa is about 100 million per milliliter, and of these about 20 percent are morphologically abnormal and less than 25 percent are nonmotile. The secretion of the seminal vesicles contributes substantially to the volume of the semen. It is rich in fructose, which is a source of energy for the highly motile spermatozoa. The alkaline secretions of the other accessory glands tend to help neutralize the acid contents of the male urethra and the vagina. Following ejaculation, the spermatozoa become actively motile; their tails perform undulating movements which propel them forward and at the same time rotate them on their long axis. The speed varies with the conditions of the environment, but it is about 2 to 3 mm a minute. It has been estimated that about 10 to 20 percent of marriages are sterile, and in about one-third to one-half of these the male is the sterile partner. For this reason, the microscopic and biochemical examination of the semen has become important in childless marriages.

TRANSPORT OF SPERMATOZOA IN THE FEMALE GENITAL TRACT

Immediately upon their arrival in the vagina the spermatozoa are in a hostile environment. The acidity of the vaginal fluid inhibits motility, and the path along which the spermatozoa must travel is against the fluid current set up by the movement of cilia in the uterus and uterine tubes, as this current flows toward the exterior. It is thought that the journey through the uterus and uterine tubes is accomplished mainly by the contraction of the muscle in the walls of these structures rather than by the motility of the spermatozoa. It is believed that the fertilizing ability of spermatozoa does not extend beyond a day or two. Once these cells enter the cervix, the alkaline secretions of the uterus and the uterine tubes help to preserve a favorable environment. As the result of experiments using excised human uteri and

tubes, it has been possible to show that spermatozoa require 70 minutes to reach the lateral ends of the tubes.

TRANSPORT OF THE OVUM THROUGH THE UTERINE TUBE

The extrusion of the ovum from its follicle within the ovary into the peritoneal cavity comprises *ovulation*. The periodic extrusion of an ovum from the ovary and the regular maturation of a group of primordial follicles is referred to as the *ovarian cycle*. As a rule only one ovum is extruded with each cycle, and the ovaries are thought to alternate with an irregular and unpredictable sequence. Ovulation occurs approximately 14 days $\pm$ 1 day before the beginning of the next menstrual bleeding. Once the ovum lies free within the peritoneal cavity, it is sucked into the open fimbriated end of the uterine tube by the currents in the peritoneal fluid caused by the beating of the cilia of the mucous membrane of the tube. The ovum is now moved along the tube by the rhythmic contractions of the muscular walls and the action of the cilia. During the passage, the ovum begins to lose its coat of cumulus cells (corona radiata). It is not known exactly for how long the ovum remains fertilizable within the tube, but the period is probably less than 1 day. If fertilization does not take place, the ovum begins to degenerate.

FERTILIZATION

This is the fusion of a spermatozoon with an ovum to form a single cell, the *zygote* (Figs. 2-1 & 2-2). Only one spermatozoon of the many millions that are deposited in the female genital tract with a single ejaculation is required to fertilize an ovum. Fertilization usually takes place in the lateral third of the uterine tube. When the motile spermatozoon

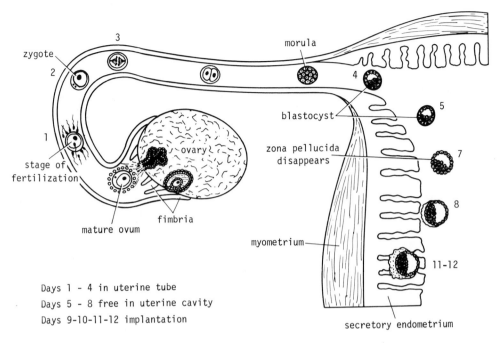

Fig. 2-1. The successive changes which take place in the ovum, zygote, and blastocyst while passing along the uterine tube and entering the uterine cavity to become implanted in the endometrium. Numbers signify days after ovulation.

reaches the zona pellucida of the ovum, the sperm head starts to penetrate this layer. It is thought that enzymes present in the acrosomal cap may assist in this process. Once the head of the spermatozoon has pierced the zona pellucida, the movement of the tail ceases, and the entire spermatozoon, including the tail, is engulfed by the cytoplasm of the ovum and drawn inward. Immediately following the penetration of the ovum by one spermatozoon, the permeability of the zona pellucida changes so that even though other competing spermatozoa become attached to the zona, they usually do not succeed in gaining entrance to the ovum. During this process, the second polar body is extruded from the ovum and the remaining 22 + X chromosomes reconstitute themselves into a nucleus called the *female pronucleus.* The nucleus of the head of the spermatozoon be-

comes swollen and forms the *male pronucleus;* the body and tail disintegrate and disappear (Fig. 2-2). The two pronuclei now meet in the center of the ovum. Two centrioles, probably derived from the anterior centriole of the spermatozoon, now appear. Meanwhile each pronucleus loses its nuclear membrane and resolves its chromatin into a complete single set of chromosomes (i.e., 23 each). Thereafter the chromosomes become organized on the spindle and the 23 paternal and 23 maternal chromosomes split longitudinally at the centromere and a normal mitotic division occurs. This is the first *cleavage division* (Fig. 2-2). Fertilization thus results in the reassociation of the male and female chromosomes and restores the full diploid number. The determination of the sex of the zygote has been achieved and cleavage has been initiated. From experi-

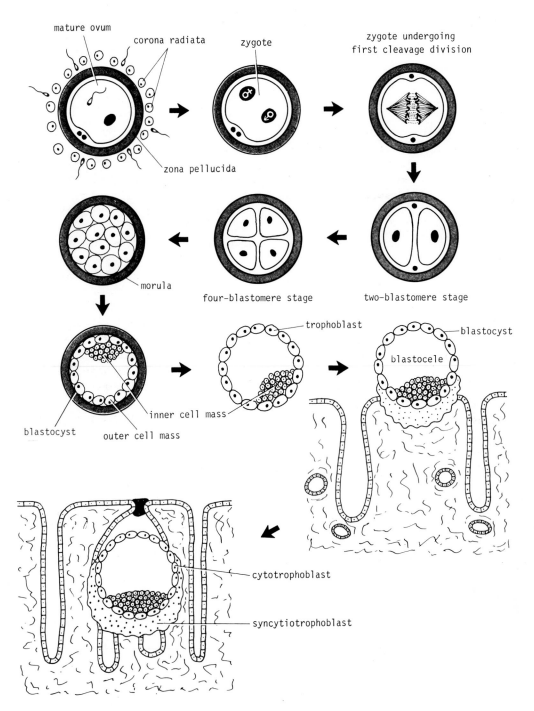

Fig. 2-2. Stages of fertilization, cleavage, and implantation.

ments, it is believed that the zygote reaches the two-cell stage at about 30 hours after fertilization.

CLEAVAGE

The term *cleavage* is given to the rapid succession of mitotic divisions which produce a large number of smaller cells called *blastomeres*. With each division, the cell size becomes smaller. Experiments in vitro show that the four-cell stage occurs at about 40 to 50 hours after fertilization. The large numbers of new cells are located internal to the zona pellucida; collectively they have the appearance of a mulberry and are known as the *morula* (Fig. 2-2). As cell division continues, the morula is slowly propelled down the uterine tube by the peristaltic waves of contraction of the muscle in its wall and the beating of the cilia of the columnar cells of the lining mucous membrane. The secretions of the glandular cells of the mucous membrane provide a fluid vehicle which helps in the transport of the morula along the tube and also provides some nourishment for the actively dividing cells. At about the twelve- to sixteen-cell stage, the morula enters the uterine cavity 5 to 8 days after ovulation. Glandular secretion from the uterine cavity passes through the zona pellucida and diffuses between the cells of the morula. At this stage the morula consists of a group of centrally placed cells, the *inner cell mass*, completely surrounded by a layer of cells, the *outer cell mass* (Fig. 2-2). It should be noted that while these various processes have been taking place, the total size of the morula has not significantly increased within the zona pellucida, since at each cell division the blastomeres were reduced in size. Cleavage is thus a fractionating process rather than a process of growth; i.e., no new protoplasm has been formed. From future development, it is known that the cells of the inner cell mass develop into the tissues of the *embryo* and those of the outer cell mass form the *trophoblast*.

FORMATION OF THE BLASTOCYST

As the fluid in the intercellular spaces within the morula gradually increases in amount, the spaces on one side of the inner cell mass become confluent, forming a single cavity, the *blastocele* (Fig. 2-2). The inner cell mass is thus attached at one pole of the morula to the inner surface of the cells of the outer cell mass. At this time the morula is known as the *blastocyst*. The zona pellucida now disappears. With further accumulation of fluid within the blastocele, the cells of the outer cell mass become flattened and are known as the *trophoblast*. While floating freely within the uterine cavity, the blastocyst receives its nourishment and oxygen requirements from the secretions of the endometrial glands. The young embryo is now ready to become attached to the uterine wall. This probably occurs between the fifth and ninth days after ovulation.

PREPARATION OF THE UTERINE ENDOMETRIUM TO RECEIVE THE BLASTOCYST

During the growth of the graafian follicle up to the stage of ovulation, estrogen alone is secreted by the ovary, and this gives rise to the *proliferative changes* in the endometrium (Fig. 2-3). On about the fifth or sixth day of the menstrual cycle, when the damage resulting from the menstrual period has been repaired, proliferative changes begin. The endometrium is initially thin and consists of a ciliated columnar epithelium that dips down into a loose stroma to form simple tubular glands. During the sixth to fourteenth days, the endometrium thickens, be-

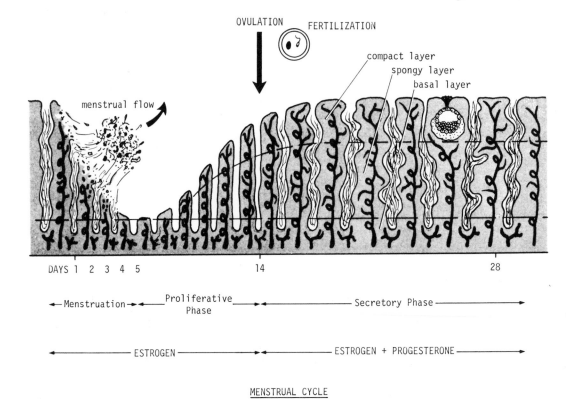

OVULATION   FERTILIZATION

compact layer
spongy layer
basal layer

menstrual flow

DAYS 1 2 3 4 5   14   28

←—Menstruation—→←—Proliferative Phase—→←———— Secretory Phase ————→

←———— ESTROGEN ————→←———— ESTROGEN + PROGESTERONE ————→

MENSTRUAL CYCLE

Fig. 2-3. Changes in the endometrium during different phases of the menstrual cycle. If fertilization occurs, the blastocyst becomes embedded in the secretory endometrium about 10 to 12 days after ovulation.

comes more vascular, and the glands elongate and become dilated in their deeper part. Once the corpus luteum is formed, it starts to secrete progesterone and the theca interna continues to produce estrogen. The combined action of these two hormones produces the *secretory changes* in the endometrium. The endometrium increases in thickness and the glands become long and tortuous and distended with secretion that is rich in glycogen, mucopolysaccharides, and lipid. The stroma cells proliferate, enlarge, and become closely packed. The arteries are very coiled and congested and are known as the *spiral arteries*.

It is thus seen that the various changes that take place in the endometrium during the second half of the menstrual cycle may be regarded as the preparation of the uterine lining for the nourishment and reception of the blastocyst.

If the ovum is fertilized, the corpus luteum continues to increase in size until the fourth month of pregnancy. During this time it actively produces progesterone, and the secretory activity of the endometrium increases. The corpus luteum is controlled by the gonadotropic hormone produced by the pituitary; it is also believed that this hormone is produced by the trophoblast cells. At the end of the fourth month, the corpus luteum starts to degenerate, and, although it is still present at the end of the pregnancy, progesterone production after the fourth month is taken over by the placenta. As the result of this mechanism, the thick endometrium is maintained throughout pregnancy.

Should fertilization not occur, the corpus luteum degenerates and the endometrium is deprived suddenly of the supporting action of estrogen and progesterone. The spiral arteries constrict and the blood supply to the superficial zone of the endometrium is cut off. After a variable time, the constricted arteries open up, the walls of the damaged vessels in the superficial part of the endometrium rupture, and blood pours into the stroma disrupting the tissue. The process leads to hemorrhage into the uterine cavity and the shedding of all but the deepest part of the endometrium. The *menstrual flow* thus consists of blood, partially disintegrated epithelium and stroma, and secretions of the endometrial glands. The deep or basal parts of the endometrium are supplied by their own arteries, the *basal arteries,* which do not undergo constriction. The epithelial cells forming the blind ends of the glands in the basal endometrium will multiply and repair the denuded surface of the endometrium and so the proliferative changes will begin once again.

It is important to note that the high level of excretion of the gonadotropic hormone in the urine during the early stages of pregnancy forms the basis for the *Aschheim-Zondek reaction* and the other diagnostic tests of pregnancy.

IMPLANTATION

The endometrium of the uterus reaches its maximum thickness (5 mm) and development during the secretory phase of the menstrual cycle (Fig. 2-3). Three distinct layers can be recognized: the superficial *compact layer,* an intermediate *spongy layer,* and a thin *basal layer.*

The blastocyst enters the uterine cavity between the fourth and ninth days after ovulation, and, with the disappearance of the zona pellucida, the outer surface of the trophoblast comes into direct contact with the endometrium and adheres to it. The adherence and attachment of the blastocyst to the endometrium are referred to as *implantation* (Figs. 2-1—2-3). Normal implantation takes place in the endometrium of the body of the uterus, most frequently on the upper part of the posterior wall near the midline. Usually the blastocyst becomes attached between the openings of the endometrial glands, but occasionally it lodges within the mouth of one of the glands. In the region of contact between the blastocyst and the endometrium, the trophoblast cells start to proliferate so that the wall of the blastocyst becomes thickened. In this area the trophoblast cells become differentiated into an inner *cytotrophoblast* (Fig. 2-2) composed of a single layer of individual cells which are contiguous to the inner cell mass and a thick outer layer, the *syncytiotrophoblast,* in which the cell boundaries are lost. The part of the trophoblast wall of the blastocyst that projects into the uterine cavity remains thin. As the result of enzymatic and physical influences by the trophoblast, the uterine epithelium in the area of attachment starts to degenerate and break down. It is believed that the trophoblast has the ability to absorb the products of cellular breakdown that are utilized to nourish the developing embryo. By the eleventh or twelfth day, the blastocyst sinks beneath the surface epithelium and becomes completely embedded in the stroma of the compact zone of the endometrium (Fig. 2-2). The defect in the endometrial surface is closed by blood clot, and later by the proliferation of the surrounding surface epithelium.

In some individuals, sufficient bleeding may occur to simulate the beginning of the menstrual period which would be expected about this time. This *implantation bleeding* is of clinical importance, since it may result in an erroneous calculation of the duration of pregnancy.

ABNORMAL PHENOMENA

Sterility

About 10 to 20 percent of marriages are sterile, and in one-third to one-half of these the male is the responsible partner. From the previous description it can be understood that for successful fertilization to occur many different cellular processes must take place normally and the male and female reproductive organs, including the external genitalia, must be functioning correctly. The ovaries and testes may be incapable of producing mature, competent ova or spermatozoa owing to hormonal, inflammatory (e.g., mumps), or genetic reasons. Ovulation may take place at irregular and infrequent intervals. A seminal analysis on a masturbation specimen may show a reduced volume of semen, a reduced number of spermatozoa, a reduced motility of the spermatozoa, or an excessive number of abnormal forms of spermatozoa. Inflammatory disease and resulting fibrosis may cause narrowing or blockage of the male and female ducts and tubes (e.g., gonorrhea, tuberculosis). The uterine cavity may be narrowed or distorted by a tumor. The presence of pathogenic bacteria in the vagina and cervix may alter the chemical composition of the secretions to such an extent that spermatozoa cannot survive. Congenital defects in the formation of the penis (hypospadias, epispadias), vagina (double vagina, imperforate vagina, intact hymen), or uterus (rudimentary uterus) may make coitus and insemination difficult or impossible. Psychological factors in the male may cause impotence or premature ejaculation. Age is an important factor in relation to fertility, and it has been found that fertility in both the male and the female diminishes after the age of 35. The general health of the partners must be considered; excessive obesity, diabetes, and chronic nephritis, for example, may be responsible for infertility.

Abnormal Implantation

Hertig has found that blastocysts do occur which show defective blastomeres and abnormal development of the trophoblast. It is not possible to estimate the number of abortions that result from this cause, but it is believed to be considerable. The blastocyst may become attached to an endometrial excrescence or polyp, and this may lead to an early death of the embryo. It has been shown that the zygote or blastocyst is susceptible to maternal infections that modify its development, e.g., German measles. Genetic defects in the zygote may also result in failure of implantation.

Abnormal Sites of Implantation

In Figure 2-4 the different abnormal sites of implantation of the fertilized ovum are shown. In order of frequency they occur as follows: (1) region of the internal os of the cervix, (2) ampulla of the uterine tube, (3) isthmus of the uterine tube, (4) angle of the uterine cavity, (5) infundibulum of the uterine tube, (6) ovary, (7) interstitial portion of the uterine tube, (8) peritoneum of the broad ligament, mesentery of the intestine or rectouterine pouch, and (9) pregnancy in a rudimentary uterine horn.

Implantation of the blastocyst outside the uterine cavity is referred to as an *ectopic pregnancy*. The blastocyst buries itself in the extra-uterine structure as the result of the destructive action of the trophoblast. If this takes place within the uterine tube, early abortion occurs with or without rupture of the tube and is accompanied by considerable hemorrhage. This usually takes place between the sixth and tenth weeks of pregnancy. Very rarely the tube slowly ruptures

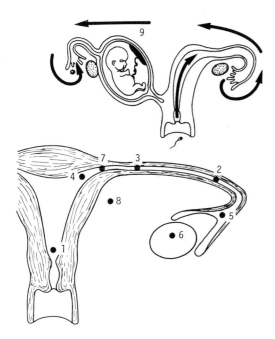

Fig. 2-4. Abnormal sites of implantation in order of frequency: (1) region of internal os of cervix, (2) ampulla of uterine tube, (3) isthmus of uterine tube, (4) angle af uterine cavity, (5) infundibulum, (6) ovary, (7) interstitial portion of uterine tube, (8) peritoneum, (9) rudimentary uterine horn (arrows indicate path taken by sperm to accomplish fertilization).

and the developing fetus enlarges into the abdominal cavity to reach full term. This is known as *tubo-abdominal pregnancy.* In ovarian pregnancy, implantation occurs in the stroma of the ovary and the ovarian tissue generally ruptures early, but cases have been recorded in which the pregnancy continued to term.

The occurrence of a *rudimentary horn of the uterus* is described in Chapter 16, where congenital anomalies of the uterus are discussed. In the great majority of cases, no canal exists between the cavity of the rudimentary horn and the cervix (Fig. 2-4). For implantation to occur, it is believed that a spermatozoon passes up the normal uterine tube, escapes into the peritoneal cavity, and

crosses over to the region of the opposite ovary, where it fertilizes the ovum. The zygote then passes into the rudimentary horn, where it is implanted. In the majority of cases, the rudimentary horn ruptures early in pregnancy. Very rarely the pregnancy advances to full term, when a spurious labor occurs and the fetus dies.

Excessive Proliferation of the Trophoblast

This may lead to the condition of *hydatidiform mole.* The trophoblastic outgrowths become converted into masses of vesicles which may be as large as grapes. This condition occurs in about one in two thousand pregnancies and is most common in certain parts of southeast Asia. The uterus may become filled with the vesicles and the fetus dies (Figs. 2-5 & 2-6). Excessively large quantities of *chorionic gonadotropin* are produced by

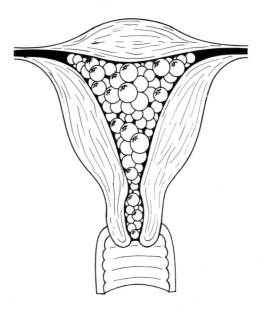

Fig. 2-5. Uterine cavity filled with vesicles (hydatidiform mole) produced by the excessive proliferation of the trophoblast.

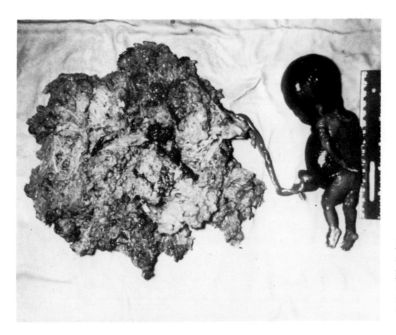

Fig. 2-6. Hydatidiform mole and aborted fetus. The trophoblastic outgrowths have become converted into masses of vesicles. (Courtesy of Dr. G. Avery.)

the trophoblast and it appears in the urine. This fact may be used in making a diagnosis.

Chorionepithelioma

This is a rare disease, and over half of the cases occur following hydatidiform mole. It presents as persistent or repeated uterine bleeding following abortion, normal pregnancy, or hydatidiform mole. A chorionepithelioma is a malignant tumor of the chorionic villi and produces chorionic gonadotropin in large quantities. The test for this hormone in the urine greatly assists in making a diagnosis.

Clinical Problems

Answers on page 429

1. A 28-year-old woman visited her gynecologist because she had failed to conceive after 4 years of marriage. She stated that she had normal and satisfying coital relations with her husband, but they were both saddened by having no children. What percentage of couples with involuntary sterility exists in the United States? What is the frequency of the various factors responsible for sterility?

2. A young married couple concerned at not having children sought advice from their physician. What general disorders or drugs do you know of that could affect the genital tract and produce sterility?

3. A 19-year-old man was recently operated on for a left-sided varicocele (dilatation of the veins draining the testis). He asked his physician whether or not the varicocele or the surgical operation was likely to produce sterility. What would you tell this patient?

4. While considering the possible causes of sterility, a physician should know the common diseases that directly involve the genital tract in both sexes. Name some of the more important diseases.

5. After reviewing a case of infertility in a 23-year-old woman, it was decided to carry out a series of examinations. Using your knowledge of anatomy and physiology, what tests would you perform?

6. What special tests could you perform on a male who you may believe is responsible for a sterile marriage?

7. A freshman medical student, concerned about the population explosion, as well as regarding a vasectomy as a matter of convenience, decided to have one performed. Just as the surgeon was about to apply the scalpel, the student hastily asked whether or not he was likely to suffer from any unpleasant side-effects following the vasectomy. He also wished to know if it would be possible for him to have another operation later to restore the continuity of the vas deferens and so allow him to reproduce. What would you have told the student?

8. A 30-year-old woman wished to remarry following the death of her husband. She had had a bilateral tubal ligation 5 years previously and was inquiring whether or not it would be possible to have an operation to become fertile again. Is it possible to reconstruct a uterine tube following its division or ligation?

9. A medical student who enjoyed the company of the opposite sex read in a medical journal an article on the "morning-after pill." He wanted to know whether or not it successfully prevented conception, and, if so, how it worked. What would you tell him?

10. A 19-year-old woman admitted to the emergency ward complained of severe spasmodic pain in the right iliac fossa. Just prior to admission, the pain had sud-denly intensified, and the patient had collapsed. On physical examination the patient was observed to have the signs and symptoms of internal hemorrhage. There was extreme tenderness in the right iliac fossa and some rigidity of the abdominal muscles. On questioning about her menstrual history, she disclosed that she had missed her last period. The attending physician made a diagnosis of a ruptured ectopic pregnancy. Using your knowledge of embryology, can you explain where implantation normally occurs? What changes take place in the uterine tube if implantation occurs in the tube?

11. A 45-year-old woman was delighted to learn that she was pregnant. Her first prenatal examination had shown her to be physically fit, and she looked forward to having a normal delivery. During the fifth month of her pregnancy she started to have vaginal bleeding, and on one occasion she noted what she thought looked like grapes mixed up with the blood. On physical examination the uterus was found to be softer than normal and was at least 1 month larger than normal for the estimated date of delivery. No fetal heart sounds could be heard, and no fetal structures were recognized on abdominal palpation. Laboratory examination of her urine showed an excessively high level of chorionic gonadotropin. What is your diagnosis?

12. A 30-year-old woman received a thorough uterine curettage for the treatment of hydatidiform mole. She was asked by her gynecologist to visit him every 2 weeks for 3 months, then every month for 1 year. At each visit she was given a thorough physical examination and her chorionic gonadotropin titers were measured. One month after her curettage she complained of further vaginal bleeding. On examination a purplish-red hemorrhagic swelling was

seen on the cervix. Her chorionic gonadotropin titer was markedly raised. A chest x-ray revealed a slight opacity in the lower lobe of the left lung. Using your knowledge of embryology, make the diagnosis.

REFERENCES

Austin, C. R. Fertilization and Transport of the Ovum. In *Mechanics Concerned with Conception,* edited by C. G. Hartman. Macmillan, New York, 1963. P. 285.

Austin, C. R. Ultrastructural Changes During Fertilization. In *Preimplantation Stages of Pregnancy,* edited by G. E. W. Wolstenholme and M. O'Connor. Little, Brown, Boston, 1965. P. 3.

Austin, C. R., and Bishop, M. W. H. Role of the Rodent Acrosome and Perforatorium in Fertilization. *Proc. Roy. Soc.* [*Biol.*] 149:241, 1958.

Bickers, W. Sperm Migration and Uterine Contractions. *Fertil. Steril.* 11:286, 1960.

Bishop, D. W., and Tyler, A. Fertilizing of Mammalian Eggs. *J. Exp. Zool.* 132:575, 1956.

Black, D. L., and Asdell, S. A. Transport Through the Rabbit Oviduct. *Amer. J. Physiol.* 192:63, 1958.

Blandau, R. J. Biology of Eggs and Implantation. In *Sex and Internal Secretions,* 3d ed., edited by W. C. Young. Williams & Wilkins, Baltimore, 1961. Vol. 2, p. 797.

Boyd, J. D., and Hamilton, W. J. Cleavage, Early Development, and Implantation of the Egg. In *Marshall's Physiology of Reproduction,* 3d ed., edited by A. S. Parkes. Little, Brown, Boston, 1952. Vol. 2, p. 1.

Enders, A. C., and Schlafke, S. J. Fine Structure of the Blastocyst. In *Preimplantation Stages of Pregnancy,* edited by G. E. W. Wolstenholme and M. O'Connor. Little, Brown, Boston, 1965. P. 29.

Green, T. H., Jr. *Gynecology: Essentials of Clinical Practice,* 2d ed. Little, Brown, Boston, 1971.

Hamilton, W. J. Phases of Maturation and Fertilization in Human Ova. *J. Anat.* 78:1, 1944.

Hamilton, W. J. Early Stages of Human Development. *Ann. Roy. Coll. Surg. Eng.* 4:281, 1949.

Harper, M. J. K., Bennett, J. P., Boursnell, J. C., and Rowson, L. E. A. An Autoradiographic Method for the Study of Egg Transport in the Rabbit Fallopian Tube. *J. Reprod. Fertil.* 1:249, 1960.

Hertig, A. T., Adams, E. C., and Mulligan, N. J. On the Pre-Implantation Stages of the Human Ovum: A Description of Four Normal and Four Abnormal Specimens Ranging from the Second to the Fifth Day of Development. *Contrib. Embryol.* 35:199, 1954.

Hertig, A. T., Rock, J., and Adams, E. C. A Description of 34 Human Ova Within the First 17 Days of Development. *Amer. J. Anat.* 98:435, 1956.

Lewis, B. V., and Harrison, R. G. A Presomite Human Embryo Showing a Yolk-Sac Duct. *J. Anat.* 100:389, 1966.

Lewis, W. H., and Hartman, C. G. Early Cleavage Stages of the Egg of the Monkey (Macacus Rhesus). *Contrib. Embryol.* 24:187, 1933.

Lloyd, C. W., and Leathem, J. H. Physiology of the Female Reproductive Tract. In *Human Reproduction and Sexual Behavior,* edited by C. W. Lloyd. Lea & Febiger, Philadelphia, 1964. P. 70.

Mann, T. *The Biochemistry of Semen.* Methuen, London, 1954.

Mann, T. Semen. In *Scientific Foundations of Obstetrics and Gynaecology,* edited by E. E. Philipp, J. Barnes, and M. Newton. Davis, Philadelphia, 1970. P. 41.

Masters, W. H., and Johnson, V. E. *Human Sexual Response.* Little, Brown, Boston, 1966.

Ohno, S., Klinger, H. P., and Atkin, N. B. Human Oogenesis. *Cytogenetics* (Basel) 1:42, 1962.

Roland, M. *Management of the Infertile Couple.* Thomas, Springfield, Ill., 1968.

Schwartz, R., Brooks, N., and Zinsser, H. H. Evidence of Chemotaxis as a Factor in Sperm Motility. *Fertil. Steril.* 9:300, 1958.

Shettles, L. B. *Ovum Humanum.* Hafner, New York, 1960.

Sobrero, A. J. Sperm Migration in the Female Genital Tract. In *Mechanisms Concerned with Conception,* edited by C. G. Hartman. Macmillan, New York, 1963. P. 173.

Szollosi, D. G., and Ris, H. Observations on Sperm Penetration in the Rat. *J. Biophys. Biochem. Cytol.* 10:275, 1961.

Turner, C. D. *General Endocrinology,* 4th ed. Saunders, Philadelphia, 1966.

Westman, A. Investigations into the Transit of Ova in Man. *J. Obstet. Gynaec. Brit. Comm.* 44:821, 1937.

Zuckerman, S., ed. *The Ovary.* Academic, New York, 1962. Vols. 1 and 2.

Further Development of the Trophoblast; the Formation and Differentiation of the Three Germ Layers

3

FURTHER DEVELOPMENT OF THE TROPHOBLAST

As has been shown in Chapter 2, the process of implantation commences about the sixth day, and by the eleventh or twelfth day the blastocyst has sunk beneath the surface epithelium of the endometrium and is embedded in the compact layer of the stroma (Fig. 3-1). The site of implantation may be recognized as a small elevated area of endometrium having a central pore filled with blood clot. Once the blastocyst begins to sink into the substance of the endometrium, more and more of its surface comes into contact with the endometrial stroma. As a result, the differentiation of the trophoblast into two layers continues until the entire trophoblast is made up of an *inner cytotrophoblast* and an *outer syncytiotrophoblast* (Fig. 3-2). Meanwhile the trophoblast continues to penetrate deeper into the endometrium, but the blastocyst remains confined to the compact layer and never lies deeper than a few millimeters from the surface. Vacuoles appear in the syncytiotrophoblast which coalesce to form large irregular spaces known as *lacunae*. The lacunae contain fluid stained with maternal blood.

DIFFERENTIATION OF THE INNER CELL MASS AND THE FORMATION OF TWO GERM LAYERS (TWELFTH DAY)

On the surface of the inner cell mass, which faces the cavity of the blastocyst, a single layer of flattened cells, the *entoderm,* appears. The remaining cells of the inner cell mass which are continuous with the trophoblast form the *ectoderm.* Between the ectoderm cells a space appears called the *amniotic cavity.* The "floor" of the amniotic cavity is formed by a single layer of columnar cells called the *embryonic ectoderm.* The remainder of the amniotic cavity is lined with *amniotic ectoderm.* Meanwhile a second cavity is formed below the entoderm, called the *primary yolk sac.* The origin of the cells that line the wall of the sac is not exactly known but it is thought that the entodermal cells are contributors. The cells destined to form the embryo are now clearly defined, in the form of a bilaminar *embryonic disc* (Figs. 3-1 & 3-2). The upper surface of the disc is formed by the columnar cells of the embryonic ectoderm, and the lower surface of the disc is formed by the flattened cells of the entoderm (Fig. 3-2).

Meanwhile the cytotrophoblast cells pro-

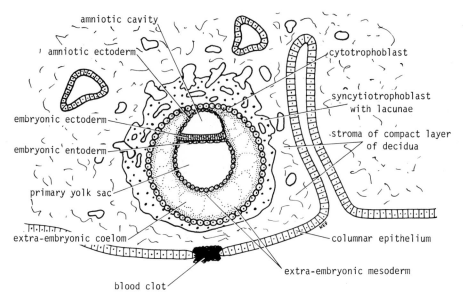

Fig. 3-1. Cross section of 11-day-old blastocyst showing the formation of two germ layers. Also shown are the amniotic cavity, the primary yolk sac, and the extra-embryonic coelom. The trophoblast has differentiated into the syncytiotrophoblast with lacunae and the cytotrophoblast.

liferate and the newly formed cells enter the fluid-filled blastocyst cavity to form a loosely arranged tissue, the *extra-embryonic meso-derm.* Later the intercellular spaces in the extra-embryonic mesoderm coalesce to form a large cavity, the *extra-embryonic coelom.* This new space surrounds the amniotic cavity and the primary yolk sac except where the extra-embryonic mesoderm remains as a connection between the embryonic disc and the trophoblast called the *connecting stalk* or *body stalk* (Fig. 3-2). The amniotic ecto-dermal cells forming the roof of the amniotic cavity gradually sever their connection with the trophoblast, and the body stalk takes over the function of firmly attaching the growing embryo to the trophoblast.

At about this time the entodermal cells become further rearranged so that a small *secondary yolk sac,* the yolk sac proper, is pinched off from the primary yolk sac in the region of the embryonic disc. The cavity of the yolk sac is completely lined with ento-derm. For purposes of description, the ento-derm may be divided into two types accord-ing to its position: *embryonic entoderm,* forming part of the embryo, and *yolk sac entoderm,* lining the remainder of the yolk sac cavity. The remnants of the primary yolk sac soon disappear.

With the formation of the extra-embryonic coelom, the extra-embryonic mesodermal cells become divided into two areas: *somato-pleuric mesoderm,* covering the ectoderm of the amniotic cavity and lining the tropho-blast, and *splanchnopleuric mesoderm,* cover-ing the entoderm of the secondary yolk sac. The trophoblast with its lining of somato-pleuric mesoderm is now known as the *chorion.*

THE PRIMITIVE STREAK AND THE FORMATION OF THE THIRD GERM LAYER

As growth proceeds, the embryonic disc, when viewed from inside the amniotic cavity, soon becomes pear-shaped and on its narrow

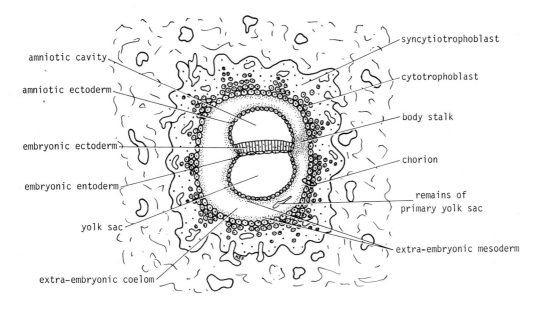

Fig. 3-2. Longitudinal section of 13-day-old blastocyst showing the formation of the body stalk as a condensation of extra-embryonic mesoderm extending from the embryonic disc to the trophoblast.

caudal end there appears an opaque streak, the *primitive streak* (Fig. 3-3). The opacity is caused by a proliferation of ectoderm cells which become heaped up to form a linear thickening. The cephalic end of the primitive streak is swollen and is known as the *primitive knot,* or *Hensen's node.* The ectodermal cells of the primitive streak undergo further proliferation and extend laterally, cephalically, and caudally between the ectoderm and entoderm of the embryonic disc. These cells form the third germ layer, the *embryonic mesoderm* (Fig. 3-3).

At first the mesodermal cells have an epithelial appearance; later many become loosely arranged, irregular in shape, and display ameboid activity. Such cells form a very loose tissue referred to as *mesenchyme.* As the mesodermal cells extend laterally, they finally reach and fuse with the extra-embryonic mesoderm of the amnion and yolk sac. At the cephalic end of the embryonic disc, the ectodermal and entodermal layers fuse over a

small area which later becomes the *buccopharyngeal membrane.* In a similar manner, at the caudal end of the embryonic disc, the ectodermal and entodermal layers fuse to form the *cloacal membrane.* The process of mesodermal extension cephalically and caudally between the ectoderm and entoderm continues until they fuse in the midline. It should be noted, however, that the mesoderm does not extend between the ectoderm and entoderm of the buccopharyngeal and cloacal membranes. At the caudal end of the embryonic disc, the mesoderm, having passed around the cloacal membrane, becomes continuous with the extra-embryonic mesoderm of the *body stalk* (Figs. 3-3 & 3-4).

FORMATION OF THE NOTOCHORD

While the primitive streak is giving rise to the embryonic mesoderm, a solid cord of cells grows cephalically from the primitive knot

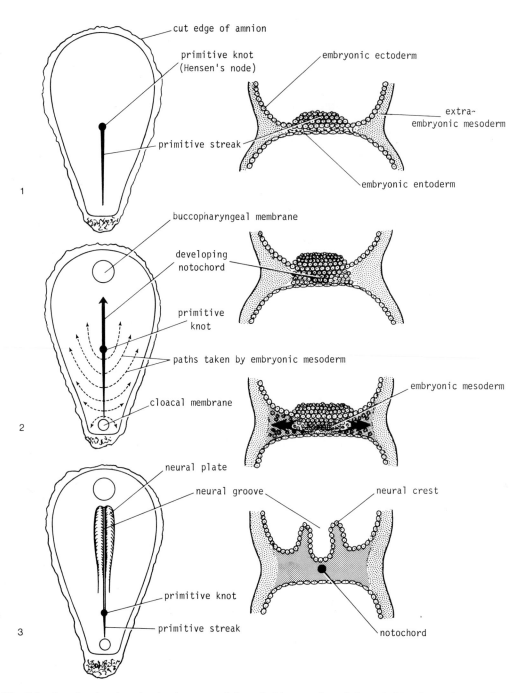

Fig. 3-3. A series showing the development of the primitive streak and the primitive knot, the notochord, and the appearance of the neural groove. The embryonic mesoderm spreads out between the ectoderm and entoderm, finally fusing with the extra-embryonic mesoderm at the edge of the embryonic disc.

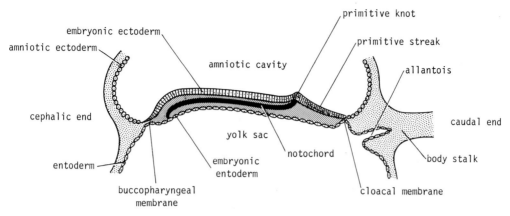

Fig. 3-4. Longitudinal section of 17-day-old embryo. Also shown are the buccopharyngeal and cloacal membranes formed by the fusion of the embryonic ectoderm with the embryonic entoderm. The notochord is shown as a forward growth of ectodermal cells from the primitive knot to the region of the buccopharyngeal membrane. The allantois, which is present in the body stalk, is an outgrowth from the entoderm of the yolk sac.

between the ectoderm and entoderm and becomes attached to the entoderm just caudal to the region of the buccopharyngeal membrane. This cord of cells is known as the *notochord* (Figs. 3-3 & 3-4). The further development of the notochord is complicated and not fully understood, and the details are not necessary for a student of medicine. The final result is the formation of a solid rod of cells around which the vertebral column and the caudal part of the base of the skull develop later.

DIFFERENTIATION OF THE GERM LAYERS

Ectoderm

Formation of Neural Tube and Neural Crest

Following the development of the primitive streak and primitive knot with the subsequent formation of the intra-embryonic mesoderm and the notochord, a further thickening of the ectoderm, the *neural plate,* appears at the cephalic end of the embryo (Fig. 3-3). This plate is situated between the buccopharyngeal membrane and the primi-

tive knot. As the result of differential growth, the primitive knot and primitive streak move caudally and at the same time the neural plate increases in length. Shortly after its appearance, the neural plate becomes depressed below the surface in the long axis of the embryo to form the *neural groove* (Figs. 3-5 & 3-6). The lateral walls of the groove are called the *neural folds.* The edge of each fold is known as the *neural crest.* As the neural groove deepens, the margins fuse in the midline to form the *neural tube.* The process of fusion begins in the region of the future embryonic neck and extends toward the cephalic and caudal ends of the embryo. It is thus seen that the neural tube communicates for a time with the amniotic cavity through the *anterior* and *posterior neuropores* (Fig. 3-7). The neural tube will ultimately give rise to the central nervous system. The cephalic end will dilate to form the forebrain, midbrain, and hindbrain; the remainder of the tube will become the spinal cord. The cells of the neural crest will form the cells of the *posterior root ganglia,* the *sensory ganglia of the cranial nerves,* the *autonomic ganglia,*

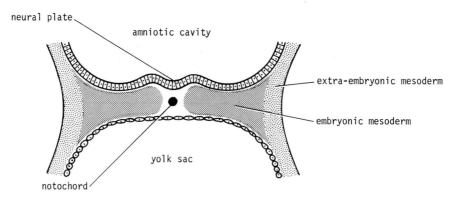

Fig. 3-5. Cross section of embryo showing fusion of embryonic mesoderm with extra-embryonic mesoderm at edge of embryonic disc. The neural plate is starting to become depressed.

Schwann cells, the cells of the *suprarenal medulla,* and *melanocytes.* It is also believed that neural crest cells give rise to mesenchymal cells in the head and neck.

Formation of Auditory and Lens Placodes

During the fourth week of development the *auditory placodes* appear as ectodermal thickenings on the side of the developing head. Each placode now sinks below the surface to form the *auditory pit.* Later the pit severs its connection with the surface and is known as the *auditory vesicle.* (For further discussion of the development of the inner ear, see Chapter 21.) Similar ectodermal thickenings appear in the face region of the embryo and are known as the *lens placodes.* These will sink beneath the surface ectoderm to form the *lens vesicles.* (For further discussion of the development of the eye, see Chapter 21.)

The remainder of the ectoderm will form the epidermis of the skin and its derivatives, nails, hair, epithelial cells of the sebaceous, sweat, and mammary glands; the mucous membrane lining the mouth, nasal cavities, and paranasal sinuses; the enamel of the teeth; the pars anterior and intermedia of the pituitary and the alveoli and ducts of the parotid salivary glands; the mucous membrane of the lower half of the anal canal; and the terminal parts of the genital tract and the male urinary tract. The ectoderm will also form the corneal epithelium, the lens of the eye, the retina, and the optic nerve.

Mesoderm

In its early stages the embryonic mesoderm is a loose feltwork of cells extending laterally, anteriorly, and posteriorly between the ectoderm and the entoderm. At the edge of the embryonic disc it is continuous with the extra-embryonic mesoderm that surrounds the yolk sac and amniotic cavity and lines the trophoblast. It soon becomes differentiated into three distinct regions: *paraxial mesoderm,* *intermediate mesoderm,* and *lateral mesoderm* (Fig. 3-8).

Paraxial Mesoderm

In its early stage this is a column of tissue situated on either side of the midline of the embryo. At about the fourth week it becomes divided into segmental blocks of tissue, the process being known as *segmentation of the mesoderm.* The blocks, or *somites,* can be seen through the amniotic or dorsal surface of the embryo. There are approximately 43

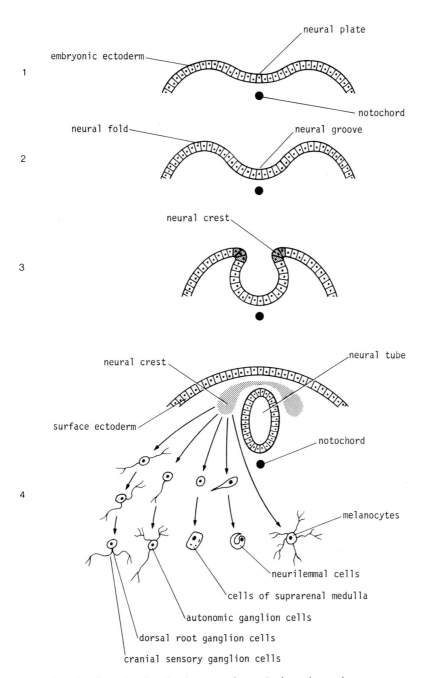

Fig. 3-6. Cross section of embryo showing development of neural tube and neural crest.

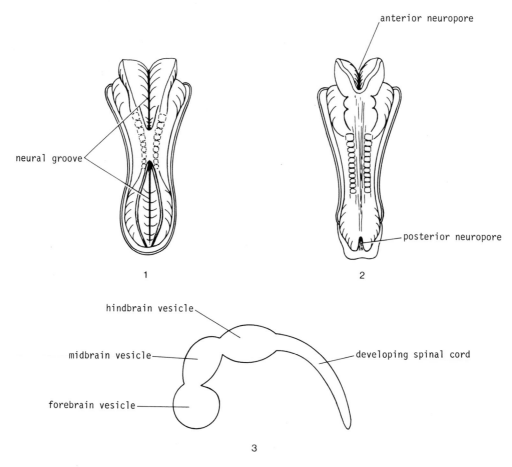

Fig. 3-7. Development of neural tube: (1) Neural groove at 22 days. (2) Almost complete closure of the neural tube (later stage). The tube still remains in communication with the amniotic cavity through the anterior and posterior neuropores. (3) Dilatation of the cephalic end of the neural tube into forebrain, midbrain, and hindbrain vesicles.

pairs of somites, which appear in a craniocaudal sequence and extend from the region of the developing hindbrain to the caudal end of the embryo. Each somite then becomes differentiated into a ventromedial part called the *sclerotome* and a dorsolateral part called the *dermomyotome* (Fig. 3-9). The mesenchymal cells of the sclerotome are loosely arranged and migrate medially to surround the notochord. There they will undergo further differentiation and take part in the formation of the bones, cartilage, and ligaments

of the vertebral column and part of the base of the skull. The dermomyotome now further differentiates into the *myotome* and *dermatome* (Fig. 3-9). The cells of the myotome will give rise to skeletal or voluntary muscle of its own segment. The mesenchymal cells of the dermatome will migrate laterally under the overlying ectoderm and assist in the formation of the dermis and subcutaneous tissues of the skin. It is important to remember that the muscles derived from a given myotome and the dermis formed from

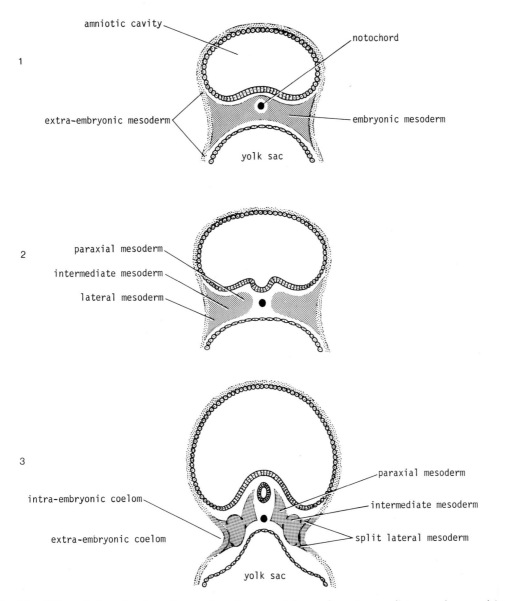

Fig. 3-8. Differentiation of embryonic mesoderm into paraxial mesoderm, intermediate mesoderm, and lateral mesoderm. The last splits into somatic and splanchnic layers. Numbers indicate progressive stages of development.

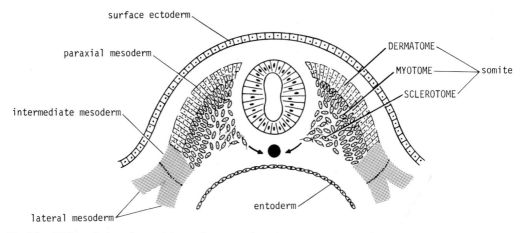

Fig. 3-9. Differentiation of paraxial mesoderm into dermatome, myotome, and sclerotome.

a given dermatome always retain the nerve supply from the segment of the spinal cord which supplies that particular somite.

Intermediate Mesoderm

This is a second column of mesodermal tissue present on both sides of the embryo and connected to the paraxial mesoderm and the lateral mesoderm (Fig. 3-9). The intermediate mesoderm will give rise to portions of the urogenital system.

Lateral Mesoderm

This is directly continuous with the extra-embryonic mesoderm beyond the margins of the embryonic disc (Fig. 3-10). This tissue splits into a *somatic* and *splanchnic* layer associated with ectoderm and entoderm, respectively, and encloses a cavity, the *intra-embryonic coelom*. The intra-embryonic coelom is continuous on each side of the embryo with the extra-embryonic coelom (Figs. 3-10 & 3-11). The intra-embryonic coeloms communicate across the midline just cranial to the buccopharyngeal membrane to form a horsehoe-shaped cavity. The portion of the coelom which lies cranial to the bucco-pharyngeal membrane will eventually form

the *pericardial cavity* (Fig. 3-12). The remainder of the intra-embryonic coelom will form the *pleural* and *peritoneal cavities*. The cells of the somatic and splanchnic layers of mesoderm will form the serous membranes of the pericardial, pleural, and peritoneal cavities.

With the bending ventrally of the developing head fold of the embryo, the pericardial cavity comes to lie ventral to the developing gut. That part of the mesoderm which initially was cranial to the pericardium now lies caudal to it and ventral to the developing gut. This mass of mesoderm, which contains parts of the somites from cervical segments 3, 4, and 5, is known as the *septum transversum* (Fig. 3-12). The latter will be used to convey blood vessels to the heart; the liver will develop in it and it will form the muscle of the diaphragm.

The embryonic mesenchyme, in addition, gives origin to the following: smooth, voluntary, and cardiac muscle; all forms of connective tissue, including cartilage and bone; blood vessel walls and blood cells; lymph vessel walls and lymphoid tissue; the serous membranes of the pericardial, pleural, and peritoneal cavities; the synovial membranes of joints and bursae; and the suprarenal cortex.

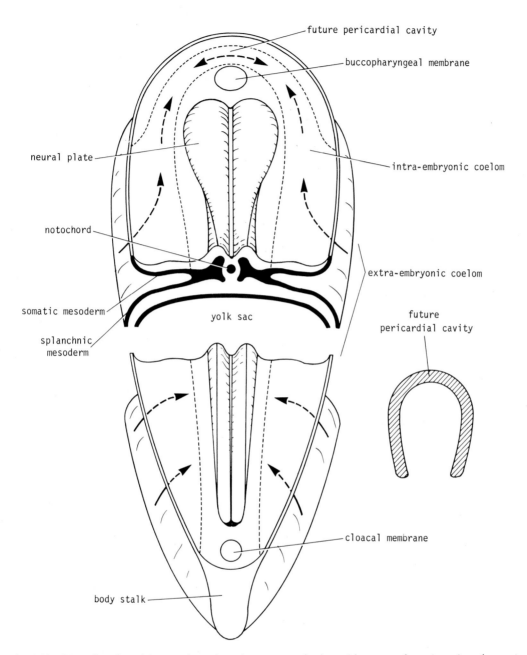

Fig. 3-10. Horseshoe-shaped intra-embryonic coelom communicating with extra-embryonic coelom (*arrows*).

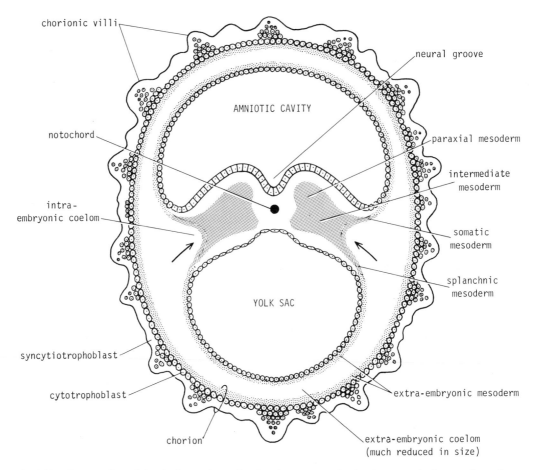

Fig. 3-11. Cross section of developing embryo showing free communication between the intra-embryonic coelom and the extra-embryonic coelom (*arrows*).

Entoderm

This is initially a flat layer of cells covering the surface of the embryonic disc that faces the yolk sac. As the embryo grows in length, the cephalic and caudal ends of the embryonic disc become bent to form a *head fold* and a *tail fold* (Fig. 3-12). With the continued growth in the width of the embryonic disc, the lateral margins become bent ventrally to form the *lateral folds.* The result is that part of the yolk sac is taken into the embryo to form the *foregut, midgut,* and *hindgut.* At first the midgut remains in open communication with the yolk sac by way of a broad tube, the *vitelline duct* or *vitello-intestinal duct* (Fig. 3-12). As the gut is drawn further into the growing embryo, the duct becomes longer and narrower and lies within the umbilical cord.

The *mouth* begins as a depression on the surface ectoderm called the *stomodeum.* This in the early stage is separated from the foregut by a plate of ectoderm plus entoderm, the *buccopharyngeal membrane.* This ruptures at the end of the third week so that the alimentary tract opens into the amniotic cavity. At the tail end of the embryo a similar

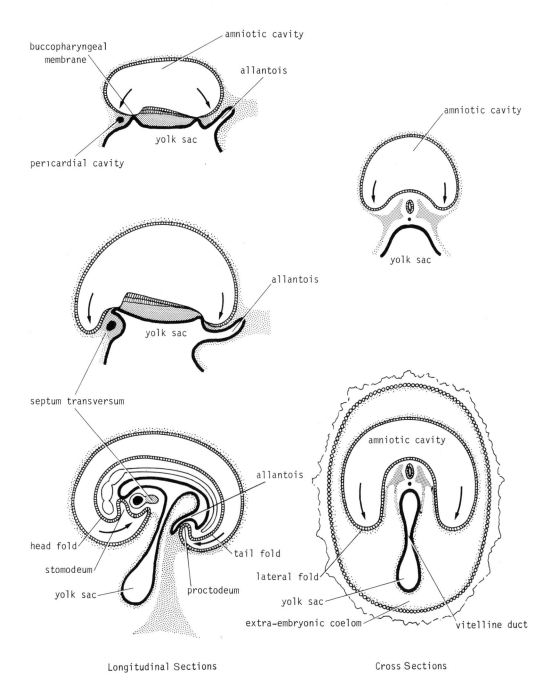

Longitudinal Sections   Cross Sections

Fig. 3-12.   Development of a head fold, a tail fold, and lateral folds.

depression, the *proctodeum,* occurs on the surface ectoderm. The hindgut is separated from the exterior by a plate of ectoderm plus entoderm known as the *cloacal membrane.* Later this breaks down to form the anal and genital orifices.

From the hindgut there arises a diverticulum called the *allantois* (Figs. 3-4 & 3-12), which grows into the body stalk. The part of the hindgut from which it arises eventually becomes the urinary bladder. The allantois becomes a fibrous cord, the *urachus,* which stretches from the apex of the bladder to the umbilicus.

The entoderm eventually gives origin to the following structures: the epithelial lining of the alimentary tract from the mouth cavity down to halfway along the anal canal and the epithelium of the glands that develop from it, namely, the thyroid, parathyroid, thymus, liver, pancreas; the epithelial lining of the respiratory tract; the epithelial lining of the pharyngotympanic tube, the middle ear (including the inner layer of the tympanic membrane), the antrum, and the mastoid air cells; the epithelial lining of the urinary bladder (excluding initially the trigone), parts of the female and male urethras, the greater vestibular glands, the glands of the prostate, and the bulbo-urethral glands; and the epithelial lining of the vagina.

Congenital Anomaly

Teratoma

This is a tumor that usually arises in or near the midline close to the vertebral column (Fig. 3-13). The common sites are within the pelvis, retroperitoneal, and mediastinal. It varies in structure from simple cysts to a mass of material composed of well-differentiated tissues. The tumor is thought to arise from undifferentiated embryonic cells which retain some or all of their totipotentiality. The common midline position has lead pathologists to suggest that teratomas arise from the primitive streak.

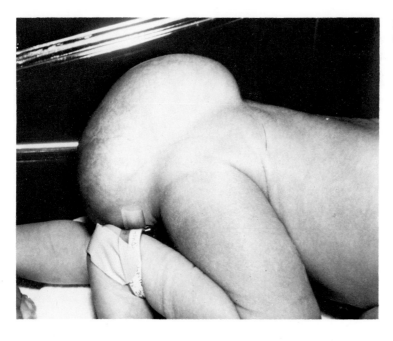

Fig. 3-13. Sacrococcygeal teratoma in a newborn infant. (Courtesy of Dr. G. Avery.)

Clinical Problems
Answers on page 431

1. A 20-year-old woman with severe mitral stenosis following acute rheumatic carditis, became pregnant and was seen by her obstetrician. In view of her marked limitation of physical activity due to her cardiac disease, he advised that the pregnancy be terminated. The duration of the pregnancy was estimated to be 8 weeks. What is your definition of the term *abortion?* Where does the blastocyst normally become implanted within the uterus? When implantation is complete, at what depth does the blastocyst lie within the uterine wall relative to the uterine lumen? What dangers are there to the mother in a therapeutic abortion by curettage?

2. A 25-year-old woman went into labor and was about to deliver what appeared to be a normal child. The head, arms, thorax, and abdomen of the child were extracted without difficulty, but considerable traction was required to deliver the pelvis. On examination of the male infant a semisolid swelling was seen on the right buttock, which extended forward to the anus. Later, a gentle rectal examination was performed, and the buttock swelling was found to extend up into the pelvis in front of the coccyx and sacrum, pushing the rectum forward. A diagnosis of sacrococcygeal teratoma was made. Following operative removal of the tumor a pathological examination revealed that it consisted of numerous cysts in among solid tissue. Pieces of skin, cartilage, bone, intestine, muscle, and nervous tissue could be identified. Using your knowledge of embryology, can you speculate as to the possible origin of this tumor?

REFERENCES

Böving, B. G.   The Biology of Trophoblast. *Ann. N.Y. Acad. Sci.* 80:21, 1959.

Brewer, J. I.   A Human Embryo in the Bilaminar Blastodisc Stage (the Edwards-Jones-Brewer Ovum). *Contrib. Embryol.* 27:85, 1938.

Hamilton, W. J.   Early Stages of Human Development. *Ann. Roy. Coll. Surg. Eng.* 4:281, 1949.

Hamilton, W. J., and Boyd, J. D.   Development of the Human Placenta in the First Three Months of Gestation. *J. Anat.* 94:297, 1960.

Hertig, A. T., and Rock, J.   Two Human Ova of the Previllous Stage, Having an Ovulation Age of Eleven and Twelve Days Respectively. *Contrib. Embryol.* 29:127, 1941.

Hertig, A. T., and Rock, J.   Two Human Ova of the Previllous Stage, Having a Developmental Age of About Seven and Nine Days Respectively. *Contrib. Embryol.* 31:65, 1945.

Hertig, A. T., Rock, J., and Adams, E. C.   A Description of 34 Human Ova Within the First 17 Days of Development. *Amer. J. Anat.* 98:435, 1956.

Heuser, C. H., Rock, J., and Hertig, A. T.   Two Human Embryos Showing Early Stages of the Definitive Yolk Sac. *Contrib. Embryol.* 31:87, 1945.

Lewis, B. V., and Harrison, R. G.   A Presomite Human Embryo Showing a Yolk-Sac Duct. *J. Anat.* 100:389, 1966.

Rock, J., and Hertig, A. T.   The Human Conceptus During the First Two Weeks of Gestation. *Amer. J. Obstet. Gynec.* 55:6, 1948.

Wislocki, G. B., and Bennett, H. S.   The Histology and Cytology of the Human and Monkey Placenta with Special Reference to the Trophoblast. *Amer. J. Anat.* 73:335, 1943.

Wislocki, G. B., and Streeter, G. L.   On the Placentation of the Macaque (Macaca Mulatta) from the Time of Implantation Until the Formation of the Definitive Placenta. *Contrib. Embryol.* 27:1, 1938.

Formation of the Decidua, the Fetal Membranes, and the Placenta

DEVELOPMENT

Formation of the Decidua

When the process of implantation is complete, the blastocyst lies in the superficial part of the compact layer of the endometrium (day 12). The stroma cells lying close to the trophoblast enlarge, become polyhedral in shape, and are filled with glycogen and lipid material. The capillaries of the endometrium become congested and dilated to form intercommunicating sinusoids. As trophoblastic erosion of the endometrium continues, the walls of the maternal blood sinusoids are broken down. Meanwhile many of the trophoblastic lacunae become confluent with one another and with the maternal blood sinusoids. In the earliest stage, the blood in the lacunae and spaces in the endometrial stroma show no circulation. Later, when the walls of the maternal arterioles and venules have become eroded by the trophoblast, a definite circulation of blood is established. It is thus seen that the secretory phase of the endometrium found in the latter half of the menstrual cycle has undergone further changes at the site of implantation. The changed endometrium is now known as the *decidua,* and the enlarged stroma cells are called *decidual cells.* The decidual cells are first confined to the immediate area of im-

plantation, but they soon appear throughout the lining of the uterus. At this stage the entire lining of the uterus is referred to as the decidua, and three different regions can be recognized: (1) the *decidua basalis,* a region lying between the blastocyst and the muscular wall of the uterus; (2) the *decidua capsularis,* a region that covers the blastocyst and separates it from the cavity of the uterus; and (3) the *decidua parietalis,* which is the remainder of the lining of the uterus (Fig. 4-1).

Fetal Membranes

These are structures that have developed from the zygote but do not form part of the embyro. They may be regarded as auxiliary organs that assist in the protection of the embryo and provide for its respiration, nourishment, and excretion while it lies within the uterine cavity. They include the yolk sac, allantois, amnion, and chorion. The placenta is a compound organ that has been elaborated by higher mammals and is included with these structures.

Yolk Sac and Allantois

The formation of the yolk sac and allantois has already been described in the section on entoderm in Chapter 3. As development pro-

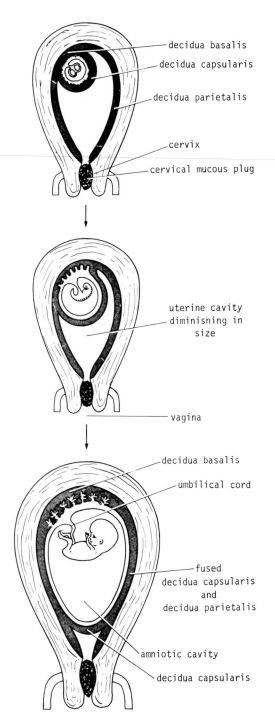

ceeds, the yolk sac becomes a pear-shaped structure which by the second month measures about 5 mm across. The sac persists throughout pregnancy and gradually shrinks in size. It never possesses any yolk and therefore plays no part in the storage of nourishment for the embryo. It is generally believed, however, that it plays an important part in the transfer of nutritive fluid from the trophoblast via the extra-embryonic mesoderm and the extra-embryonic coelom to the embryo. In the early embryo, the splanchnic mesoderm covering the yolk sac differentiates, with the formation of blood cells and blood vessels. This first occurs in isolated areas called *blood islands*. Later these vessels join to form a vascular network in the wall of the yolk sac, which communicates with the developing blood vessels within the embryo by way of the paired *vitelline arteries and veins*. The vitelline arteries arise from the dorsal aortae, and later when part of the yolk sac is taken into the embryo to form the gut, these arteries supply the midgut and ultimately fuse to form the *superior mesenteric artery* (for the fate of the vitelline veins see Chap. 8). Once the placental circulation has been established, the yolk sac circulation loses its importance.

The allantois arises as a diverticulum from that part of the yolk sac that forms the hindgut. It grows into the body stalk and thus gains a covering of mesenchyme. Later, with the incorporation of the body stalk into the umbilical cord, it is seen there as a narrow tube (Fig. 4-2). The blood vessels in the wall of the allantois eventually enlarge and become the *umbilical vessels*. The allantois becomes a fibrous cord, the *urachus,* which

Fig. 4-1. The developing conceptus expanding into the uterine cavity. The three different regions of the decidua can be recognized. By the fourth month the uterine cavity is obliterated by the fusion of the decidua capsularis with the decidua parietalis.

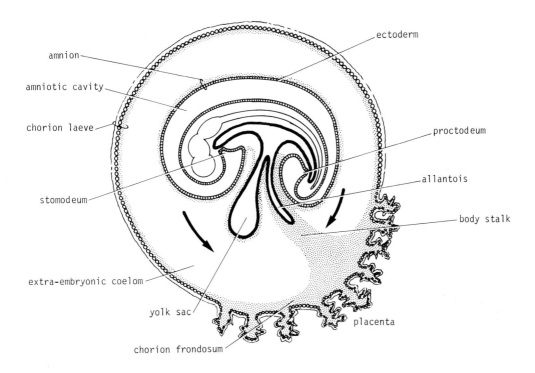

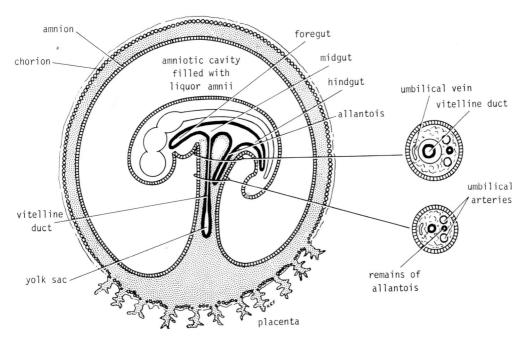

Fig. 4-2.   The formation of the umbilical cord.

extends from the apex of the urinary bladder to the umbilicus.

Amnion

This membrane forms the wall of the amniotic cavity and is attached to the periphery of the embryonic disc, which serves as a "floor" to the amniotic cavity. The amnion is a thin, tough, transparent, nonvascular membrane formed of ectoderm on the inside and extra-embryonic mesoderm on the outside (Fig. 4-2). The amniotic cavity contains a pale straw-colored watery fluid, the *liquor amnii*. In the early stage, it is thought that the liquor is produced only by the cells forming the wall of the amnion. Later, when the kidneys of the embryo start to function, urine is added to the fluid so that eventually the kidneys become the major source of the liquor amnii. Once the buccopharyngeal membrane ruptures, liquor enters the intestinal tract of the embryo where it is absorbed into the bloodstream and passes by way of the placenta into the mother's blood. The volume of liquor gradually increases as the pregnancy progresses and at term averages 1 liter. The liquor circulates and does not stagnate. During the later months of pregnancy, it has been estimated that the turnover of water in the liquor is at a rate of one-third of the volume each hour.

As the embryo develops, it bulges into the amniotic cavity, and the liquor surrounding it protects it from injury and allows it freedom of movement. With continued growth of the embryo, the amniotic cavity gradually expands and comes to obliterate the extra-embryonic coelom (Fig. 4-2). The result is that the amnion and chorion become fused while the body stalk and yolk sac become approximated to form the *umbilical cord*. By this means the umbilical cord acquires an outer covering of amnion.

At the beginning of labor, a protuberance of fused amnion and chorion is pushed down into the canal of the cervix as the result of a rise in pressure in the liquor caused by uterine contraction. With each succeeding uterine contraction, the fluid wedge, or "bag of waters," is forced more and more down the cervical canal (Fig. 24-4). As the membranes stretch and descend, they tear away from the uterine wall and push out the plug of mucus which closes the cervical canal, and this, together with slight bleeding, is referred to as the "show." Later the membranes rupture and the liquor escapes as the *"waters."* By this time the advancing head of the fetus has entered the cervix and plugs the canal. It is not until the end of labor that the remaining liquor amnii escapes, and it comes with a gush after delivery of the child's body.

The liquor amnii is 98 to 99 percent water. The solids consist of small quantities of protein, glucose, and inorganic salts. The function of the liquor amnii is to provide the fetus with a protective cushion against external injury and localized pressure from the uterine contractions in labor. It also serves as a medium in which the fetus can move easily, and it provides the fetus with fluid to drink and keeps it at an even temperature. As has been mentioned above, the bag of waters plays an important part in the early stages of labor as a hydrostatic wedge.

Chorion

The chorion consists of the trophoblast and the lining of extra-embryonic mesoderm. During the process of implantation (see Chap. 2) lacunae appear in the syncytiotrophoblast, which later become confluent. As the result of erosion of the decidual blood vessels, maternal blood enters the lacunae. Between day 9 and day 20, the chorion undergoes intense growth and differentiation. Cords of cytotrophoblast cells migrate into the irregular processes of the syncytial layer (Fig. 4-3). At this stage the processes are known as *primary villi*. Each villus now has an inner core of cytotrophoblast and an outer covering of syncytiotrophoblast. These villi

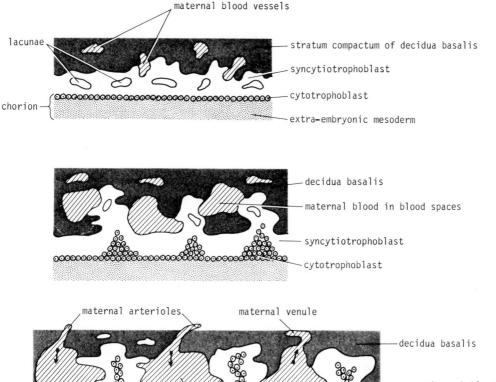

maternal blood vessels

lacunae

stratum compactum of decidua basalis

syncytiotrophoblast

cytotrophoblast

chorion

extra-embryonic mesoderm

decidua basalis

maternal blood in blood spaces

syncytiotrophoblast

cytotrophoblast

maternal arterioles   maternal venule

decidua basalis

syncytiotrophoblast

cytotrophoblast

maternal blood   intervillous   primary villus   extra-embryonic
                        space   mesoderm

Fig. 4-3. The development of the primary chorionic villi.

lie between the large blood spaces formed by the confluence of the trophoblastic lacunae and the excavated areas of the decidua. The blood-filled spaces are known as *intervillous spaces*. The extra-embryonic mesoderm of the chorion now invades the cytotrophoblastic core of each primary villus which becomes known as a *secondary villus* (Fig. 4-4). At this stage, the cytotrophoblast cells and the syncytiotrophoblast proliferate until they con-

tact the stroma of the decidua. With further proliferation, they come to line all the intervillous spaces. Some of the villi project freely into the blood spaces and are not attached to the decidua.

By the end of the third week, the mesenchymal cells that form the core of each secondary villus differentiate and small blood capillaries appear. These soon link with the capillaries in the wall of the chorion and the

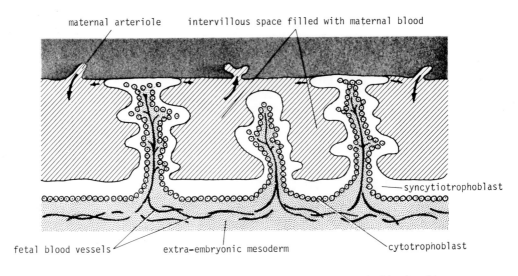

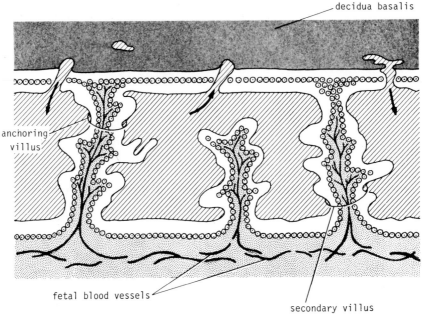

Fig. 4-4. The development of the secondary chorionic villi.

newly formed blood vessels in the body stalk. At about the same time young blood vessels are forming in the embryo, and soon the umbilical veins will convey blood from the chorion along the body stalk and into the primitive heart tube of the embryo. From the latter, two arteries called the *dorsal aortae,* which run caudally along the posterior body wall of the embryo, will return blood to the body stalk and chorionic villi by large branches called the *umbilical arteries.* In this manner simple intra-embryonic and extra-embryonic vascular systems are established.

At first the whole outer surface of the chorion possesses villi, though they are less well developed on the side of the decidua capsularis. As the embryo continues to enlarge, it encroaches further on the uterine cavity. The decidua capsularis becomes stretched and thin while the villi in the corresponding part of the chorion gradually atrophy. On the other hand, the villi opposite the decidua basalis and in the region of the body stalk increase in size and complexity, and the chorion in this region is known as the *chorion frondosum*. When the villi under the decidua capsularis disappear completely, the chorion in this region is smooth and is called the *chorion laeve*.

With further growth of the embryo, the decidua capsularis comes into contact with the decidua parietalis and fuses with it (Fig. 4-1). The decidua capsularis later degenerates so that the chorion comes into direct contact with the decidua parietalis. The uterine cavity is now obliterated except at the cervix. The cervix does not develop a decidua, but its glands enlarge and secrete mucus to form the *cervical plug*. The cervical plug closes off the uterine cavity from the exterior and is not shed until the beginning of labor.

Umbilical Cord

As the tail fold of the embryo becomes further developed, the embryonic attachment of the body stalk to the caudal end of the embryonic disc comes to lie on the ventral aspect of the embryo. The body stalk is now in close proximity to the remains of the yolk sac (Fig. 4-2). Meanwhile the amniotic cavity has expanded within the extra-embryonic coelom so that the amnion and chorion fuse. The amnion thus comes to enclose the body stalk and yolk sac with their vessels to form the tubular *umbilical cord*. The space bounded by the junction of the amnion with the ventral body wall of the embryo will become the *umbilicus*. The mesenchymal core of the cord becomes converted into a loose connective tissue called *Wharton's jelly*. Embedded in this are the remains of the yolk sac, the vitelline duct, the remains of the allantois, and the umbilical vessels.

The umbilical vessels consist of two arteries which carry deoxygenated blood from the fetus to the chorion. In the adult, these arteries are represented by the *obliterated umbilical arteries*, branches of the internal iliac arteries. The two umbilical veins convey oxygenated blood from the chorion to the fetus. The right vein, however, disappears at an early stage. In the adult, the left umbilical vein is represented by the *ligamentum teres*, which runs from the umbilicus to join the left branch of the portal vein in the porta hepatis and the vitelline veins are represented in the abdominal cavity by part of the *inferior vena cava*, the *hepatic veins*, the *liver sinusoids*, the *portal vein*, and the *superior mesenteric vein*. In the region of the cord close to the fetus, there remains a small part of the extra-embryonic coelom. This will be used temporarily to accommodate the developing gut, which will be later withdrawn into the abdominal cavity.

The umbilical cord is a twisted tortuous structure that measures about ¾ inch (2 cm) in diameter. It increases in length until, at the end of pregnancy, it is about 20 to 24 inches (50 to 60 cm) long, i.e., about the same length as the child.

At birth, the cord is tied off close to the umbilicus. It is advisable to leave about 2 inches of cord between the umbilicus and the ligature, since a piece of intestine may be present as an umbilical hernia in the remains of the extra-embryonic coelom. Following application of the ligature, the umbilical vessels constrict and thrombose. Later the stump of the cord sloughs off and the umbilical scar tissue becomes retracted and slowly assumes the shape of the *umbilicus* or *navel*.

Placenta

The placenta is the organ that carries out respiration, excretion, and nutrition for the embryo, and it is fully formed during the fourth month. Before considering the structure of the mature placenta, it is of interest to

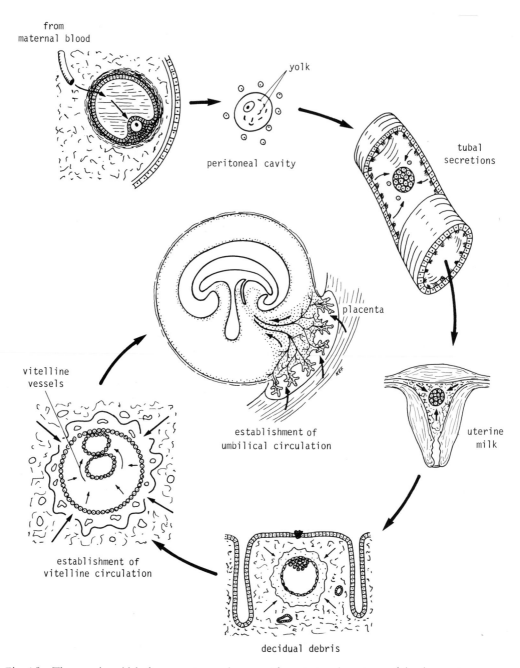

from
maternal blood

yolk

peritoneal cavity

tubal
secretions

placenta

establishment of
umbilical circulation

uterine
milk

vitelline
vessels

establishment of
vitelline circulation

decidual debris

Fig. 4-5.   The ways by which the conceptus receives nourishment at various stages of development.

reconsider briefly the different ways by which the ovum has been nourished from the time of ovulation to the end of the third month of pregnancy (Fig. 4-5).

Nourishment of the Ovum and the Embryo

The oocyte, while growing in the graafian follicle, receives its nourishment from the blood vessels of the ovary via the theca interna, granulosa cells, and zona pellucida. Immediately following ovulation, it probably relies on the small reserves of yolk granules in its cytoplasm. Once the oocyte enters the uterine tube, it is bathed in secretions produced by the lining cells of the tube, and it is possible that substances present in the secretions are of benefit to the oocyte. On entering the uterine cavity, the zona pellucida disappears and morula lies free within the secretion (*uterine milk*) produced by the highly developed endometrium. This secretion is rich in glycogen, mucopolysaccharides, and lipid, and it provides an excellent medium for the rapidly dividing cells in the blastocyst.

During implantation of the blastocyst, the syncytiotrophoblast gradually erodes the decidua and provides cytolytic products from the breakdown of stroma cells, blood cells, glandular epithelium, capillary walls, and glandular secretions. This rich food source is rapidly absorbed by the syncytiotrophoblast and diffuses to the developing embryonic disc. With the continued eroding action of the trophoblast and the formation of large blood-filled spaces around the blastocyst, the conceptus becomes surrounded by a pool of circulating maternal blood. At this time the vitelline veins are established in the wall of the yolk sac and aid in the transport to the embryo of nutritive materials that have diffused through the trophoblast, the extra-embryonic mesoderm, and the extra-embryonic coelom to the yolk sac.

At this stage, the embryo and its membranes are rapidly enlarging and can no longer depend entirely on the diffusion process across the extra-embryonic coelom. The chorion now undergoes considerable development with the formation of branching villi that are bathed by maternal blood circulating through the intervillous spaces. The umbilical vessels become established in the body stalk and connect the capillaries in the chorionic villi with the heart and blood vessels in the embryo. At the same time, the chorionic villi of the chorion frondosum undergo extensive development and further invade the decidua basalis. The concentration of highly developed villi at one pole of the conceptus greatly improves the efficiency of transport of nourishment to the embryo, since the chorion frondosum develops immediately adjacent to the attachment of the body stalk with its large umbilical vessels conveying blood to and from the embryo. The embryo has now reached the end of the third month of development, and the placenta is about to be established.

Establishment of the Placenta

Biologically the placenta is an organ developed by mother and child in symbiosis and consisting of fetal and maternal parts. The fetal part is formed by the *chorion frondosum;* the maternal part is formed by the stratum compactum and the intervillous spaces of the decidua basalis (Fig. 4-6).

Fetal Part of the Placenta

The villi of the chorion frondosum enlarge and become elaborately branched; they project into the intervillous spaces. Other villi are attached directly to the decidua and have the additional function of insuring anatomical fixation of the growing embryo to the uterine wall; for this reason, they are called *anchoring villi*. At the tip of such a villus the syncytiotrophoblast and the cells of the cytotrophoblast grow directly onto the decidua

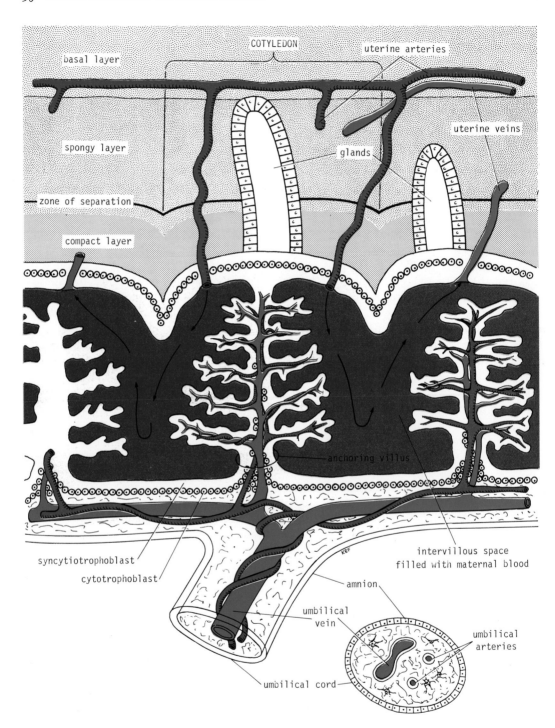

Fig. 4-6. The fetal and maternal parts of the placenta. The heavy solid line indicates the zone in the stratum spongiosum where separation occurs during the third stage of labor.

and spread over the surface of the decidua basalis so that the whole of the maternal blood space is lined with trophoblast cells. Frequently small clumps of trophoblast cells can be found in the decidua some distance from the villi; these are referred to as *wandering trophoblast cells*. Each villus has to begin with an outer covering of syncytiotrophoblast and an inner layer of cytotrophoblast. During the fourth month, the layer of cytotrophoblast begins to regress, leaving only a syncytial covering. At the center of each villus is a connective tissue core containing blood vessels. At the base of the villus are found the arterioles and venules, but these taper to capillaries in the fine branches of the villi. It is thus seen that in the mature placenta the fetal blood is separated from the maternal blood only by the endothelium of the capillaries and the single layer of syncytiotrophoblast. In the wall of the chorion, the blood vessels anastomose with one another and the larger vessels converge to the attachment of the umbilical cord. The edge of the fetal part of the placenta is continuous with the chorion laeve.

Maternal Part of Placenta

During the invasion of the stratum compactum of the decidua basalis by the syncytiotrophoblast, large areas were excavated to form irregular spaces, the intervillous spaces (Figs. 4-3—4-5). The lacunae of the syncytiotrophoblast form a small part of these spaces. As the intervillous spaces develop, they become lined with trophoblast as described previously. Maternal spiral arterioles containing oxygenated blood open into the spaces at intervals and bathe the outer surfaces of the bushy villi of the fetal part of the placenta. Venules drain the maternal blood from the spaces, and this process is aided by the mild contractions of the uterus. The *marginal sinus* is the name given to the most peripheral part of the intervillous space, i.e., that part that lies close to the edge of the placenta. It has no particular significance.

In some areas, parts of the stratum compactum remain as solid projections, or septa, which project into the intervillous space. Such septa, called *placental septa,* mark off the territory of a major villous tree and in so doing divide the placenta into distinct lobules or *cotyledons*. In all, there may be fifteen to thirty cotyledons incompletely separated from each other by the placental septa. At the edge of the maternal part of the placenta, the decidua basalis is continuous with the decidua parietalis.

Gross Appearance of the Placenta

By the fourth month of pregnancy, the placenta is a well-developed organ. As the pregnancy continues, the placenta increases in area and thickness. The increase in the placental area accompanies the steadily expanding uterus. In fact, the placental attachment occupies one-third of the internal surface of the uterus throughout the remainder of the pregnancy. The increase in placental thickness is a result of the elongation of the villi.

At full term, the placenta has a flattened circular shape, with a diameter of about 8 inches (20 cm), a thickness of about 1 inch (2.5 cm), and weighs about 1 lb. (500 gm). It thins out at the edges, where it is continuous with the fetal membranes (Fig. 4-7). The fetus is suspended from the placenta by the umbilical cord.

At birth, a few minutes after the delivery of the child, the placenta separates from the uterine wall and is expelled from the uterine cavity as the result of the contractions of the uterine musculature. The line of separation occurs through the spongy layer of the decidua basalis.

The outer *maternal surface* of the freshly shed placenta is dark red in color and oozes blood from the torn maternal vessels. When held between the finger and thumb, it has a

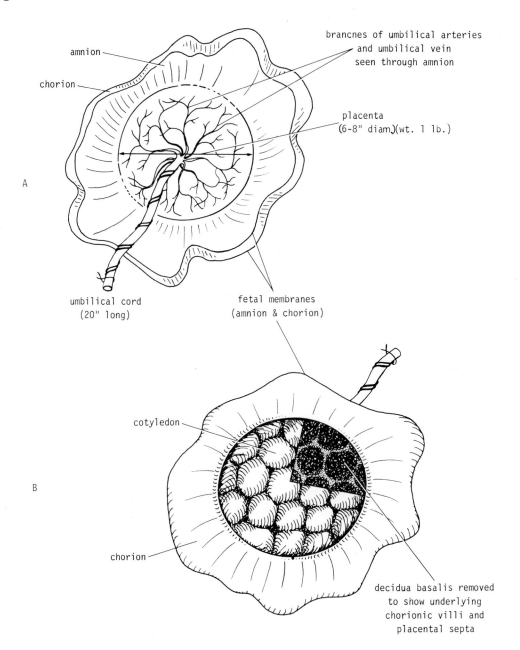

amnion

chorion

brancnes of umbilical arteries
and umbilical vein
seen through amnion

placenta
(6-8" diam.)(wt. 1 lb.)

A

umbilical cord
(20" long)

fetal membranes
(amnion & chorion)

cotyledon

B

chorion

decidua basalis removed
to show underlying
chorionic villi and
placental septa

Fig. 4-7. The mature placenta as seen from the fetal surface (A) and the maternal surface (B).

sponge-like consistency. The outer surface is rough, and margins of the lobules or cotyledons may be recognized (Fig. 4-7).

The *fetal surface* is smooth and shining and is raised in ridges by the umbilical vessels which radiate from the attachment of the umbilical cord near its center. This surface is covered by amnion, which is fused with the underlying chorion.

The fetal membranes, which surround and enclose the liquor amnii, are continuous with the edge of the placenta and are the amnion and chorion laeve and a small amount of adherent decidua parietalis.

Placental Circulation

Maternal Circulation in the Placenta

Maternal blood enters the intervillous spaces by the spiral arteries of the decidua basalis and leaves by means of numerous thin-walled decidual veins. The total capacity of the intervillous spaces is relatively large and contains about 175 ml of maternal blood. It has been determined that in the mature placenta the blood flow is about 500 ml per minute. The spiral arteries squirt the fresh maternal blood onto the bushy embyronic villi and the blood is drained away by the venules. The periodic uterine contractions aid this process by squeezing the intervillous spaces and forcing the blood into the venules and uterine veins.

Fetal Circulation in the Placenta

The deoxygenated fetal blood reaches the chorionic villi via the two umbilical arteries and their branches. The blood flows through the arterioles and small capillaries in the frond-like branches of the villi. Oxygenated blood now returns to the fetus via the venules and veins, which join one another and drain into the umbilical vein. The volume of blood flowing through the fetal villi has been estimated to be about 400 ml per minute. In the mature placenta the fetal blood is separated from the maternal blood in the villi by the very thin syncytiotrophoblast, the mesenchymal stroma, and the endothelial lining of the capillaries. These layers constitute the *placental membrane* or *placental barrier,* and the total area of this membrane corresponds to about 14 square meters.

Functions of the Placenta

The functions of the placenta fall into several groups. (1) *Respiration:* Oxygen supplied by the mother diffuses across the placental membrane into the fetal blood. This process is aided by the fact that fetal hemoglobin has a greater affinity for oxygen than maternal hemoglobin. Carbon dioxide passes readily in the opposite direction. The placenta thus serves as an efficient lung for the fetus. (2) *Nutrition:* Water, inorganic salts, carbohydrates, fats, proteins, and vitamins can all pass in different forms from the maternal to the fetal blood. (3) *Excretion:* Products of fetal metabolism can cross the placenta into the maternal circulation, the placenta functioning like a kidney. (4) *Protection:* Foreign particulate matter such as bacteria is unable to cross the barrier unless the placenta itself becomes actively involved in the inflammatory process. (5) *Endocrine:* Hormones, including progesterone, estrogen, and gonadotropin, are produced in large amounts.

Detailed Structure of the Placental Membrane

This structure separates the fetal blood in the chorionic villi from the maternal blood in the intervillous spaces. In the early stage, it measures about 0.025 mm in thickness and consists of the fetal capillary endothelium, the stroma of the villus, the cytotrophoblast, and the syncytiotrophoblast. After the fifth month of pregnancy, the cytotrophoblast cells disappear, the syncytiotrophoblast becomes greatly thinned, and the stroma of the villi is much reduced. In the later months of pregnancy, the membrane is only about 0.002 mm thick. Toward the end of pregnancy, fibrinoid material is deposited on the maternal surface of the chorionic villi; this tends to thicken the placental membrane.

It has been shown by using tracer substances that the permeability of the placental membrane alters with histological changes. It reaches its maximum during the thirty-sixth week and rapidly declines during the last few weeks of pregnancy. Electron microscopic examination of the syncytiotrophoblast shows that numerous microvilli are present on its free surface, which greatly increases the surface area for diffusion. The presence of vacuoles and pinocytotic vesicles also indicates that macromolecules and fluid are transferred across the membrane by means other than simple diffusion. Histochemical investigations of the placental membrane have revealed the presence of the enzymes cholinesterase, acid and alkaline phosphatase, and proteolytic and glycolytic enzymes, all of which are probably involved in the transfer process.

Transfer Across the Placental Membrane

1. DIFFUSION. Simple diffusion is the method used to transfer molecules of small size across the membrane, for example, gases, water, free amino acids, simple sugars, some hormones and vitamins, and inorganic substances.

2. ACTIVE TRANSPORT. It has been shown that the concentrations of calcium, inorganic phosphorus, and free amino nitrogen are slightly higher in fetal blood than in maternal blood. This raises the possibility of some transport mechanism in addition to simple diffusion. The level of fructose in fetal blood is considerably higher than that in maternal blood. It is possible that the placenta manufactures fructose from glucose. Vitamin C appears to be selectively absorbed across the placenta. Substances of very high molecular weight, such as protein, are known to cross the membrane, and it is now generally agreed that pinocytosis is the method of transfer. It is believed that antigens and antibodies are also transferred by this means. It is known

that maternal antibodies that have a high molecular weight—for such diseases as diphtheria, scarlet fever, tetanus, smallpox, and measles—are actively transferred across the barrier so that the child will receive passive immunity to such infections for a variable period after birth. Enzyme systems, demonstrated histochemically to be present, probably participate in the transmission of substances actively across the placental membrane.

Some researchers have suggested the existence of small openings in the membrane which may be sufficiently large to permit the passage of very large protein molecules or erythrocytes. The evidence supporting the existence of such holes, however, is unconvincing. In Rh-incompatibility, fetal erythrocyte antigens cross the membrane and result in antibody production by the mother against the Rh antigens. The maternal antibodies then cross the membrane and cause breakdown of the erythrocytes of the fetus with consequent severe anemia, jaundice, and even fetal death.

Drugs and the Placental Membrane

Most drugs have a low molecular weight, so the majority cross the membrane by simple diffusion. Antibiotics such as sulfonamides and penicillin pass across in small amounts, as do alcohol and nicotine. Morphine, barbiturates, and general anesthetics, when given to the mother, do cross into the fetal circulation and depress the respiratory center of the fetus. Particular attention must be paid to this fact at the time of delivery, since the child may have difficulty in breathing immediately after birth. Certain drugs taken by the mother are definitely harmful for the fetus. Thalidomide, for example, a popular tranquilizing drug given to mothers some years ago during the early months of pregnancy, crossed the placental membrane and caused numerous defects in fetal growth.

The Placenta as an Endocrine Gland

The placenta produces estrogens, progesterone, and gonadotropin. As the result of extraction procedures, it has been found that they are mainly present in the fetal part of the placenta. It is probable that the syncytiotrophoblast produces the steroid hormones, and the cytotrophoblast, the gonadotropin necessary for the maintenance of the maternal part of the placenta.

ANOMALIES

Fetal Membranes

Yolk Sac and Allantois

For anomalies of the yolk sac and the vitelline duct, see Chapter 12. For anomalies of the allantois see patent urachus, Chapter 15.

Amnion and Liquor Amnii

HYDRAMNIOS. The average amount of liquor in the last trimester of a normal pregnancy varies from 500 to 1,500 ml. In the condition of hydramnios, as much as 6 liters or more may be present. The condition occurs in about 1 in 225 pregnancies. The cause of over half the cases is not known. Fetal conditions that are commonly associated with the abnormality are twins, anencephaly, and esophageal atresia. In case of anencephaly, it is believed that the cerebrospinal fluid is secreted into the amniotic cavity; also it is common to find that anencephalic fetuses cannot swallow, so that the liquor is not absorbed into the intestinal tract. The latter fact may also explain the high incidence of hydramnios in esophageal atresia. Diabetes mellitus is the most common maternal disease associated with hydramnios; even in controlled diabetic mothers, it occurs in one in four pregnancies.

OLIGOHYDRAMNIOS. The condition is unusual, and in almost all cases is associated with absent renal function in the fetus. Rarely the condition may occur as the result of premature rupture of the membranes with prolonged leakage of amniotic fluid. Only a few ounces of viscid liquor are present. The fetus usually has multiple deformities caused by the almost direct pressure of the uterine wall on the skull, limbs, and trunk.

AMNIOTIC ADHESIONS. These may occur in association with oligohydramnios or they may occur with a normal volume of liquor amnii. The adhesions may stretch between the fetal skin and the amnion or between meninges and the amnion.

Chorion

Hydatidiform mole and chorionepithelioma have been described in Chapter 2.

The Placenta

Abnormalities of Size and Shape (Fig. 4-8)

PLACENTA MEMBRANACEA. This thin placenta lines the greater part of the uterine cavity. The chorionic villi of the chorion laeve persist so that the chorion laeve and the chorion frondosum both take part in the formation of the placenta. This type may require manual removal during labor.

PLACENTA BIPARTITA OR TRIPARTITA. The placenta has two or three incomplete lobes and the umbilical vessels pass from one lobe to the other before joining the umbilical cord.

PLACENTA DUPLEX, TRIPLEX, OR MULTIPLEX. The placenta has two or more separate lobes and the umbilical cord branches sending vessels to each lobe.

PLACENTA SUCCENTURIATA. The placenta has one or two small accessory lobes completely separate from the main placenta, and blood vessels pass from the small lobe to the main lobe along the membranes. Clinically, this type must be recognized, since the small accessory lobe or lobes may be left behind in the uterus.

PLACENTA FENESTRATA. The placenta has failed to develop over a small area. The

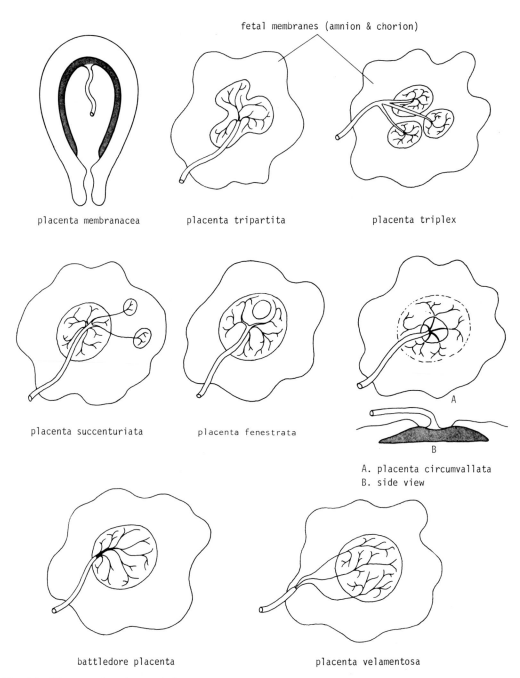

fetal membranes (amnion & chorion)

placenta membranacea   placenta tripartita   placenta triplex

placenta succenturiata   placenta fenestrata

A. placenta circumvallata
B. side view

battledore placenta   placenta velamentosa

Fig. 4-8. The anomalous forms of placenta.

defect is filled with fetal membranes and has the appearance of a window.

PLACENTA CIRCUMVALLATA. The placenta has a central depression on its fetal surface to the margins of which the fetal membranes are attached.

BATTLEDORE PLACENTA. The umbilical cord is attached to the margin of the placenta.

PLACENTA VELAMENTOSA. The umbilical cord is attached to the membranes some dis-tance from the margin of the placenta. The umbilical vessels pass along the membrane to reach the margin.

Weight and Position

The placenta normally weighs about 1 lb. (500 gm). Very small placentas are found in women suffering from chronic hypertension. Excessively large placentas occur with *fetal hydrops,* a condition of the fetus with severe

TYPE I

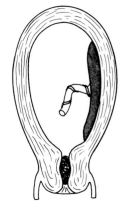

lateral placenta praevia

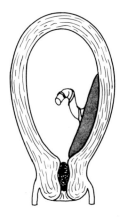

lateral placenta praevia

TYPE II

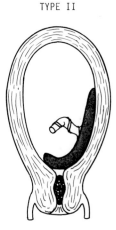

marginal placenta praevia

TYPE III

central placenta praevia

Fig. 4-9. The different types of placenta praevia.

hemolytic disease resulting from serological incompatibility of mother and baby (e.g., presence of Rhesus antigens; see Chap. 17).

Normally the placenta is situated in the upper half of the uterus. Should implantation occur in the lower half of the body of the uterus, the condition is called *placenta praevia* and is of great clinical importance. Twin pregnancy may favor its development, since two fetuses require a larger placenta than one. The three types of placenta praevia are shown in Figure 4-9, which is self-explanatory. Severe painless hemorrhage occurring from the twenty-eighth week onward is the clinical sign of placenta praevia and is caused by expansion of the lower half of the uterine wall at this time, and by its tearing away from the placenta.

Placental Infarction

This is found to some degree in more than half of the placentas at birth. Palpable solid areas can be identified close to the decidual surface. Initially coagulation of maternal blood occurs around a group of villi, and the vessels within the villi become engorged. At this stage the infarct is red. Later the villi undergo necrosis and fibrose, and the infarct becomes white in color. Massive infarction of the placenta can lead to death of the fetus. In most cases the cause is unknown, but in some it may be caused by trauma applied to the mother's abdomen producing shearing forces on the placental uterine junction, which locally interferes with the maternal circulation.

Clinical Problems

Answers on page 432

1. Following the diagnostic procedure of dilatation and curettage of a uterus for dysfunctional uterine bleeding, the histopathologist informed the gynecologist that the uterine scrapings had the appearance of the decidua. What is the decidua? May the decidua be divided up into different areas? What are the main parts of the placenta?

2. A woman aged 21, who was 7 months pregnant, complained of breathlessness and swelling of the feet and ankles. She also said she experienced abdominal discomfort and felt very large. On examination, her abdomen looked excessively distended and the fundus of the uterus was at a higher level than normal. The uterus was tender on palpation, and the fetal parts could not be easily felt through the anterior abdominal wall. The fetal heart sounds could not be heard. The fetus could be moved around the uterus

with excessive ease. Using your knowledge of embryology, what diagnosis would you make? What is the normal volume of amniotic fluid near term? What is the origin of the amniotic fluid? What common congenital anomalies are associated with this condition?

3. A pregnant woman phoned her obstetrician and told him that she thought her labor had started. She had just observed a small quantity of blood-stained mucus emerging from her vagina. She was also experiencing irregular pains in her back and abdomen. Using your knowledge of embryology, can you explain the appearance of the blood-stained mucus?

4. While traveling to the hospital in an ambulance a pregnant woman at term started to experience regular labor pains in her abdomen and back. At the height of one of the pains the attendant noticed a sudden flow of straw-colored fluid from

the vagina. Using your knowledge of embryology, can you explain the appearance of this straw-colored fluid? Can you explain the term *hydrostatic wedge* in relation to the process of dilatation of the cervix?

5. On physical examination of the abdomen of a woman 34 weeks pregnant, the circumference of the abdomen was found to be much less than normal. What are the possible explanations for this observation?

6. A medical student was asked in an obstetrics examination to define the term *oligohydramnios*. He was then asked whether or not it is commonly encountered in obstetric practice and what common congenital anomalies may be found in the fetus in such a condition. How would you have answered these questions?

7. A nurse attending the birth of a child was alarmed at seeing green-colored amniotic fluid escaping from the vagina when the fetal membranes ruptured. What is the normal color of liquor amnii? What is the cause of the green coloration? What would you do in the same circumstances?

8. Is it ever desirable to examine the amniotic fluid during pregnancy? If so, where would you withdraw the fluid from the mother?

9. Name the blood vessels present in the umbilical cord. Would it be possible for drugs to be injected into these vessels if it was felt necessary to stimulate the child at birth? Into which vessel would you inject?

10. At birth, the umbilical cord is tied off with a ligature about 2 in. from the umbilicus. Why is it advisable to leave about 2 in. of the cord between the ligature and the umbilicus? Knowing the structure of the cord, do you think that a fine strong ligature might sever the cord? Would you recommend the use of a second ligature or a clamp to be applied

to the cord on the placental side of the first ligature and the division of the cord between the points of ligation? If so, why? Can you think of any complications that may involve the stump of the cord? Does the umbilical scar ever give way?

11. How long is the normal umbilical cord at term? Do you think that an excessively long or an excessively short cord could give rise to problems during parturition? Can you explain a knotted umbilical cord?

12. During the third stage of labor, the placenta and fetal membranes are expelled from the uterus. The obstetrician must carefully examine the placenta and the membranes to make sure that no part of them has been retained in the uterus. What is the approximate diameter and thickness of a normal placenta? Describe the appearance of the maternal and fetal surfaces of a full-term placenta. Is it possible to separate the amnion from the chorion?

13. Why is it important that an obstetrician know the various anomalous forms of the placenta?

14. A medical student was astounded to learn that the placenta is an endocrine gland. What hormones are produced by the placenta, and what are their main functions?

15. Describe the functions of the placenta. How may the efficiency of this organ be impaired?

16. Name three harmful organisms and three harmful drugs that could pass from the mother through the placenta to the fetus.

17. A 23-year-old woman was admitted to the emergency room with severe vaginal bleeding. She was 35 weeks pregnant. On questioning she stated that she had slight bleeding a week previously, but this had stopped spontaneously. There was absolutely no pain associated with the bleeding. On examining the abdomen it was

found that the fetal head was high, and it was not possible to make it enter the pelvis. The uterus had a normal consistency and was not tender. On examination of the genital organs, no cause for the bleed-

ing could be determined. A diagnosis of placenta praevia was made. What is placenta praevia? What is the cause of the bleeding? Why is the bleeding painless?

REFERENCES

Amoroso, E. C. Placentation. In *Marshall's Physiology of Reproduction,* 3d ed., edited by A. S. Parkes. Little, Brown, Boston, 1952. Vol. 2, p. 127.

Amoroso, E. C., and Porter, D. G. The Endocrine Functions of the Placenta. In *Scientific Foundations of Obstetrics and Gynaecology,* edited by E. E. Philipp, J. Barnes, and M. Newton. Davis, Philadelphia, 1970. P. 556.

Arey, L. B. *Developmental Anatomy,* 7th ed. Saunders, Philadelphia, 1966.

Assali, N. S., Rauramo, L., and Peltonen, T. Measurement of Uterine Blood Flow and Uterine Metabolism. VIII. Uterine and Foetal Blood Flow and Oxygen Consumption in Early Human Pregnancy. *Amer. J. Obstet. Gynec.* 79:86, 1960.

Baird, D. *Combined Textbook of Obstetrics and Gynaecology,* 8th ed. Livingstone, Edinburgh, 1969.

Baker, J. B. E. The Effects of Drugs on the Foetus. *Pharmacol. Rev.* 12:37, 1960.

Boe, F. Vascular Morphology of the Human Placenta. *Sympos. Quant. Biol.* 19:29, 1954.

Bourne, G. L. *The Human Amnion and Chorion.* Lloyd-Luke, London, 1962.

Bourne, G. L. The Membranes. In *Scientific Foundations of Obstetrics and Gynaecology,* edited by E. E. Philipp, J. Barnes, and M. Newton. Davis, Philadelphia, 1970. P. 181.

Böving, B. G. Endocrine Influences on Implantation. In *Recent Progress in the Endocrinology of Reproduction.* Academic, New York, 1959. P. 205.

Boyd, J. D. Morphology and Physiology of the Utero-Placental Circulation. In *Gestation: Transactions of the Second Conference,* edited by C. A. Villee. The Josiah Macy, Jr., Foundation, New York, 1956. P. 132.

Boyd, J. D., and Hamilton, W. J. The Giant Cells of the Pregnant Human Uterus. *J. Obstet. Gynaec. Brit. Comm.* 67:208, 1960.

Boyd, J. D., and Hamilton, W. J. Cytotrophoblast Contribution to Syncytium. *J. Anat.* 100:451, 1966.

Boyd, J. D., and Hamilton, W. J. Placental Septa. *Z. Zellforsch* 69:613, 1966.

Cassmer, O. Hormone Production of the Isolated Human Placenta. *Acta Endocr.* (Kobenhavn) (Suppl.) 45:1, 1959.

Dancis, J. The Placenta. *J. Pediat.* 55:85, 1959.

Dawes, G. S. *Foetal and Neonatal Physiology.* Year Book, Chicago, 1968.

Flexner, L. B., Cowie, D. G., Hellman, L. M., Wilde, W. S., and Vosburgh, G. J. Permeability of Human Placenta to Sodium in Normal and Abnormal Pregnancies and Supply of Sodium to Human Fetus as Determined with Radioactive Sodium. *Amer. J. Obstet. Gynec.* 55:469, 1948.

Gadd, R. L. The Liquor Amnii. In *Scientific Foundations of Obstetrics and Gynaecology,* edited by E. E. Philipp, J. Barnes, and M. Newton. Davis, Philadelphia, 1970. P. 254.

Hagerman, D. C., and Villee, C. A. Transport Functions of the Placenta. *Physiol. Rev.* 40:313, 1960.

Hamilton, W. J., and Boyd, J. D. Development of the Human Placenta in the First Three Months of Gestation. *J. Anat.* 94:297, 1960.

Hamilton, W. J., and Boyd, J. D. Specializations of the Syncytium of the Human Chorion. *Brit. Med. J.* 1:1501, 1966.

Hamilton, W. J., and Boyd, J. D. Development of the Human Placenta. In *Scientific Foundation of Obstetrics and Gynaecology,* edited by E. E. Philipp, J. Barnes, and M. Newton. Davis, Philadelphia, 1970. P. 185.

Keele, C. A., and Neil, E. *Samson Wright's Applied Physiology,* 11th ed. Oxford University Press, New York; London, 1965.

Malmnäs, C. *Immunity in Pregnancy.* Almquist and Wiksells, Stockholm, 1958.

Moya, F., and Thorndike, V. Passage of Drugs Across the Placenta. *Amer. J. Obstet. Gynec.* 84:1778, 1962.

Page, E. W. Physiology of Pregnancy. *Clin. Obstet. Gynec.* 3:277, 1960.

Plentl, A. A. The Origin of Amniotic Fluid. In *Gestation: Transactions of the Fourth Confer-*

ence, edited by C. A. Villee. The Josiah Macy, Jr., Foundation, New York, 1958. P. 71.

Ramsey, E. M. Vascular Patterns in the Endometrium and the Placenta. *Angiology* 6:321, 1955.

Ramsey, E. M. Distribution of Arteries and Veins in the Mammalian Placenta. In *Gestation: Transactions of the Second Conference,* edited by C. A. Villee. The Josiah Macy, Jr., Foundation, New York, 1956. P. 299.

Reynolds, S. R. M. Formation of Fetal Cotyledons in the Hemochorial Placenta. *Amer. J. Obstet. Gynec.* 94:425, 1966.

Serr, D. M., Sadowsky, A., and Kohn, G. The Placental Septa. *J. Obstet. Gynaec. Brit. Comm.* 65:774, 1958.

Symposium on Placenta. *Amer. J. Obstet. Gynec.* 84:1541, 1962.

Villee, C. A. *The Placenta and Fetal Membranes.* Williams & Wilkins, Baltimore, 1960.

Walker, C. W., and Pye, B. G. The Length of the Human Umbilical Cord. *Brit. Med. J.* 1:546, 1960.

Wilkin, P. G. Organogenesis of the Human Placenta. In *Organogenesis,* edited by R. L. DeHaan and H. Ursprung. Holt, Rinehart & Winston, New York, 1965. P. 743.

Wislocki, G. B., and Dempsey, G. W. The Chemical Histology of the Human Placenta and Decidua with Reference to Mucopolysaccharides, Glycogen, Lipids and Acid Phosphatase. *Amer. J. Anat.* 83:1, 1948.

Wislocki, G. B., and Dempsey, G. W. Electron Microscopy of the Human Placenta. *Anat. Rec.* 123:133, 1955.

In man, multiple births are relatively uncommon. The highest number recorded has been seven* (septuplets), and it is extremely rare to have more than four (quadruplets). In the United States the incidence of *twins*† is about 1 in 95 births, triplets about 1 in 10,750 births, and quadruplets about 1 in 909,090 births. The risks to the mother and baby are greater in multiple pregnancies than in single pregnancies. There are essentially two types of multiple pregnancies: *monozygotic* and *dizygotic* (trizygotic, etc.).

MONOZYGOTIC PREGNANCY

About one-quarter of multiple pregnancies are monozygotic. This condition occurs when one fertilized ovum splits to form eventually two or more babies which will be identical. The precise time at which this occurs is unknown. If it occurs at the two-cell stage, the resulting fetuses will have completely separate chorionic sacs and placentas. If it occurs at the stage of the blastocyst, with division of the inner cell mass into two or more masses, the fetuses will be in a single chorionic sac or even in a common amnion (Fig. 5-1).

Coming as they do from one ovum, such children will have identical genetic backgrounds and will have physical and mental similarities. The later the division occurs in development, the more identical will the babies be. Monozygous babies are of the same sex and blood groups.

On rare occasions the splitting of the inner cell mass may be incomplete. This may result in incomplete splitting of the primitive streak and the embryonic disc, which leads to *conjoined twins* (Figs. 5-2 & 5-3). The union may vary from slight skin fusion to a *double monster,* in which trunks, organs, and limbs are shared. In the case of *Siamese twins,* a skin bridge or liver bridge commonly connects the two babies. If the splitting into two parts is grossly unequal, one of the fetuses may monopolize the placental blood and the other one, if it survives, may become dependent on the cardiovascular system of its partner. In recent years it has been possible to separate conjoined twins by surgical means, provided each baby is not entirely dependent on the other for one of its major systems.

---

* Higher numbers have recently been reported in the lay press following the administration of pituitary FSH and chorionic gonadotropic hormone for the treatment of sterility.

† The term *twinning* may be defined as the nearly simultaneous birth of two babies (twins) by one mother.

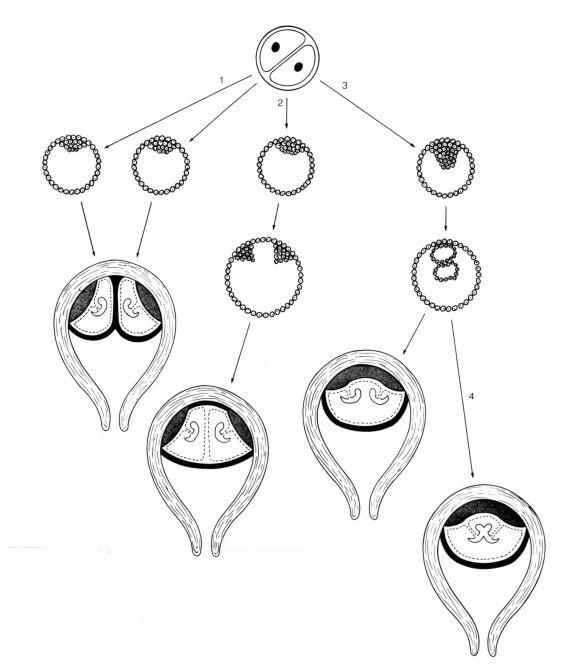

Fig. 5-1. Possible relations of the fetal membranes in monozygotic twins: (1) Splitting occurs at the two-blastomere stage and each fetus has its own placenta, amnion, and chorion. (2) Splitting occurs later, at the inner cell mass stage, and each fetus has its own placenta and amnion but a common chorion. (3) Splitting occurs at the inner cell mass stage but later than at stage 2, after the formation of one amniotic cavity. The fetuses have a common placenta, a common amniotic cavity, and a common chorion. (4) Splitting occurs at the inner cell mass at a later stage than at stage 2, but the split is incomplete. The fetuses have a common placenta, a common amniotic cavity, and a common chorion. (Unfortunately the fetuses are joined and in many cases they also share the same major organs.)

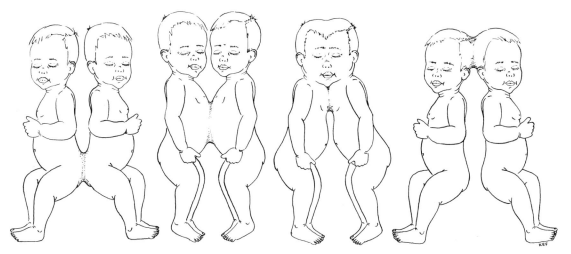

Fig. 5-2. Different types of conjoined twins that can occur in a monozygotic form of multiple pregnancy.

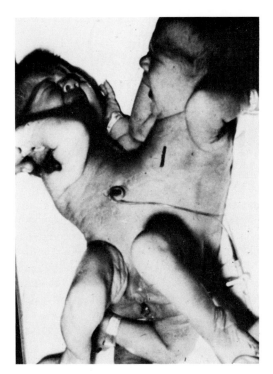

Fig. 5-3. Conjoined twins. (Courtesy of Dr. M. Platt.)

DIZYGOTIC PREGNANCY

About three-quarters of multiple pregnancies are dizygotic. The cause of dizygotic pregnancy is the shedding of two ova at approximately the same time in one ovarian cycle and the fertilization by two different spermatozoa. Each ovary may produce an ovum or two ova may come from one ovary either from a single graafian follicle or from two separate follicles. In twins the two zygotes implant separately and two separate placentas may form with two chorions and two amnions (Fig. 5-4); or the placentas may fuse to form one placenta and the membranes may be arranged so that there is a septum composed of four layers between the fetuses. The circulations of the fused placentas do not mix. If one fetus should die, it may become compressed between the uterine wall and the membranes of the surviving fetus.

Multiple ovulation is believed to be a hereditary character. Dizygotic pregnancy has a great ethnic difference in incidence. For example, in Japan it is rare (1.3 per 1,000 births), while in Nigeria the rate is 39.9 per 1,000 births. Height, age, standard of living of the mother, and the number of previous

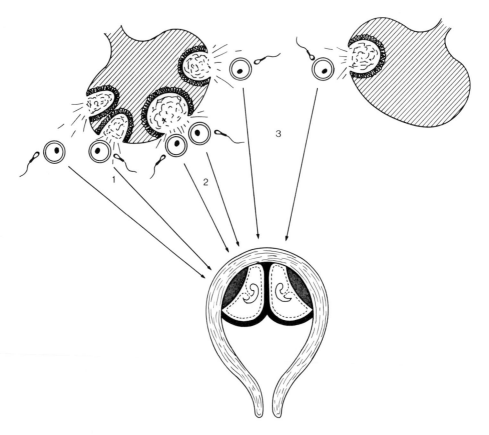

Fig. 5-4. Possible ways by which dizygotic twins may occur: (1) Two ova ovulate from two graafian follicles in one ovary at about the same time. They are fertilized by two spermatozoa. (2) Two ova ovulate from a single graafian follicle in one ovary at the same time. They are fertilized by two spermatozoa. (3) One ovum ovulates from each ovary at about the same time. They are fertilized by two spermatozoa.

pregnancies all seem to play a part. Tall, older, multiparous women from the upper social classes are more likely to have multiple dizygotic pregnancies than others. It is interesting to note that artificial stimulation of the ovaries in the treatment of amenorrhea or anovular menstruation may result in multiple pregnancies. The use of the pituitary follicle-stimulating hormone (FSH), followed by the chorionic gonadotropic hormone or treat-

ment with the synthetic nonsteroid *clomiphene,* may cause the maturation and liberation of several ova that may become fertilized.

Coming as they do from different ova, the babies will have different genetic constitutions and will be no more alike than babies from separate pregnancies, and they may or may not be of the same sex.

Clinical Problems
Answers on page 435

1. A 21-year-old pregnant woman asked her obstetrician what her chances were of having twins. Her mother had had twins and so had her grandmother. How would you answer her inquiry? Do you think it is necessary to ask this woman whether her mother and grandmother had identical or dissimilar sets of twins? Does the incidence of multiple pregnancies on the father's side of the family have any effect on the chances of having twins?

2. A fourth-year medical student was asked by an obstetrician whether a 40-year-old mother was more likely to have a multiple pregnancy than a 20-year-old mother. What would you say in answer to the question?

3. Do you think there are any racial differences in the incidence of multiple pregnancies? Does parity have any influence on the frequency of twinning?

4. What is the etiological relationship between identical twins, conjoined twins, and a double-headed monster?

5. What is the approximate incidence of twins and triplets in the United States? Do you know of any therapeutic measures which could increase the incidence of multiple births?

6. A 28-year-old expectant mother was told by her obstetrician that she was going to have twins. The father, after recovering from the shock, asked the physician whether or not the mortality for twins was higher than for a single birth and the risks greater for the mother who has twins. How would you have answered these questions?

7. If, during the management of a multiple pregnancy, one fetus should die, what becomes of the dead fetus? Does the live fetus suffer any ill effects?

8. An obese 23-year-old primigravid woman was successfully delivered of two fine babies. On learning that she had twins, she was very annoyed and could not understand why her obstetrician had not made the diagnosis before she went into labor. Using your knowledge of embryology, how would you diagnose twins in a pregnant woman? Is it sometimes difficult to make the diagnosis? If so, why?

9. What type of twins would you diagnose if the following were present: (a) two chorions? (b) one sex? (c) one placenta? (d) two amnions? (e) one amnion? (f) two sexes? (g) two placentas? (h) one chorion?

REFERENCES

Baird, D. *Combined Textbook of Obstetrics and Gynaecology,* 8th ed. Livingstone, Edinburgh, 1969.

Corner, G. W. The Observed Embryology of Human Single Ovum Twins and Other Multiple Births. *Amer. J. Obstet. Gynec.* 70:933, 1955.

Fogel, B. J., Nitowsky, H. M., and Gruenwald, P. Discordant Abnormalities in Monozygotic Twins. *J. Pediat.* 66:64, 1965.

Gedda, L. *Twins in History and Science.* Thomas, Springfield, Ill., 1961.

Hamilton, W. J., Brown, D., and Spiers, B. G. Another Case of Quadruplets. *J. Obstet. Gynaec. Brit. Comm.* 66:409, 1959.

Nance, W. E.   Twins: An Introduction to Gemellology. *Medicine* 38:403, 1959.

Newman, H. H.   *Multiple Human Births: Twins, Triplets, Quadruplets and Quintuplets.* Doubleday, Doran, New York, 1940.

Newman, H. H., Freeman, F. N., and Holzinger, K. J.   *Twins: A Study of Heredity and Environment.* University of Chicago Press, Chicago, 1937.

Oettle, A. G.   Paternal Influence in Polyzygotic Births. *J. Obstet. Gynaec. Brit. Emp.* 60:775, 1953.

Potter, E. L.   Twin Zygosity and Placental Form in Relation to the Outcome of Pregnancy. *Amer. J. Obstet. Gynec.* 87:566, 1963.

Price, B.   Primary Biases in Twin Studies. *Amer. J. Hum. Genet.* 2:293, 1950.

Salerno, L. J.   Monoamniotic Twinning. *Obstet. Gynec.* 14:205, 1959.

Smith, S. M., and Penrose, L. S.   Monozygotic and Dizygotic Twin Diagnosis. *Ann. Hum. Gen.* 19:273, 1955.

White, C., and Wyshak, G.   Inheritance in Human Dizygotic Twinning. *New Eng. J. Med.* 271:1003, 1964.

The prenatal growth of the developing child may be divided into three main periods:

Period I.　　*The preembryonic period* extends from the fertilization of the ovum to the formation of the embryonic disc with three germ layers. This is from *week 1* to *week 3,* inclusive.

Period II.　　*The embryonic period* is a time of rapid growth and differentiation, and of the formation of all the major organs of the body. This extends from *week 4* to *week 8,* inclusive.

Period III.　　*The fetal period* is characterized by growth and further development of the organs and systems established during the embryonic stage. This extends from *week 9* to the *tenth lunar month,* inclusive.

ESTIMATION OF AGE DURING THE PRENATAL PERIOD

To estimate accurately the age in the prenatal period, it would be necessary to have the precise coital and menstrual history of the mother. This information is extremely difficult to obtain, since the majority of pregnant women do not present themselves to the obstetrician until their pregnancies are fairly well advanced, by which time any recollection of the precise date of coitus is usually vague. The embryologist commonly uses two methods to estimate the age of the fetus: (1) he measures the crown-rump (C.R.) length, i.e., from the vertex of the skull to the breech, and (2) in embryos between week 4 and week 5, inclusive, he records the age by the number of somites present. It should be pointed out that there is considerable variation in the rate of development from one individual to another, so that a precise estimate of age of the fetus is impossible.

An obstetrician uses the date of the commencement of the last menstrual cycle as the point of reference, which most women have no difficulty in remembering. This point of reference is sufficiently accurate for the estimation of the approximate date of delivery (see Chap. 24), but in women with irregular menstrual cycles the estimate may be very inaccurate. There is thus no absolutely precise method of estimating the age of the fetus during the prenatal period. For information on age, size, and weight of the fetus, see Table 6-1.

Table 6-1. Size and weight of the human embryo and fetus at various ages

Age of Conceptus (weeks)	Crown-Rump Length (mm)	Weight (gm)
4	5	0.02
5	8	—
8	23	1
12	56	14
16	112	105
20	160	310
24	203	640
28	242	1,080
32	277	1,670
36	313	2,400
Full term	350	3,300

Source: Arey, 1966

Before considering the growth and development of the fetus, it would seem desirable to review here the main landmarks of development during the embryonic period, i.e., week 4 to week 8, inclusive. Table 6-2 presents a timetable of normal human development during the prenatal growth period.

MAJOR DEVELOPMENTAL CHANGES DURING THE EMBRYONIC PERIOD

Fourth Week (Fig. 6-1). The embryo has become elongated and curved upon itself with the formation of a head fold and a tail fold. The lateral body folds are also well developed so that the embryo is no longer a flat pear-shaped disc, but is tubular. Most of the body systems have appeared and are in rudimentary form. The neural tube, which will form the brain and spinal cord, is present; the laryngotracheal groove and lung buds, which will become the respiratory system, have appeared. The eyes, nose, and ears are present in rudimentary form. The yolk sac has largely been taken into the embryo to form the intestinal system and already the esophagus, stomach, liver, and pancreatic buds are differentiating. The thyroid and thymus glands have started to develop. The heart is beating, and a primitive circulatory system is established connecting the capillary plexuses of the yolk sac and chorion with the embryo. The extremities are seen as bud-like projections on the surface of the embryo. The chorion, with its villi, has become greatly developed, and the placenta has started to form. The embryo measures about 5 mm (0.2 in.) C.R. length.

Fifth Week. The parathyroids, spleen, genital ridges, and external genitalia have begun to form. The stomach starts to rotate and the midgut forms a loop. The face is forming, and the limb buds show some differentiation into limb, forelimb, hand, or foot. The embryo measures about 8 mm (0.3 in.) C.R. length.

Eighth Week (second month). The head has greatly increased in size and is nearly as large as the rest of the body. The neck region has become established. The central nervous system undergoes rapid growth with the expansion of the forebrain vesicle. Neuromuscular development is now sufficient to permit movements of the fetus. The body is covered with a thin skin. The epidermis is established and the fetus is covered with a layer of *periderm,* or *epitrichium.* The facial features are more distinct and the eyes are directed more forward instead of laterally; the nose is more prominent. Centers of ossification are appearing in the bones. The limbs are more developed, and the digits on the hands and feet are separate. Of the two sets of limb buds, the upper appears first and undergoes differentiation sooner. The external genitalia, with the formation of the genital tubercle and genital swellings, have developed further, but no definite sex characteristics have appeared. The embryo measures

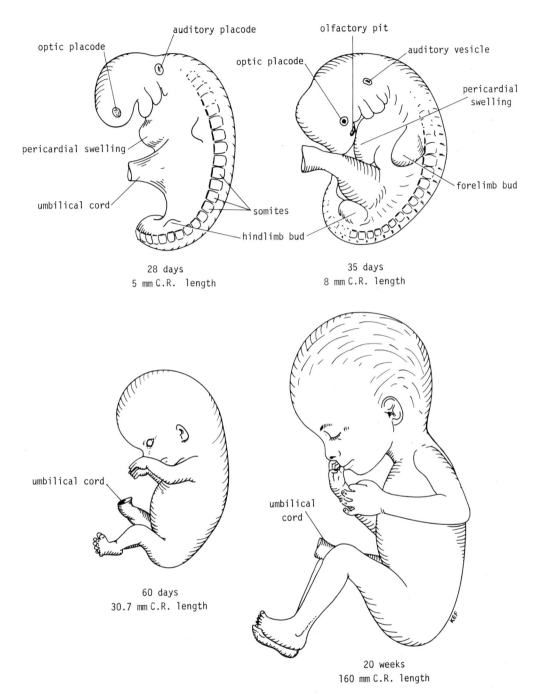

Fig. 6-1. Two embryos and two fetuses at different stages of development.

Table 6-2. Timetable of Normal Human Development

Age (weeks)	Gross Appearance	Cardiovascular	Digestive	Respiratory	Urogenital	Nervous System	Sense Organs	Musculoskeletal
1st	Fertilization. Cleavage of zygote. Blastocyst enters uterine cavity. Trophoblast, inner cell mass.							
2d	Zona pellucida disappears. Blastocyst enlarges. Implantation. Syncytiotrophoblast and cytotrophoblast formed. Primary chorionic villi. Formation of embryonic disc, ectoderm, endoderm, amnion, and yolk sac. Extra-embryonic mesoderm. Extra-embryonic coelom. Primitive streak. Mesoderm and notochord.							
3d	Head and tail folds.	Primitive vascular system established. Heart tube.	Buccopharyngeal membrane breaks down. Allantois begins to form.			Neural plate. Neural folds. Partial fusion of neural folds.		Somites appear.

			Foregut. Midgut. Hindgut.					
4th	Body narrow and tubular; C-shaped. Connection with yolk sac very narrowed; limb buds appear. Placenta begins to form.	Heart is enlarged and beating. Partitioning of atrium begins. Hemopoiesis in yolk sac.	Esophagus, stomach, liver, and pancreatic buds.	Laryngo-tracheal tube, trachea, lung buds.	Meso-nephros rapidly forming.	Neural tube. Three primary vesicles of brain.	Optic placode and auditory vesicle present.	Most somites formed. Myotome, sclerotome, and dermatome.
5th	Head increases greatly in size. Face is forming. Limb buds show limb, forelimb, hand or foot.	Cardiac septa developing. Atrio-ventricular cushions fusing.	Stomach starts to rotate. Midgut forms loop. Uro-rectal septum.	Lobes of lung formed.	Genital ridges. External genitalia.	Telen-cephalon. Dienceph-alon. Mesen-cephalon. Metencepha-lon. Myelen-cephalon. Cerebral hemisphere.	Lens vesicle. Auditory vesicle.	Condensation of mesen-chyme to form cartilage and muscle.
6th	Head dominant. Oral and nasal cavities confluent.	Heart now has definitive form. Foramen primum closes.	Upper lip forming. Dental laminae. Palatal processes.	Bronchi dividing.	Parame-sonephric ducts. Sex cords start to develop	Flexures of brain obvious.	Naso-lacrimal duct.	Chondrification. Intramembranous ossification.

Timetable of Normal Human Development (continued)

Age (weeks)	Gross Appearance	Cardiovascular	Digestive	Respiratory	Urogenital	Nervous System	Sense Organs	Musculoskeletal
6th cont'd	Curvature of embryo diminished. Fingers and toes recognizable.	Aortico-pulmonary septation. Hematopoiesis in liver.	Pleuro-peritoneal canals close. Midgut loop herniates. Cecum and appendix. Vitello-intestinal duct atrophies.		in testis. Cloaca divided.			
8th	Head nearly as large as rest of body. Facial features more distinct. Eyes directed more anteriorly. Neck established. Limbs more developed. Digits of hands and feet separated. Fetus covered with epitrichium. Retrogression of tail.	Ventricular septum completed in week 7.	Enamel organs. Small intestine rotating in umbilical cord. Cloacal membrane has broken down.	Bron-chioles dividing.	Genital tubercle and genital swellings further developed. Still sexless. Meso-nephros fully developed. Meta-nephric duct branch-ing to form collect-ing tu-bules.	Rapid growth of CNS. Expansion of forebrain vesicle.	Eyes con-verging. Eyelids develop-ing. External nares plugged. Auricle of ex-ternal ear forming.	Fetal muscular movement commences. Enchondral ossification. Smooth muscle.

12th	Rapid growth in fetal length. Head still relatively large. Eyes look anteriorly. External ears on side of head. Eyelids fused. Lanugo present. Nails. Sex recognition possible.	Hematopoiesis in liver and spleen.	Nasal septum and palate fusion complete. Midgut loop returns to abdominal cavity. Fetus swallowing amniotic fluid.	Lungs are of definitive shape.	Testes and ovaries recognizable. Kidneys have started to secrete urine. External genitalia sufficiently developed to identify sex. Testes close to future deep inguinal ring.	Brain and spinal cord well developed. Cauda equina. Filum terminale.	Eyelids fuse. Nasal septum fuses with palate.	
16th	Further rapid growth in fetal length. Head still relatively large. Eyes widely separated	Hematopoiesis in bone marrow commences.	Ascending and descending colon retroperitoneal. Meconium		Mesonephros involuted. Definitive lobulated kidney present. External	Cerebellum prominent. Myelination begins in spinal cord.	Eyes, ears, and nose in final positions.	Joint cavities.

Timetable of Normal Human Development (continued)

Age (weeks)	Gross Appearance	Cardiovascular	Digestive	Respiratory	Urogenital	Nervous System	Sense Organs	Musculoskeletal
16th cont'd	but eyelids fused. Auricles of ear high up on side of head. Fetus looks human.		starts to accumulate.		genitalia well developed.			
20th	Lanugo covers entire body. Vernix caseosa present. Hair present on head. Mother detects quickening.	Fetal heart beat heard with stethoscope.	Meconium reaches rectum.					Distinct movements of limbs felt by mother (quickening).
24th	Skin wrinkled and red. Head still relatively large. Face child-like. Eyebrows and eyelashes present. Eyelids open.			Pulmonary alveoli appear.		Myelination begins in brain.	Eyelids reopen.	Movements stronger.

28th	Skin wrinkled. Subcutaneous fat appearing. Fetal contours more rounded. Hair on head longer.		Testes in inguinal canal.			
32d	Fetus looks wrinkled and scraggy. Lanugo hair has disappeared from face. Vernix caseosa thick. Nails reach end of fingers.					
36th	Fetus looks plumper and rounder.		Left testis in scrotum.	Cerebral fissures and convolutions rapidly developing.		Movements much stronger.
40th	Fetus fully developed. More subcutaneous fat present. Lanugo hairs disappear. Nails project beyond ends of fingers and toes.	Bronchioles and alveoli still developing.	Both testes in scrotum. Kidneys lie opposite L2.	Lower end of spinal cord L3.	Paranasal sinuses are rudimentary.	Bones of skull are firm. Circumference of skull larger than rest of body.

about 23 mm (0.9 in.) C.R. length and weighs about 1 gm.

MAJOR DEVELOPMENTAL CHANGES DURING THE FETAL PERIOD

This period is characterized by the rapid growth of the body, while there is minimal further morphological differentiation of the tissues.

Twelfth Week (third month). The fetus grows rapidly, nearly doubling its length. The head remains relatively large and is about one-third of the C.R. length. The forehead is high and prominent, and as a result of broadening of the face the eyes look directly anteriorly. The external ear, which was low down on the side of the head, is now located opposite the jaw. The eyes have lids that now fuse and do not reopen until the seventh month. The first rudiments of fine hair, called *lanugo,* appear over the forehead and eyebrow region. Nails are present on the dorsal aspect of the tips of the fingers. The midgut has been withdrawn into the abdomen from the extra-embryonic coelom in the umbilical cord. The kidneys have started to secrete urine. The buccopharyngeal membrane has ruptured during the third week, and the fetus now starts to swallow amniotic fluid. The external genitalia are sufficiently developed to identify the sex of the fetus. The fetus measures about 56 mm (2.2 in.) C.R. length and weighs about 14 gm (0.5 oz.).

Sixteenth Week (fourth month). A rapid increase in size takes place and the fetus now looks definitely human; individual differences can be recognized. The head is still proportionately large, but the face is relatively broad and the eyes are widely separated. The eyelids remain fused. The mandible is sufficiently developed so that the fetus exhibits a chin. The auricles of the ear now rise to a higher level on the side of the head. The external genitalia are well developed and the identification of the sex of the fetus presents no difficulty. The fetus measures about 112 mm (4.5 in.) C.R. length and weighs about 105 gm (3.7 oz.).

Twentieth Week (fifth month). The fine lanugo hair covers the entire body and the sebaceous glands are actively secreting sebum. The sebum mixes with the surface epithelium to form a greasy, cheesy substance called the *vernix caseosa,* which covers the skin from now until birth. Hair appears on the head. Fetal movements are sufficiently strong that they may be detected by the mother. This early detection of movement by the mother is called *quickening.* The fetal heart beat may be heard through a stethoscope placed on the mother's abdomen. The fetus measures about 160 mm (6.5 in.) C.R. length and weighs about 310 gm (10.8 oz.).

Twenty-fourth Week (sixth month). The skin is characteristically very wrinkled and red at this time. This is probably a result of the rapid growth of the skin and lack of subcutaneous fat; the red myohemoglobin of the muscle shows through the translucent skin. The head is still large in size as compared to the rest of the body. The face is more childlike, the eyebrows and eyelashes are present, and the eyelids have opened. The fetus measures about 200 mm (8.1 in.) C.R. length and weighs about 640 gm (1 lb. 4 oz.). The majority of fetuses born at this time die shortly after birth.

Twenty-eighth Week (seventh month). The fetus still looks old and wrinkled. However, subcutaneous fat has started to be deposited so that the fetal contours will become rounded. The hair on the head is longer. The fetus measures about 240 mm (9 in.) C.R. length and weighs about 1,080 gm (2 lb. 6 oz.). If born at this stage, the fetus will probably survive, with careful attention. At birth the baby will move and cry quite vigorously.

Thirty-second Week (eighth month). The fetus still looks wrinkled and scraggy, but further subcutaneous fat has been deposited. The lanugo hair has disappeared from the face and the hair on the head is longer. The vernix caseosa now thickly covers the skin and probably protects it from maceration by the liquor amnii. The fingernails reach the ends of the fingers, but the toenails do not yet reach the ends of the toes. The fetus measures about 280 mm (11 in.) C.R. length and weighs about 1,670 gm (3 lb. 11 oz.). If born at this time, the fetus has a good chance of survival if given careful attention.

Thirty-sixth Week (ninth month). The subcutaneous fat is much thicker and the child loses its wrinkled appearance and looks plumper and rounder. In the male, the left testis has usually descended into the scrotum. The fetus now measures about 310 mm (12.55 in.) C.R. length and weighs about 2,400 gm (5¼ lb.). If born at this time, the fetus has an excellent chance of survival.

Fortieth Week (tenth month). During the tenth month, the fetus reaches full development and further subcutaneous fat is deposited. The lanugo hairs disappear and the nails project beyond the ends of the fingers and toes. In the male, both testes are in the scrotum. The bones of the skull are firm and the circumference of the skull is larger than that of any other part of the body, which is an important factor to be considered in childbirth. The baby measures about 350 mm (14 in.) C.R. length and weighs about 3,300 gm (7¼ lb.). The birth weight varies quite considerably, but healthy babies weigh from about 2,500 gm (5½ lb.) to 5,000 gm (11 lb.).

Clinical Problems
Answers on page 436

1. A 25-year-old-woman was delivered of a premature baby weighing about 3½ lb. The child looked small and wrinkled and was covered with lanugo hair except on the face. The skin was covered with a cheesy-looking material. The fingernails reached the ends of the fingers, but the toenails did not reach the ends of the toes. The child had a lusty cry and a good color. What is the definition of premature? What is the name of the cheesy material covering the skin? What is the approximate period of gestation? Do you think the child had a good chance of survival?
2. What are the differences between the embryonic period and the fetal period?
3. Can you think of any cause for a baby born at full term to be excessively small and underweight?

REFERENCES

Arey, L. B. *Developmental Anatomy,* 7th ed. Saunders, Philadelphia, 1966.
Davis, C. L. Description of a Human Embryo Having 20 Paired Somites. *Contrib. Embryol.* 15:1, 1923.

Hamilton, W. J., and Mossman, H. W. *Human Embryology,* 4th ed. Williams & Wilkins, Baltimore, 1972.
Heuser, C. H., and Corner, G. W. Developmental Horizons in Human Embryos: Description of

Age Group X, 4 to 12 Somites. *Contrib. Embryol.* 36:29, 1957.

Scammon, R. E., and Calkins, H. A. *Development and Growth of the External Dimensions of the Human Body in the Foetal Period.* University of Minnesota Press, Minneapolis, 1929.

Streeter, G. L. Developmental Horizons in Human Embryos: Age Group XI, 13–20 Somites, and Age Group XII, 21–29 Somites. *Contrib. Embryol.* 30:211, 1942.

Streeter, G. L. Developmental Horizons in Human Embryos: Age Group XIII, Embryos 4 or 5 mm. Long and Age Group XIV, Indentation of Lens Vesicle. *Contrib. Embryol.* 31:26, 1945.

Streeter, G. L. Developmental Horizons in Human Embryos: Age Groups XV, XVI, XVII, and XVIII, Being the Third Issue of a Survey of the Carnegie Collection. *Contrib. Embryol.* 32:133, 1948.

Willier, B. H., Weiss, P. A., and Hamburger, V. *Analysis of Development.* Saunders, Philadelphia, 1955.

DEVELOPMENT

The Primitive Vascular System

At the third week of development, the embryo can no longer nourish itself adequately by the process of simple diffusion of food materials across the extra-embryonic coelom. A primitive vascular system is now established. Clusters of mesenchymal cells in the yolk sac wall, chorion, and body stalk start to proliferate and form *blood islands* (Figs. 7-1 & 7-2). The peripheral cells of each island become flattened and form the endothelial lining of the vessels. Intercellular clefts appear between the centrally located cells, and these become detached and free and form the *primitive blood cells*. Meanwhile fluid has been accumulating between the blood cells and forms the blood *plasma* (Fig. 7-3). As more blood islands form, they enlarge and fuse with each other, and the endothelial-lined spaces become arranged to form capillary plexuses. In the wall of the yolk sac, these plexuses are known as the *area vasculosa,* and as they join one another they eventually envelop the whole sac. Gradually certain of the capillaries enlarge to form main blood vessels, and in this manner the *vitelline vessels* are formed in the wall of the yolk sac and the *umbilical vessels* are formed in the chorion

and body stalk. These extra-embryonic blood vessels now join blood vessels inside the embryo that have developed from the mesenchyme in a similar manner. A primitive extra-embryonic and intra-embryonic vascular system has now been established (Fig. 7-4).

Formation of the Heart Tube

Scattered clusters of cells arise in the mesenchyme at the cephalic end of the embryonic disc, cephalic to the buccopharyngeal membrane and the neural plate. These isolated groups of cells now form a plexus of endothelial vessels that fuse to form *right* and *left endocardial heart tubes*. These soon fuse to form a single median *endocardial heart tube*. As the head fold develops, the pericardial cavity (see page 34) and the endocardial tube rotate on a transverse axis through almost 180 degrees, so that they come to lie ventral to the foregut and caudal to the buccopharyngeal membrane. The septum transversum (Chap. 3) is now situated between the pericardial cavity and the stalk of the yolk sac. The heart tube starts to bulge into the dorsal surface of the pericardial cavity (Fig. 7-5). As the tube sinks further into the pericardial cavity, it becomes suspended from its dorsal wall by a mesentery, the

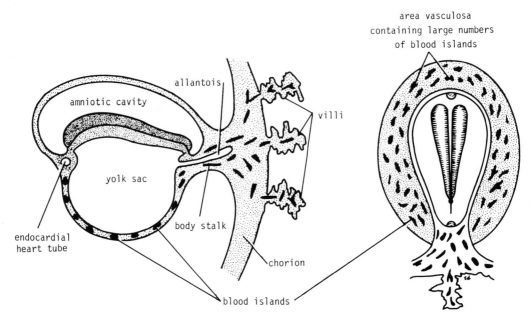

Fig. 7-1. Longitudinal section of embryo showing the appearance of blood islands in the splanchnic mesoderm of the wall of the yolk sac. Similar islands are appearing in the body stalk. These will ultimately join and form, with the capillaries in the chorionic villi, the extra-embryonic circulation.

Fig. 7-2. Embryonic disc as seen from above. The amnion has been cut away and removed.

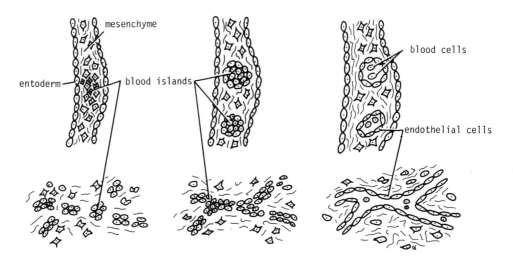

Fig. 7-3. Differentiation of mesodermal cells in a blood island to form endothelial lining cells and blood cells.

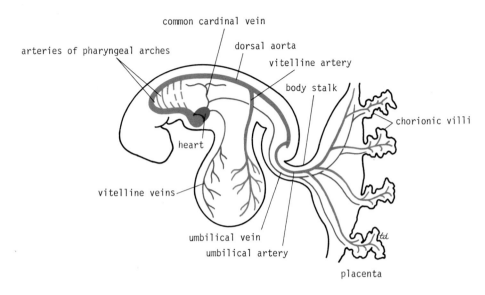

common cardinal vein

arteries of pharyngeal arches

dorsal aorta

vitelline artery

body stalk

chorionic villi

heart

vitelline veins

umbilical vein

umbilical artery

placenta

Fig. 7-4. Intra-embryonic and extra-embryonic circulations.

dorsal mesocardium. Meanwhile the endocardial tube becomes surrounded by a thick layer of mesenchymal cells forming the *myoepicardial mantle.* Later the cells of this mantle will differentiate into the muscle cells of the *myocardium* and the mesothelial cells of the *epicardium.* The dorsal mesocardium now disappears, leaving the heart tube attached to the pericardium only at its cephalic and caudal ends. The primitive heart has been established and is situated ventral to the pharynx. The cephalic end of the heart is the arterial end, and the caudal end is the venous end. The heart begins to beat during the third week.

The arterial end of the primitive heart is continuous beyond the pericardium with a large vessel, the *aortic sac.* The sac gives off two branches, each of which runs dorsally in the first pharyngeal arch on each side; the branches then run caudally along the posterior wall of the embryo as the two *dorsal aortae.* Five additional arteries next appear on each side caudal to the first and join the aortic sac to the dorsal aortae, each running

in a respective pharyngeal arch. In lower animals, the aortic sac is represented by two vessels, the ventral aortae.

The venous end of the primitive heart tube receives the vitelline veins from the yolk sac, the umbilical veins from the placenta, and the common cardinal veins from the body wall (Fig. 7-6).

Further Development of the Heart Tube

The heart tube now undergoes differential expansion so that several dilatations, separated by grooves, result. From the arterial to the venous end these dilatations are called the *bulbus cordis,* the *ventricle,* the *atrium,* and the right and left horns of the *sinus venosus.* It should be noted that in the earliest stages the atrium and the right and left horns of the sinus venosus are situated outside the pericardium, and later, as development proceeds, they become drawn into the pericardial cavity. The bulbus cordis and ventricular parts of the tube now start to elongate more rapidly than the other parts of the tube, and

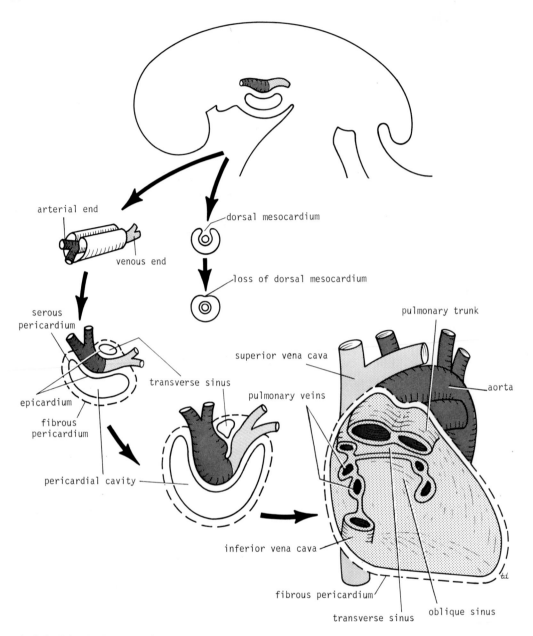

Fig. 7-5. The development of the endocardial tube in relation to the pericardial cavity.

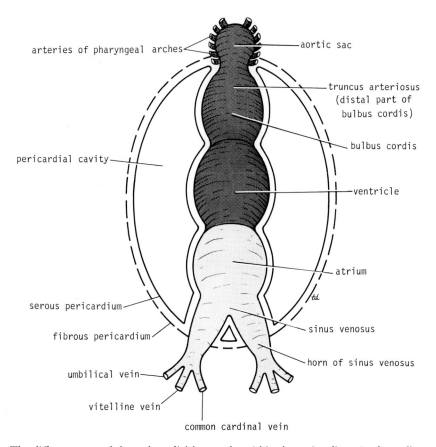

arteries of pharyngeal arches

aortic sac

truncus arteriosus
(distal part of
bulbus cordis)

bulbus cordis

pericardial cavity

ventricle

atrium

serous pericardium

sinus venosus

fibrous pericardium

horn of sinus venosus

umbilical vein

vitelline vein

common cardinal vein

Fig. 7-6. The different parts of the endocardial heart tube within the pericardium. In the earliest stages, the atrium and the sinus venosus lie outside the pericardial cavity.

since the arterial and venous ends are fixed by the pericardium, the tube begins to bend (Fig. 7-7). With a continued rapid increase in length, the bend soon becomes a U-shaped loop with its convexity directed anteriorly and to the right. Later it becomes a compound S-shaped curve with the atrium lying posterior to the ventricle; in addition, the venous and arterial ends are brought close together as in the adult. Meanwhile the passage between the atrium and the ventricle narrows to form the *atrioventricular canal.* The atrium, ventricle, and bulbus cordis now expand rapidly and undergo some change in position. The atrium expands transversely and appears on either side of the bulbus

cordis. As these changes are taking place, there is a gradual caudal migration of the pericardium and heart tube. In the earliest stage they are situated in the neck region at the level of the third and fourth somites. Later they are found opposite the derivatives of the seventeenth to twentieth somites.

Development of the Atria and Fate of the Sinus Venosus

The primitive atrium becomes divided into two, i.e., the right and left atria in the following manner (Fig. 7-8): The atrioventricular canal becomes widened transversely. At the same time cellular proliferations occur on the

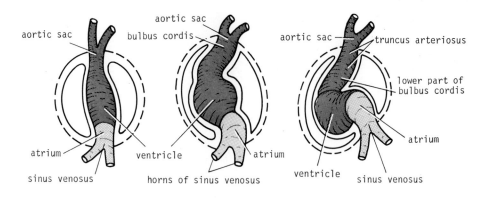

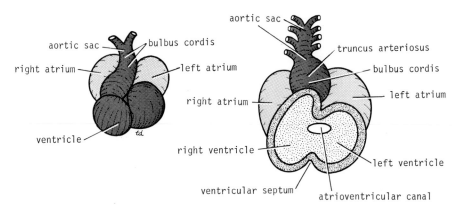

Fig. 7-7. The bending of the heart tube within the pericardial cavity.

ventral and dorsal walls of the canal producing elevations called the *ventral* and *dorsal atrioventricular cushions* (endocardial cushions). These soon fuse so that the atrioventricular canal is divided into right and left halves by a septum known as the *septum intermedium.* Meanwhile a septum, the *septum primum,* develops from the roof of the primitive atrium and grows down to fuse with the septum intermedium. Before fusion occurs, the opening between the lower edge of the septum primum and the septum intermedium is referred to as the *foramen primum.* The atrium is now divided into right and left parts. Before complete obliteration of the foramen primum has taken place,

degenerative changes take place in the central portion of the septum primum and a foramen appears, the *foramen secundum,* so that the right and left atrial chambers again communicate. Another thicker septum, the *septum secundum,* grows down from the atrial roof on the right side of the septum primum. The lower edge of the septum secundum overlaps the foramen secundum in the septum primum, but it does not reach the floor of the atrium and does not fuse with the septum intermedium. The space between the free margin of the septum secundum and the septum primum is now known as the *foramen ovale.*

Before birth, the foramen ovale allows the

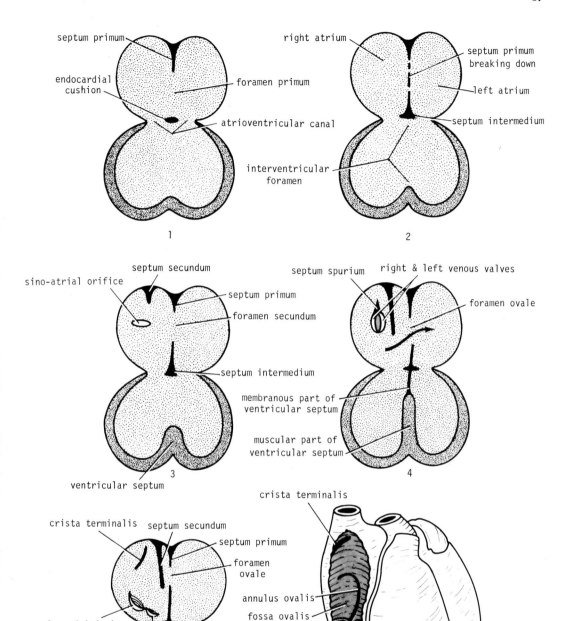

Fig. 7-8. The division of the primitive atrium into right and left atria by the appearance of the septa. The sino-atrial orifice and the fate of the venous valves is also shown, as is the appearance of the ventricular septum.

passage of oxygenated blood that has entered the right atrium from the inferior vena cava to pass into the left atrium. The lower part of the septum primum serves as a flap-like valve and prevents blood moving from the left atrium into the right atrium. At birth, owing to raised blood pressure in the left atrium, the septum primum is pressed against the septum secundum and fuses with it, and the foramen ovale is closed. The two atria are thus separated from each other. The lower edge of the septum secundum seen in the right atrium becomes the *annulus ovalis,* and the depression below this is called the *fossa ovalis* (Fig. 7-8).

Sinus Venosus

During the formation of the endocardial heart tube, the right and left endocardial tubes fuse together. The caudal ends of these tubes are the last to fuse, however, and the horns of the sinus venosus remain unfused. The sinus venosus at first opens into the primitive atrium. The right horn of the sinus venosus now grows much more rapidly than the left horn. As a consequence of this, the sino-atrial orifice moves to the right and opens into that part of the atrium which will become the right atrium. The transversely oriented oval sino-atrial orifice then becomes oriented in a vertical direction and the margins project into the right atrium as *right* and *left venous valves* (Fig. 7-8). The cranial edges of these valves later fuse to form a projection, the *septum spurium.* The sino-atrial opening now becomes dilated so that the right horn of the sinus venosus is taken into and becomes part of the right atrium. The septum spurium remains as the *crista terminalis;* in this way the crista represents the line of demarcation between the atrium proper, the interior of which is roughened by the *musculi pectinati,* and the smooth-walled sinus. The left venous valve regresses and the right venous valve becomes the *valve of the* *inferior vena cava* and the *valve of the coronary sinus.*

Originally the right and left horns of the sinus venosus received blood from the vitelline veins, the umbilical veins, and the common cardinal veins. As development proceeds, the terminal parts of the left umbilical and the left vitelline veins become obliterated, and the left sinus horn remains small. Later the left horn of the sinus becomes the *coronary sinus.*

In the left atrium, the root of the pulmonary vein is absorbed into the wall of the atrium. This process of absorption continues until all four large tributaries of the pulmonary vein open into the left atrium by separate openings. As the result of this, the part of the left atrial wall in the vicinity of the entrance of the pulmonary veins is smooth, while the remainder is roughened by the musculi pectinati. The *right* and *left auricular appendages* later develop as small diverticula from the right and left atria, respectively.

Development of the Ventricles and Fate of the Bulbus Cordis

During the fourth week, a muscular partition begins to project upward from the floor of the primitive ventricle. This *ventricular septum* first appears as the result of an indentation of the muscular wall that is represented on the external surface as a sulcus (Fig. 7-8). Later there is active growth of this muscular septum which extends upward as a crescentic plate. The space bounded by the crescentic edge of the septum and the endocardial cushions is called the *interventricular foramen.* The primitive ventricle has now been divided into right and left ventricles that communicate with each other through the interventricular foramen and with the cavity of the bulbus cordis.

Meanwhile, spiral subendocardial thickenings, the *bulbar ridges,* appear in the distal part of the bulbus cordis. By the eighth week,

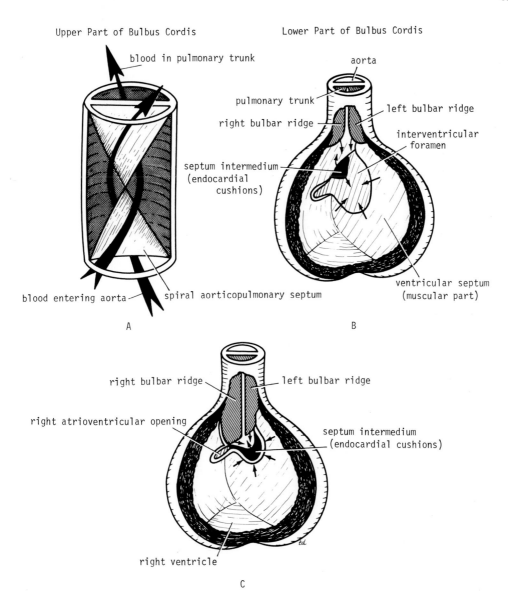

Upper Part of Bulbus Cordis Lower Part of Bulbus Cordis

blood in pulmonary trunk

aorta

pulmonary trunk

right bulbar ridge

left bulbar ridge

interventricular foramen

septum intermedium (endocardial cushions)

blood entering aorta spiral aorticopulmonary septum

ventricular septum (muscular part)

A B

right bulbar ridge left bulbar ridge

right atrioventricular opening

septum intermedium (endocardial cushions)

right ventricle

C

Fig. 7-9. The division of the bulbus cordis by the spiral aorticopulmonary septum into the aorta and pulmonary trunk: (A) The spiral septum in the truncus arteriosus (upper part of bulbus cordis). (B) Lower part of bulbus cordis. Formation of spiral septum by fusion of the bulbar ridges which then grow down and join the septum intermedium and the muscular part of the ventricular septum. (C) The area of the ventricular septum which is formed from the fused bulbar ridges and the septum intermedium is called the *membranous part* of the ventricular septum.

the bulbar ridges have grown and fused to form a *spiral aorticopulmonary septum* (Fig. 7-9).

The interventricular foramen closes as the result of proliferation of the bulbar ridges and the fused endocardial cushions (septum intermedium). This newly formed tissue grows down and fuses with the crescentic upper edge of the muscular ventricular septum and forms the *membranous part of the septum* (Fig. 7-9). The closure of the interventricular foramen not only shuts off the path of communication between the right and left ventricles but also ensures that the right ventricular cavity is in communication with the pulmonary trunk and the left ventricular cavity is in communication with the aorta. In addition, the right atrioventricular opening now connects exclusively with the right ventricular cavity and the left atrioventricular opening with the left ventricular cavity.

The distal part of the bulbus cordis is known as the *truncus arteriosus* and is divided by the spiral aorticopulmonary septum to form the roots and proximal portions of the aorta and pulmonary trunk. With the establishment of right and left ventricles, the proximal portion of the bulbus cordis becomes incorporated into the right ventricle as the definitive *conus arteriosus* or *infundibulum,* and into the left ventricle as the *aortic vestibule.*

Development of the Cardiac Valves

Semilunar Valves of the Aorta and Pulmonary Arteries

Following the formation of the aorticopulmonary septum, three swellings appear at the orifices of both the aorta and pulmonary artery. Each swelling consists of a covering of endothelium over loose connective tissue. Gradually the swellings become excavated on their upper surfaces to form the semilunar valves (Fig. 7-10).

Atrioventricular Valves

After the formation of the septum intermedium the atrioventricular canal becomes divided into right and left atrioventricular orifices. Raised folds of endocardium appear at the margins of these orifices (Fig. 7-10). These folds are invaded by mesenchymal tissue which later becomes hollowed out from the ventricular side. Three valvular cusps are formed about the right atrioventricular orifice and constitute the *tricuspid valve,* and two cusps are formed about the left atrioventricular orifice to become the *mitral valve.* The newly formed cusps enlarge, and their mesenchymal core becomes differentiated into fibrous tissue. The cusps remain attached at intervals to the ventricular wall by muscular strands. Later the muscular strands become differentiated into *papillary muscles* and *chordae tendineae.*

Cardiac Muscle and the Conducting System of the Heart

Early in development the endocardial tube becomes surrounded by a thick layer of mesenchyme called the *myo-epicardial mantle.* This later differentiates to form the cardiac muscle and fibrous tissue of the heart and the visceral layer of the serous pericardium, the epicardium. The muscle coat or myocardium differentiates into an outer compact layer of muscle and a spongy layer, the loosely arranged trabeculae of which project into the cavity of the heart. The endocardium dips into the spaces between the trabeculae and lines them. In the atria and auricles, the original trabeculae remain as the *musculi pectinati* and in the ventricles as the *trabeculae carneae,* papillary muscles, and chordae tendineae.

The myocardium of the atria is at first continuous with that of the ventricles, but later it becomes separated by fibrous tissue in the region of the atrioventricular canal, and

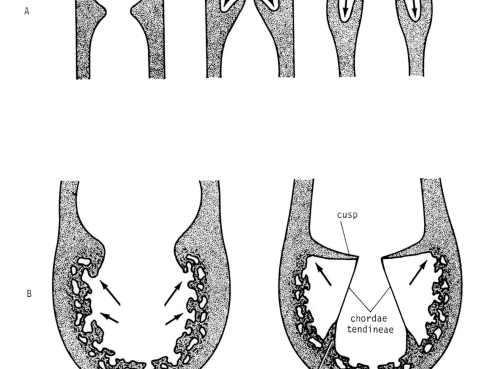

Fig. 7-10. (A) The formation of the semilunar valves of the aorta and pulmonary arteries. (B) The formation of the cusps of the atrioventricular valves.

only a small link remains. The connecting strand of muscle undergoes further differentiation and forms the *atrioventricular bundle,* a part of the conducting system of the heart. The *sino-atrial node,* the *atrioventricular node,* and the *Purkinje fibers* develop as a local differentiation of cardiac muscle. The conducting system is first seen in late embryonic or early fetal life. The cells are located just external to the endocardium. It is believed that the myocardium starts to contract during the third week. At first the rhythmic contractions are purely muscular in origin. Several weeks later the rhythm may be modified by the nervous system when the nerves invade the heart.

Coronary Circulation and the Innervation of the Heart

Just distal to the aortic valves, the two coronary arteries arise as outgrowths from the developing aorta. The superficial part of the cardiac muscle is drained into veins which join the left horn of the sinus venosus. Later the left horn becomes the *coronary sinus.*

Several weeks after the heart has started to beat, afferent and efferent nerve fibers grow into the heart from the sympathetic and parasympathetic parts of the autonomic nervous system.

Development of the Pericardium

The portion of the intra-embryonic coelom that crosses the midline of the embryo cranial to the buccopharyngeal membrane will form the pericardial cavity (Fig. 3-10). The formation of the head fold and the rotation of the pericardium and the endocardial heart tube have been described above. The pericardial cavity comes to lie ventral to the pharynx. With further development, the endocardial tube invaginates the dorsal surface of the pericardial cavity and becomes suspended within it by the *dorsal mesocardium*. Later, during the fourth week, the dorsal mesocardium disappears so that the endocardial tube is only attached to the pericardium at its arterial and venous ends. As the endocardial tube rapidly increases in length and becomes bent, the arterial and venous ends remain close together. The pericardial cavity is lined by parietal serous pericardium derived from somatic mesoderm, and the future heart and roots of the great vessels are covered with epicardium (visceral serous pericardium) derived from the myo-epicardial mantle of splanchnic mesoderm. The area of the pericardial cavity that lies between the arterial and venous ends of the heart tube is known as the *transverse sinus*. The different great veins, namely, the superior and inferior venae cavae, and the four pulmonary veins as they become established, change their position relative to one another, and the lines of reflection of the serous pericardium follow this change of position; as a result of this, the *oblique sinus* is brought into being. The pericardial cavity at first communicates with the peritoneal cavity by means of the *pericardioperitoneal canals*. Later these canals become closed off. The fibrous pericardium is formed from a condensation of the surrounding mesenchymal tissue and from the septum transversum.

CONGENITAL ANOMALIES

Gross Anomalies

ACARDIA. Absence of the heart may occur in twins that have one placenta. Such a monster is either separate or a conjoined member of twins.

ECTOPIA CORDIS. The heart is exposed on the anterior thoracic wall and is usually associated with an open pericardium and widely separated sternal halves.

DEXTROCARDIA. This is a condition in which the heart and its apex are directed toward the right. This anomaly is a result of the reversal of the loop of the endocardial tube. Although this may occur on its own, it is usually associated with transposition of all the thoracoabdominal viscera. Transposition of the aorta and pulmonary trunk may occur alone in an otherwise normal heart. This is a result of the spiral aorticopulmonary septum being formed in the wrong direction so that the aorta exits from the right ventricle and the pulmonary trunk exits from the left ventricle.

Internal Anomalies

Atrial Defects

After birth the raised pressure in the left atrium causes the septum primum to be forced over and to fuse with the septum secundum in such a way that the foramen ovale becomes completely closed. In 25 percent of hearts, a small opening persists, but this is usually of such a minor nature that it is of no clinical significance. Occasionally the opening is much larger (Fig. 7-11A) and results in oxygenated blood in the left atrium passing over into the right atrium with consequent overworking of the right side of the heart; this may even cause cyanosis. Wide patency of the septum is commonly associated with other important congenital

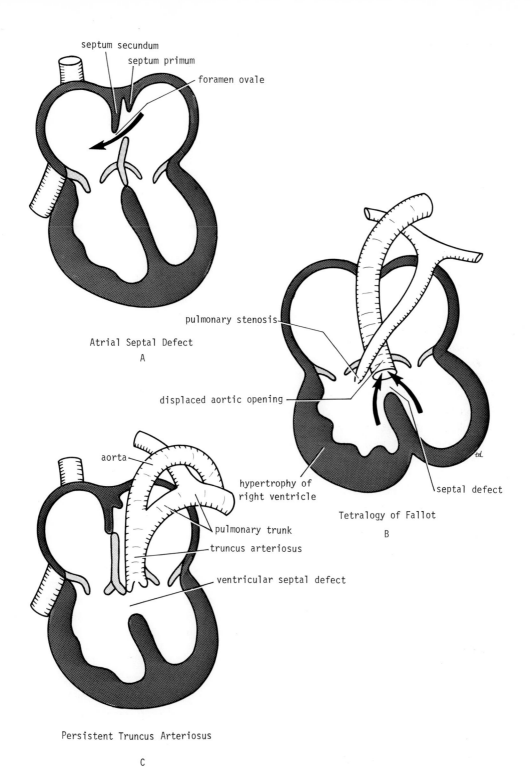

septum secundum
septum primum
foramen ovale

Atrial Septal Defect
A

pulmonary stenosis

displaced aortic opening

hypertrophy of
right ventricle

septal defect

Tetralogy of Fallot
B

aorta

pulmonary trunk

truncus arteriosus

ventricular septal defect

Persistent Truncus Arteriosus

C

Fig. 7-11. Three important congenital anomalies of the heart.

anomalies, for example, pulmonary stenosis or transposition of the great arterial trunks. In nearly half the cases of wide patency alone, death results from right-sided congestive heart failure.

Very rarely the foramen primum may persist or the entire atrial septum may be absent. Both of these conditions are more serious than patency of the foramen ovale. When there is only one atrium and two ventricles, the mortality is high.

Ventricular Septal Defects

Localized *ventricular septal defects,* though less frequent than atrial septal defects, are quite common. Normally, the ventricular septum is formed from two sources: the inferior muscular part grows up from the floor of the primitive ventricle and the membranous part is formed as the result of fusion of the lower ends of the bulbar ridges and the septum intermedium (endocardial cushions). The complete ventricular septum is formed when the membranous part fuses with the muscular part. Ventricular septal defects are almost invariably found in the membranous part of the septum. They are oval or circular in shape and measure from 1 to 2 cm in diameter. The blood passes through the defect from left to right, causing enlargement of the right ventricle. Cyanosis is rare, and there are no symptoms. Small septal defects are relatively benign, but large defects can shorten life if surgery is not performed.

Complete absence of the ventricular septum is rare. In these cases the heart is three-chambered, and if surgery is not possible the majority of such infants die before reaching adult life.

Defects of the Bulbus Cordis

Normally the bulbus cordis becomes divided into the aorta and pulmonary trunk by the formation of the spiral aorticopulmonary septum. This septum is formed by the fusion of the bulbar ridges. If the bulbar ridges fail to fuse correctly, unequal division of the bulbus cordis may occur with narrowing of the pulmonary trunk and resulting interference with the right ventricular outflow. The following defects may be present: (1) large ventricular septal defect; (2) stenosis of the pulmonary trunk that may occur at the infundibulum of the right ventricle or the pulmonary valve, or actually involve the pulmonary trunk; and (3) exit of the aorta immediately above the ventricular septal defect. The resulting high blood pressure in the right ventricle causes hypertrophy and enlargement of the right ventricle. These three defects, together with the enlargement of the right ventricle, are known as the *tetralogy of Fallot* (Fig. 7-11B). The defects cause congenital cyanosis and considerably limit activity, shortening life to but a few years.

Occasionally cases occur in which the aorta is dextraposed and partially overlaps the ventricular septum; consequently, there is a high ventricular septal defect. There is no pulmonary stenosis and no right ventricular hypertrophy. Therefore, two of the four features of the tetralogy of Fallot are absent.

Persistent truncus arteriosus (Fig. 7-11C) results when the upper part of the bulbus cordis (the truncus arteriosus) does not become divided into the aorta and pulmonary trunk because of failure of the spiral aorticopulmonary septum to develop. In this condition, only one artery arises from the heart, and the pulmonary arteries originate from this single trunk. A large ventricular septal defect is usually present.

Defects of the Aortic Valve

AORTIC STENOSIS. The edges of the valve cusps are often fused together forming a diaphragm with an eccentric orifice. The cusps are usually thickened and are often of unequal size and deformed. This condition is caused by a failure of the mesenchyme to break down and form separate cusps of equal size.

SUBAORTIC STENOSIS. This is usually caused by the presence of a band of fibrous tissue that lies approximately 1 cm below the aortic valves. This results from a persistence of mesenchymal tissue, which normally degenerates as the valve is formed.

Defects of the Pulmonary Valve

PULMONARY STENOSIS. As an isolated malformation with no defect of the ventricular septum, this anomaly is rare. There are two types: (1) stenosis of the pulmonary valve and (2) stenosis of the infundibulum of the right ventricle.

1. *Pulmonary valve stenosis.* This is similar to the condition of aortic valve stenosis in that the valve cusps are fused together to form a dome which has a central perforation.

2. *Infundibular stenosis.* This condition is caused by a failure of the lower end of the bulbus cordis to expand to form a normal-sized infundibulum. This defect usually occurs in association with the tetralogy of Fallot.

Defects of the Tricuspid Valve

TRICUSPID ATRESIA. This consists of complete absence of the right atrioventricular valve, lack of development or total absence of the right ventricle, defective development of the ventricular septum, and either normally positioned or transposition of the aorta and pulmonary trunk, with or without pulmonary stenosis or atresia. A defect of the atrial septum is always present.

DOWNWARD DISPLACEMENT OF THE TRICUSPID VALVE. The tricuspid valve cusps are attached to the ventricular wall below the atrioventricular annulus to which the tricuspid valve is normally attached.

Defect of the Mitral Valve

MITRAL ATRESIA. The mitral valve cusps are completely fused, and the valve is represented by a dimple in the floor of the left atrium. The left ventricle is poorly developed and small. The atrial septum is usually defective.

Clinical Problems
Answers on page 436

1. Following delivery of a male child the obstetrician noticed that the heart beat could be clearly seen through the anterior wall of the chest in the midline. Once respiration was established, the skin over the anterior wall of the chest became indrawn with each inspiratory effort. The child was otherwise perfectly normal. What is your diagnosis?

2. A 5-year-old girl was operated on for acute abdominal pain in the left iliac fossa. The surgeon found the appendix, cecum, and ascending colon situated on the left side of the posterior abdominal wall instead of on the right side. The patient was suffering from an acute appendicitis. Further examination revealed that other abdominal organs presented a mirror image of the normal. What is the name for this condition? How does this condition affect the position of the heart?

3. A 6-year-old girl was examined by a pediatrician. The child had a normal color and no symptoms. On physical examination a slight systolic murmur was heard with the stethoscope along the left margin of the sternum. X-ray examination revealed slight cardiac enlargement to the right,

with enlargement of the pulmonary artery along the left border of the heart. The lung fields showed a great increase in pulmonary vasculature. Cardiac catheterization revealed an increased oxygen saturation in the right atrium. A diagnosis of atrial septal defect was made. How would you explain the presence of an atrial septal defect? Are there different types of atrial septal defect? Can the condition seriously endanger the life of the patient?

4. A 4-year-old boy was examined by a pediatrician and found to have the symptoms and signs of a large ventricular septal defect. The child was short for his age, and slightly cyanotic, with clubbing of the fingers and toes. He had a history of repeated attacks of pneumonia and right-sided heart failure. How would you explain the presence of a ventricular septal defect? In which part of the septum is the defect usually found—the membranous part or the muscular part? Is cyanosis a common sign in patients with a small ventricular septal defect?

5. A 3-year-old boy with cyanosis was examined by a pediatrician. On questioning of the mother it was learned that the child had become cyanotic during his first year. Since that time, sudden attacks of breathlessness had occurred on exertion. On two occasions during an attack of breathlessness the child had lost consciousness. The mother had noticed that he tended to breathe more easily in the squatting position and tended to sleep more easily with the knees drawn up. On examination the child was found to be cyanotic, and there was evidence of clubbing of the fingers and toes. The child was thinner and shorter than normal. The thorax showed a left parasternal bulge due to the underlying right ventricular hypertrophy. A loud systolic murmur was present along the left border of the sternum. Following angiocardiography a diagnosis of tetralogy

of Fallot was made. What does this syndrome consist of? Why do you think the child did not become cyanotic immediately after birth? Why is the child breathless on exertion? Why does the child assume the squatting position?

6. A 2-month-old male child with deep cyanosis had failed to develop at a normal rate, was breathless at rest, and became more cyanotic on crying. Physical examination revealed signs of congestive heart failure. Cardiac catheterization showed evidence of shunting at the site of the atrial septum. A diagnosis of transposition of the aorta and pulmonary trunk was made. Using your knowledge of embryology, can you explain how transposition of the great vessels occurs? Why was the child cyanotic? Is it important to have an atrial septal defect in this condition? What is the prognosis?

7. An 8-year-old boy was examined by a pediatrician because of breathlessness. On physical examination he was found to be cyanotic and had clubbing of the fingers. The heart, and especially the right ventricle, was enlarged. A loud systolic murmur could be heard over the sternum. Following cardiac catheterization and cineangiography a diagnosis of persistent truncus arteriosus was made. Using your knowledge of embryology, explain this condition. What is the prognosis?

8. A 7-year-old boy was examined by a pediatrician. It was a routine examination of an apparently normal, healthy child. A harsh systolic murmur was heard over the aortic valve in the second right intercostal space. A chest x-ray film revealed hypertrophy of the left ventricle. A diagnosis of congenital aortic stenosis was made. How do you explain congenital aortic stenosis embryologically?

9. A 5-year-old boy was found on routine examination to have a loud systolic murmur at the second left intercostal space.

There was no history of breathlessness or of excessive fatigue on exertion. X-ray examination showed enlargement of the right ventricle. Cardiac catheterization revealed an increase in right ventricular pressure. A diagnosis of congenital pulmonary stenosis was made. How can you explain congenital pulmonary stenosis embryologically?

REFERENCES

Abrahams, D. G., and Wood, P. Pulmonary Stenosis with Normal Aortic Root. *Brit. Heart J.* 13:519, 1951.

Baffes, T. G., Johnson, F. R., Pott, W. J., and Gibson, S. Anatomic Variations in Tetralogy of Fallot. *Amer. Heart J.* 46:657, 1953.

Barnard, C. N., and Schrire, V. *The Surgery of the Common Congenital Cardiac Malformations.* Stapless Press, London, 1968.

Bass, A. D., and Moe, G. K. *Congenital Heart Disease.* American Association for the Advancement of Science, Washington, D.C., 1960.

Book, J. A. Heredity and Heart Disease. *Amer. J. Public Health* 50:1, 1960.

Boyd, J. D. Development of the Heart. In *Handbook of Physiology,* Section 2, Circulation, Vol. III, edited by W. F. Hamilton. American Physiological Society, Washington, D.C., 1965. P. 2511.

Brinton, W. D., and Campbell, M. Necropsies in Some Congenital Diseases of the Heart, Mainly Fallot's Tetralogy. *Brit. Heart J.* 15:335, 1953.

Byron, F. Ectopia Cordis. *J. Thorac. Surg. Cardiovasc.* 7:717, 1948.

Campbell, M., and Kauntze, R. Congenital Valvular Stenosis. *Brit. Heart J.* 15:179, 1953.

Collett, R. W., and Edwards, J. Persistent Truncus Arteriosus. *Surg. Clin. N. Amer.* 29:1245, 1949.

DeVries, P. A., and Saunders, J. B. Development of Ventricles and Spiral Outflow Tract in Human Heart. *Contrib. Embryol.* 37:87, 1962.

Dexter, L. Atrial Septal Defects. *Brit. Heart J.* 18:209, 1956.

Harris, J. S., and Farber, S. Transposition of the Great Cardiac Vessels. *Arch. Path.* (Chicago) 28:427, 1939.

Kirklin, J. W., and Karp, R. B. *The Tetralogy of Fallot.* Saunders, Philadelphia, 1970.

Kramer, T. C. The Partitioning of the Truncus and Conus and the Formation of the Membranous Portion of the Interventricular Septum in the Human Heart. *Amer. J. Anat.* 71:343, 1942.

Licata, R. H. The Human Embryonic Heart in the Ninth Week. *Amer. J. Anat.* 94:73, 1954.

Monie, J. W., and DePape, A. D. J. Congenital Aortic Atresia. *Amer. Heart J.* 40:595, 1950.

Navaratnam, V. Development of Nerve Supply to the Human Heart. *Brit. Heart J.* 27:640, 1965.

Odgers, P. N. B. The Formation of the Venous Valves, the Foramen Secundum and the Septum Secundum in the Human Heart. *J. Anat.* 69:412, 1935.

Odgers, P. N. B. The Development of the Pars Membranacea Septi in the Human Heart. *J. Anat.* 72:247, 1939.

Patten, B. M. Persistent Interatrial Foramen Primum. *Amer. J. Anat.* 107:271, 1960.

Rogers, H. M., and Edwards, J. E. Cor Triloculare Biventriculare. *Amer. Heart J.* 45:623, 1953.

Taussig, H. B. *Congenital Malformations of the Heart.* Specific Malformations, Vol. II. Harvard University Press, Cambridge, 1960.

Van Mierop, L. H. S., Alley, R. D., Kausel, M. W., and Stranahan, A. The Anatomy and Embryology of Endocardial Cushion Defects. *J. Thorac. Cardiovasc. Surg.* 43:71, 1962.

White, P. D. *Heart Disease,* 4th ed. Macmillan, New York, 1951.

Wood, P. *Diseases of the Heart and Circulation,* 3d ed. Lippincott, Philadelphia, 1968.

The Arterial and Venous Systems; the Fetal Circulation

DEVELOPMENT

The Arterial System

Formation of the Aortic Arch Arteries

In Chapter 7 the formation of the single endocardial heart tube and its ultimate differentiation into the definitive heart are described. The truncus arteriosus (distal part of the bulbus cordis) is continuous beyond the pericardium with a large vessel, the *aortic sac*. The sac gives off two branches, each of which runs dorsally in the first pharyngeal arch on each side; the branches then pass caudally in the posterior wall of the embryo as the two *dorsal aortae*. Five additional arteries next appear on each side caudal to the first and join the aortic sac to the dorsal aortae, each running in a respective pharyngeal arch and curving around the developing pharynx. The period of development of the aortic arch arteries takes place throughout the fourth week, but it should be noted that they are not all present at any one time. In the meantime, the two dorsal aortae fuse throughout much of their lengths to form the *descending thoracic aorta* and the *abdominal aorta* (Fig. 8-1).

Fate of the Aortic Arch Arteries

The *ascending aorta* below the right pulmonary artery, and the main pulmonary trunk, are derived from the truncus arteriosus (Fig. 8-1). The aorta, from the level of the right pulmonary artery up to the level of the left common carotid artery, is derived from the aortic sac. The *brachiocephalic artery* is also formed from the aortic sac. The remainder of the *arch of the aorta* is formed from the left fourth aortic arch artery and the left dorsal aorta (Fig. 8-1).

The fourth right aortic arch artery becomes the root of the right *subclavian artery,* which is also derived in sequence from a small part of the right dorsal aorta and the right seventh segmental artery. The third aortic arch artery on both sides becomes the *common carotid artery,* and this sends off a bud of mesenchyme which becomes the *external carotid artery.* The remainder of the third aortic arch artery and part of the dorsal aorta form the internal carotid artery on each side.

The first, second, and fifth aortic arch arteries involute early and disappear completely. The right and left *pulmonary arteries* are formed from the sixth aortic arch arteries. The distal part of the right sixth aortic arch artery disappears, while the remainder of the left sixth aortic arch artery becomes the *ductus arteriosus,* which, after the baby is born, becomes the *ligamentum arteriosum.* It is thus seen that parts of the dorsal aortae disappear, while other parts remain and contribute to the large definitive arteries of the

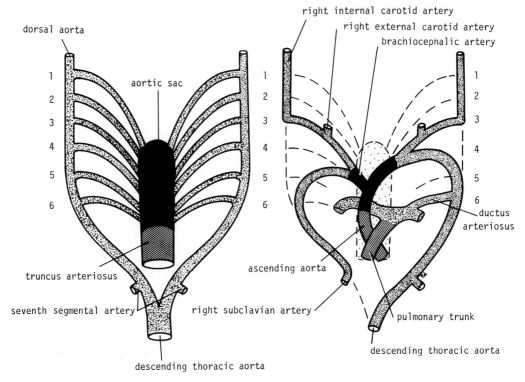

Fig. 8-1. Formation and fate of the aortic arch arteries.

neck and thorax. The descending thoracic aorta below the level of the fourth thoracic vertebra is formed from the fusion of the dorsal aortae.

With the formation of the neck, the heart descends from the region in front of the pharynx and enters the thorax. As a result of this, the carotid and brachiocephalic arteries elongate, and the root of the left subclavian artery shifts to a higher position on the aortic arch. A further consequence of the development of the neck and descent of the heart is that the branches of the vagus nerve to the larynx are pulled up as the neck elongates. On the left side, the sixth aortic arch artery persists as the ductus arteriosus, so that the *left recurrent laryngeal nerve* becomes hooked around the ductus, which becomes the ligamentum arteriosum (Fig. 8-2). On the right side, the fifth and sixth aortic arch arteries

disappear, and the *right recurrent laryngeal nerve* is pulled higher up into the neck and hooks around the fourth aortic arch artery, which becomes the right subclavian artery.

Branches of the Dorsal Aortae

Prior to the fusion of the dorsal aortae during the fourth week, each artery gives off a dorsal, a lateral, and a ventral branch to each segment of the embryo. After the aortae have fused, the segmental vessels remain and become distributed as follows (Fig. 8-3):

1. *Dorsal intersegmental arteries.* These arise from each side of the dorsal aorta from the base of the skull to the sacral region (Fig. 8-3). Each artery gives off a posterior branch which passes posteriorly between successive vertebral transverse processes and supplies the spinal cord and its meninges and the skin

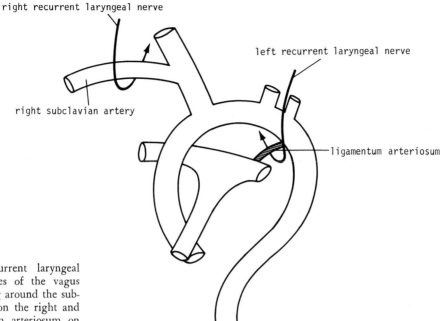

right recurrent laryngeal nerve

right subclavian artery

left recurrent laryngeal nerve

ligamentum arteriosum

Fig. 8-2. Recurrent laryngeal nerves, branches of the vagus nerves, hooking around the subclavian artery on the right and the ligamentum arteriosum on the left.

and muscles of the back. The main stem of the artery extends into the body wall following the course of the anterior primary ramus of the spinal nerve.

In the neck, the dorsal intersegmental arteries become linked together to form a longitudinal artery on each side called the *vertebral artery.* All their original stems then atrophy and disappear except the caudal one, which remains as the origin of the vertebral artery from the subclavian artery. The *thyrocervical trunk* and other longitudinally running arteries are formed in a similar manner.

In the thorax, the dorsal intersegmental arteries remain as the intercostal arteries. In the lumbar region, they also remain as the lumbar arteries. The fifth lumbar intersegmental arteries become considerably enlarged to form the *common iliac arteries.* In the sacral region, the intersegmental arteries are small and the dorsal aorta is much reduced in size and forms the *middle sacral artery.*

2. *Lateral splanchnic arteries.* These arise from each side of the dorsal aorta and supply the intermediate mesoderm and its derivatives (Fig. 8-3). Branches therefore pass to the pronephroi, mesonephroi, and metanephroi. In the adult they form the *renal, suprarenal, phrenic,* and *testicular* or *ovarian arteries.*

3. *Ventral splanchnic arteries.* Early in development, these arteries are distributed to the yolk sac as paired vitelline arteries and to the allantois as paired umbilical arteries (Fig. 8-4). Other segmentally arranged arteries pass to the gut and yolk sac, but later most of these disappear following fusion of the dorsal aortae. Three arterial trunks remain in addition to the large umbilical arteries: These are the celiac artery, which is distributed to the foregut; the *superior mesenteric artery,* which is distributed to the midgut; and the *inferior mesenteric artery,* which is distributed to the hindgut.

The umbilical arteries, with the growth in length of the embryo, migrate caudally and join the fifth lumbar intersegmental arteries. Later the origin of the umbilical arteries

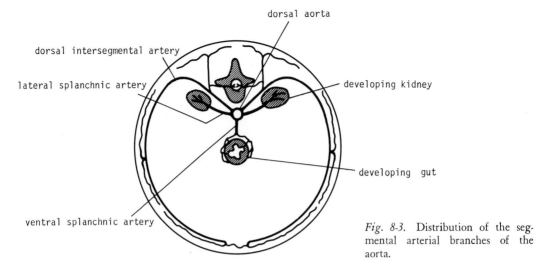

Fig. 8-3. Distribution of the segmental arterial branches of the aorta.

from the aorta is lost, so that they finally appear as branches of the internal iliac artery on each side. After birth, the first part of the umbilical artery becomes the *superior vesical artery,* and the remainder becomes the *obliterated umbilical artery* and forms a fibrous ligament, the *lateral umbilical ligament.*

Arteries of the Upper Limb

At the site of each adult vessel, a capillary network of small blood vessels appears in the upper limb bud. As development proceeds, the seventh aortic arch artery, which forms the *subclavian artery,* joins this network. Enlargement of certain pathways through this network now takes place so that the subclavian artery is continued as the *axillary, brachial,* and *anterior interosseous arteries.* Later the *ulnar* and *radial arteries* develop as branches of this main vascular axis and the anterior interosseous becomes reduced in size. The radial artery is at first a branch of the brachial artery high up in the arm. As it

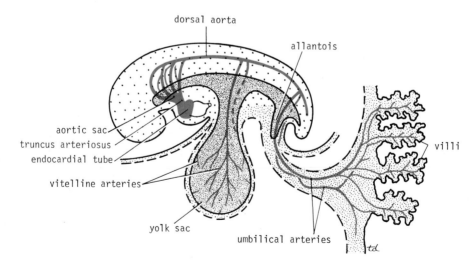

Fig. 8-4. The developing arterial system and its relationship to the gut, yolk sac, and allantois.

crosses the elbow joint, it receives a communicating branch from the brachial artery. Later the part of the radial artery above the elbow disappears.

Arteries of the Lower Limb

The blood vessels arise as a capillary network in a manner similar to that described for the upper limb. At the beginning, the vascular axis is formed by the *inferior gluteal artery,* the *artery to the sciatic nerve,* the *popliteal artery,* and the *peroneal artery.* Later the *femoral artery* develops from the external iliac artery and grows down and joins the vascular axis in the popliteal region. The upper part of the vascular axis disappears, leaving the inferior gluteal artery. The *anterior* and *posterior tibial arteries* arise as branches of the popliteal artery.

The Venous System

It has been shown in Chapter 7 that in the embryo the right and left horns of the sinus venosus each receives a vitelline vein from the yolk sac, an umbilical vein from the capillaries of the chorionic villi, and a common cardinal vein from the tissues of the embryo. The further development of each of these veins will now be considered (Fig. 8-5).

1. *Vitelline veins.* The vitelline veins enter the body of the embryo alongside the stalk of the yolk sac. They then pass cranialward, enter the mass of mesoderm, the septum transversum, and finally drain into the right or left horn of the sinus venosus (Fig. 8-6). Between the yolk sac and the septum transversum, the paired vitelline veins become connected by anastomoses that are closely related to the developing duodenum. Within the septum transversum, the vitelline veins become broken down into intercommunicating sinusoids as the result of invasion of the interior of the septum transversum by the rapidly proliferating cords of liver cells. As the result of rotation of the stomach and duodenum, and the disappearance of segments of the vitelline veins, the following vascular pattern emerges (Fig. 8-6):

a. The terminal part of the *inferior vena cava* is formed from that part of the right vitelline vein that passes from the septum transversum to the right horn of the sinus venosus.

b. The *hepatic veins* are formed from the remains of the right vitelline vein within the septum transversum.

c. The *portal vein* develops from the anastomotic network around the duodenum.

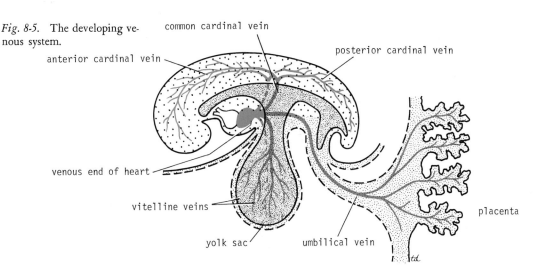

Fig. 8-5. The developing venous system.

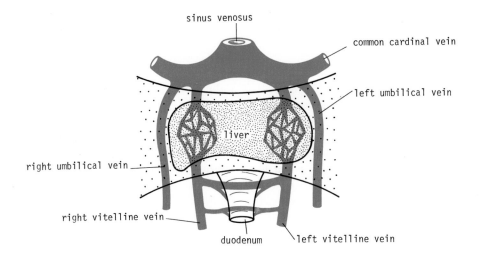

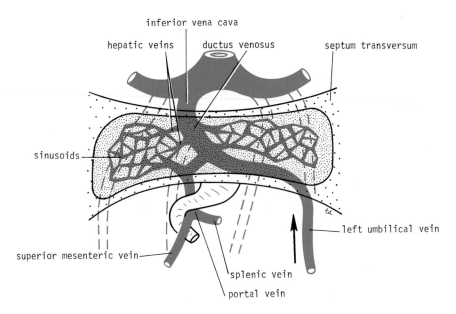

Fig. 8-6. Fate of the vitelline and umbilical veins. Note the relationship of these veins to the developing liver, duodenum, and septum transversum.

d. The *liver sinusoids* are in part developed from the remains of the right and left vitelline veins within the septum transversum.

2. *Umbilical veins.*   The umbilical veins enter the embryo through the body stalk. They then pass cranially, enter the lateral part of the septum transversum, and finally drain into the right or left horn of the sinus venosus (Fig. 8-6). As the rapidly proliferating cords of liver cells extend laterally, they not only break down the vitelline veins to form hepatic sinusoids but they break up the umbilical veins into sinusoids as well. The parts of both umbilical veins between the septum transversum and the sinus venosus disappear. The remainder of the right umbilical vein also disappears. As development proceeds and there is an increase in the placental circulation, a direct communication opens up between the right vitelline vein and the left umbilical vein. This channel has a wide diameter and enables the oxygenated blood coming to the embryo via the left umbilical vein to bypass the small hepatic sinusoids and enter directly the part of the right vitelline vein that will become the inferior vena cava. This channel is known as the *ductus venosus.* After birth, the ductus venosus becomes obliterated and fibrosed and forms the *ligamentum venosum,* and the left umbilical vein forms a similar ligament in the free margin of the falciform ligament called the *ligamentum teres.* This extends from the umbilicus to the porta hepatis of the liver.

3. *Cardinal veins.*   The *anterior cardinal veins* drain the cephalic end of the embryo and the *posterior cardinal veins* drain the caudal end of the embryo (Fig. 8-5). The anterior and posterior cardinal veins join to form the *common cardinal veins,* which then enter the horns of the sinus venosus on each side. The ultimate development and fate of the cardinal veins are very complicated, and a detailed knowledge of this is unnecessary for a medical student. The anterior cardinal vein will eventually form the cranial venous sinuses, the cerebral veins, and the large deep veins of the head and neck. The superior vena cava is formed from the terminal portion of the right anterior cardinal vein and the right common cardinal vein.

The posterior cardinal veins are reinforced by other longitudinal connecting venous channels, and together they form the *inferior vena cava* and the *azygos system of veins.*

Fetal Circulation

The placenta is an organ for the passage of nutrients, oxygen, water, hormones, and antibodies from the mother to the fetus. It also allows hormones, nitrogenous waste products, and carbon dioxide to pass from the fetus to the mother. The mechanisms involved in these physiological exchanges have been discussed in Chapter 4.

The fetal blood, having circulated through the capillaries of the placental villi, returns to the fetus through the umbilical vein about 80 percent saturated with oxygen (Fig. 8-7). The oxygenated blood then passes toward the liver, but the greater volume of it bypasses the liver and travels to the inferior vena cava by way of the *ductus venosus;* the remainder is distributed to the liver sinusoids by offshoots of the umbilical vein, and this in turn passes to the inferior vena cava by the hepatic veins. At the same time, the ductus venosus receives poorly oxygenated blood from the gut by way of the left branch of the portal vein. In addition, the inferior vena cava already contains venous blood from the caudal regions of the fetus. As a result of this admixture of blood from these various sources, the inferior vena cava contains blood about 67 percent saturated with oxygen.

Before considering the further passage of the fetal blood, it is necessary to examine the anatomical arrangement of the inferior vena

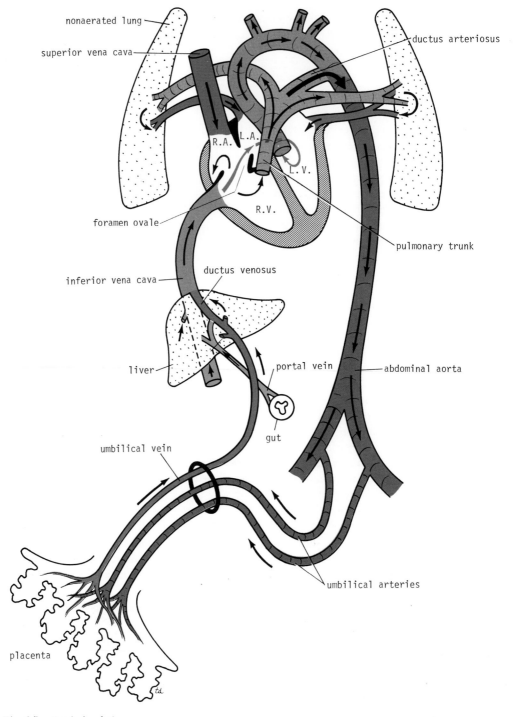

Fig. 8-7. Fetal circulation.

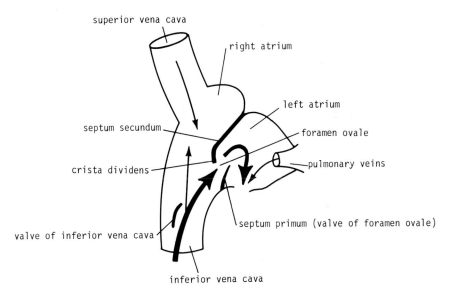

Fig. 8-8. Relationship between the opening of the inferior vena cava and the foramen ovale.

cava and its relationship with the right and left atria in the fetal heart (Fig. 8-8). In the fetus, the opening of the inferior vena cava into the right atrium lies directly opposite the *foramen ovale*. Thus, blood entering the heart through the inferior vena cava is directed through the foramen ovale and enters the left atrium. This process is assisted by the presence of the valve of the inferior vena cava.

The oxygenated fetal blood, on reaching the foramen ovale, is divided into two streams by the *crista dividens,* which is the lower margin of the septum secundum. The greater volume of blood enters the left atrium and the remainder, joined by venous blood from the superior vena cava and coronary sinus, passes from the right atrium into the right ventricle.

The oxygenated blood in the left atrium is joined by a relatively small volume of blood from the nonaerated fetal lungs. The left atrial blood then passes into the left ventricle and out into the aorta. The oxygen saturation of this blood is now about 62 percent. This is distributed chiefly to the arteries of the head and neck and upper extremities. It is there-

fore apparent that the cephalic region of the fetus receives blood that is richer in oxygen than the caudal regions of the body.

The right ventricular blood passes into the pulmonary trunk. Only a small portion of this passes into the unexpanded lungs, since the vascular resistance is high. Most of the blood bypasses the lungs by being directed through the wide channel, the *ductus arteriosus,* into the descending thoracic aorta (Fig. 8-7).

The now relatively poorly oxygenated blood passes down the descending thoracic and abdominal aortae and supplies the thoracic and abdominal viscera and the lower limbs. The fetal blood then returns to the placenta through the right and left umbilical arteries, and the circulation is repeated.

For changes which take place in the circulation at birth, see Chapter 25.

CONGENITAL ANOMALIES

The Arterial System

Anomalies of the ascending aorta and pulmonary trunk have already been considered

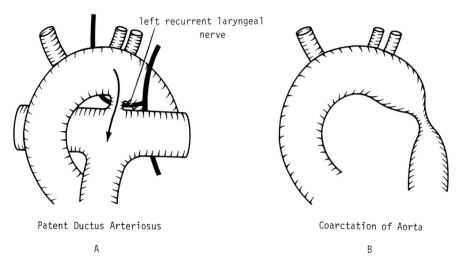

Fig. 8-9. Two important congenital anomalies of the arterial system.

under the section on congenital anomalies of the heart (Chap. 7).

PATENT DUCTUS ARTERIOSUS. This is the most frequently seen congenital anomaly of the great vessels (Fig. 8-9). The ductus arteriosus represents the distal portion of the sixth left aortic arch and connects the left pulmonary artery to the descending aorta. During fetal life, it has practically the same diameter as the pulmonary trunk and aorta, and blood passes through it from the pulmonary artery to the aorta. After birth, it normally constricts, later closes and becomes the *ligamentum arteriosum*. One week after birth its lumen is 2 mm or less in diameter. By the end of the first month, the majority have closed. It is now believed that a rise in arterial oxygen tension is an important factor in bringing about the initial contraction of the smooth muscle in the wall of the ductus. Congestion and hemorrhage of the vasa vasorum, aided by edema of the tunica intima, may initiate the process of fibrosis. In children born with respiratory distress, the delay in closure of the ductus arteriosus is probably a result of hypoxemia. Persistent patent ductus arteriosus results in aortic blood passing into the pulmonary artery, which raises the pressure in the pulmonary circulation and causes hypertrophy of the right ventricle. This, together with the possibility of causing bacterial infection of the wall of the pulmonary artery, means that patent ductus arteriosus endangers life and thus it should be ligated and divided surgically.

COARCTATION OF THE AORTA. This is a narrowing of the aorta just proximal to, opposite, or distal to the site of attachment of the ligamentum arteriosum (Fig. 8-9). It is a condition that arises after birth and is believed to be the result of an unusual quantity of ductus arteriosus muscle tissue incorporated in the wall of the aorta. As a result of this, when the ductus arteriosus contracts, the ductal muscle in the aortic wall also contracts and the aortic lumen becomes narrowed. Later, when fibrosis takes place, the aortic wall is also involved and permanent narrowing occurs. Clinically, the cardinal sign of aortic coarctation is absent or diminished femoral pulses. In an attempt to compensate for the diminished volume of blood reaching the lower part of the body, an enormous collateral circulation opens involving the internal thoracic, subclavian, and posterior intercostal arteries. The condition may be treated surgically.

DOUBLE AORTA AND RIGHT AORTIC ARCH. These anomalies are rare conditions resulting from the persistence of aortic arch arteries, which normally disappear. In the case of the right aortic arch, the development of the left arch does not take place. The *subclavian* and *carotid arteries* may also show variations in development caused by the persistence of sections of aortic arch arteries, which normally disappear, and by the disappearance of other sections, which normally remain. The *coro-*

nary arteries occasionally arise by a common trunk from the aorta or very rarely from the pulmonary trunk.

The Venous System

In view of the development of complicated patterns of veins from the cardinal veins, it is not surprising that an occasional deviation from the normal is seen in the formation of the large veins. For example, an absent or double inferior vena cava may occur. A left superior vena cava or two superior venae cavae rarely are formed.

Clinical Problems
Answers on page 438

1. An 8-year-old girl was being routinely examined by a pediatrician when he heard a continuous machinery-like murmur in the second left intercostal space. The murmur occupied both systole and diastole. The child was not cyanotic, the heart was of normal size, and there was no clubbing of the fingers. X-ray examination of the chest revealed slight enlargement of the left atrium, left ventricle, and pulmonary trunk. A diagnosis of patent ductus arteriosus was made. Using your knowledge of embryology, can you explain this condition? How does the ductus arteriosus develop? What is the prognosis in this condition?

2. A 10-year-old boy was examined by a pediatrician and found to have absent pulses of both femoral arteries and a higher blood pressure in both upper limbs than in both lower limbs. What is the diagnosis? If the patient is not treated, why is there an increased risk of cerebral hemorrhage,

cardiac failure, or bacterial endocarditis after childhood?

3. A 4-month-old baby died of heart failure. At the postmortem examination the left coronary artery was seen to arise normally from the ascending aorta, but the right coronary artery arose from the pulmonary trunk. Can you explain this rare anomaly? Why does heart failure occur in these cases?

4. At the postmortem examination of a 70-year-old man it was found that he possessed a left superior vena cava in addition to a normal right superior vena cava. Can you explain this finding?

5. A fourth-year medical student was asked by a pediatrician what factors are responsible for the closure of the foramen ovale in the atrial septum at birth. He was also asked if oxygenated or deoxygenated blood normally passes through the foramen ovale during fetal life. How would you answer these questions?

REFERENCES

Adams, F. H., and Lind, J. Physiologic Studies on the Cardiovascular Status of Normal Newborn Infants with Special Reference to the Ductus Arteriosus. *Pediatrics* 19:431, 1957.

Auer, J. The Development of the Human Pulmonary Veins and Its Major Variations. *Anat. Rec.* 101:581, 1948.

Barclay, A. E., Franklin, K. J., and Pritchard, M. M. L. *The Foetal Circulation*. Blackwell, Oxford, Eng., 1944.

Barcroft, J. *Researches on Prenatal Life*. Blackwell, Oxford, Eng., 1946.

Barcroft, J. Foetal and Neonatal Physiology. *Brit. Med. Bull.* 17:247, 1961.

Baron, D. H. The Sphincter of the Ductus Venosus. *Anat. Rec.* 82:398, 1942.

Barry, A. The Aortic Arch Derivatives in the Human Adult. *Anat. Rec.* 111:221, 1951.

Congdon, E. D. Transformation of the Aortic-Arch System During the Development of the Human Embryo. *Contrib. Embryol.* 14:47, 1922.

Dawes, G. S. *Foetal and Neonatal Physiology*. Year Book, Chicago, 1968.

Edwards, J. E., Christensen, N. A., Cladgett, O. T., and McDonald, J. R. Pathologic Considerations in Coarctation of the Aorta. *Mayo Clin. Proc.* 23:324, 1948.

Ekstrom, G., and Sandblom, P. Double Aortic Arch: Embryonic Development. *Acta Chir. Scand.* 102:183, 1951.

Griswold, H. E., and Young, M. D. Double Aortic Arch. *Pediatrics* 4:751, 1949.

Holmes, R. L. Some Features of the Ductus Arteriosus. *J. Anat.* 92:304, 1958.

Kovalcik, V. The Response of the Isolated Ductus Arteriosus to Oxygen and Anoxia. *J. Physiol.* 169:185, 1963.

Lind, J., and Wegelius, C. Human Fetal Circulation: Changes in the Cardiovascular System at Birth and Disturbances in the Postnatal Closure of the Foramen Ovale and Ducts Arteriosus. *Symp. Quant. Biol.* 19:109, 1954.

McClure, F. W., and Butler, E. G. The Development of the Vena Cava Inferior in Man. *Amer. J. Anat.* 35:331, 1925.

Neil, C. A. Development of Pulmonary Veins. *Pediatrics* 18:880, 1956.

Rudolf, A. M., and Heyman, M. A. The Circulation of the Fetus in Utero: Methods for Studying Distribution of Blood Flow, Cardiac Output and Organ Blood Flow. *Circ. Res.* 21:163, 1967.

Winter, F. S. Persistent Left Superior Vena Cava. *Angiology* 5:90, 1954.

Wood, P. *Diseases of the Heart and Circulation*, 3d ed. Lippincott, Philadelphia, 1968.

DEVELOPMENT

The Face

Early in development, the face of the embryo is represented by an area bounded cranially by the neural plate, caudally by the pericardium, and laterally by the mandibular process of the first pharyngeal arch on each side (Fig. 9-1). In the center of this area is a depression in the ectoderm known as the *stomodeum*. In the floor of the depression is the *buccopharyngeal membrane*. By the fourth week, the buccopharyngeal membrane breaks down so that the stomodeum communicates with the foregut.

The further development of the face is dependent upon the coming together and fusion of a number of important processes, the *frontonasal process,* the *maxillary processes,* and the *mandibular processes.* The frontonasal process begins as a proliferation of mesenchyme on the ventral surface of the developing brain, and this grows toward the stomodeum. Meanwhile, the maxillary process grows out from the upper end of each first arch and passes medially, forming the inferior border of the developing orbit. The mandibular processes of the first arches now approach one another in the midline inferior

to the stomodeum and fuse to form the lower jaw and lower lip.

The *olfactory pits* appear as depressions in the inferior edge of the advancing frontonasal process, dividing it into a *median nasal process* and two *lateral nasal processes* (Fig. 9-1). The rounded lateral angles of the median nasal process are called the *globular processes.* With further development, the maxillary processes grow medially and fuse with the lateral nasal processes and with the globular processes. The globular processes now fuse in the midline and form the *philtrum* of the upper lip and the *premaxilla.* The maxillary processes extend medially, forming the upper jaw and the cheek, and finally bury the globular processes and fuse in the midline. The various processes which go to form the face unite during the second month.

The Lips

The *upper lip* is formed by the growth medially of the maxillary processes of the first pharyngeal arch on each side (Figs. 9-1— 9-4). Ultimately the maxillary processes meet in the midline and fuse with each other and with the fused globular processes of the

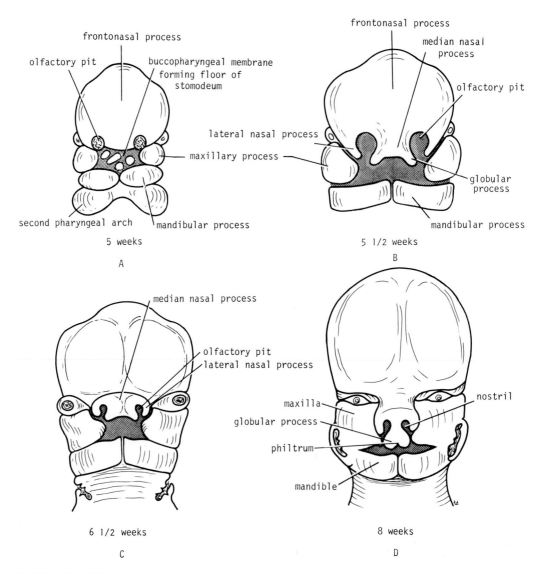

Fig. 9-1. The different stages in the development of the face.

median nasal process. The lateral parts of the upper lip are, therefore, formed from the maxillary processes, and the median part, or *philtrum,* from the median nasal process, with contributions from the maxillary processes.

The *lower lip* is formed from the mandibular process of the first pharyngeal arch on each side (Figs. 9-1—9-4). These processes grow medially inferior to the stomodeum and fuse in the midline and form the entire lower lip.

Each lip separates from its respective gum as the result of the appearance of a linear thickening of ectoderm, the *labiogingival lamina,* which grows down into the underly-

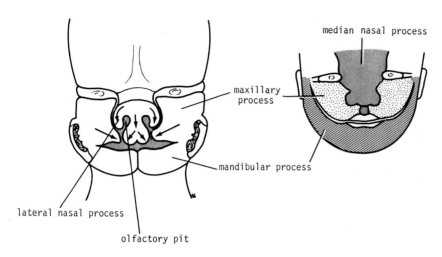

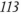

Fig. 9-2. The formation of the nose and nostrils.   *Fig. 9-3.* The formation of the lips and nose.

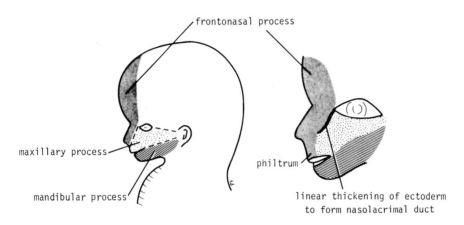

Fig. 9-4. The developing face, side view. The linear ectodermal thickening will sink into the underlying mesoderm and form the nasolacrimal duct, the lacrimal sac, and the lacrimal ducts.

ing mesenchyme and later degenerates. A deep groove thus forms between the lips and the gums. In the midline, a short area of the labiogingival lamina remains and tethers each lip to the gum and forms the *frenulum*.

At first the *mouth* has a broad opening, but later this diminishes in extent because of the fusion of the lips at the lateral angles. The muscles of the lips are derived from the second pharyngeal arch (see Chap. 10).

The Palate

In early fetal life, the nasal and mouth cavities are in communication, but later they become separated by the development of the *palate* (Figs. 9-5 & 9-6). The premaxilla, which carries the *incisor teeth,* is formed by a fusion of the globular processes of the median nasal process. Posterior to the premaxilla, the maxillary process on each side

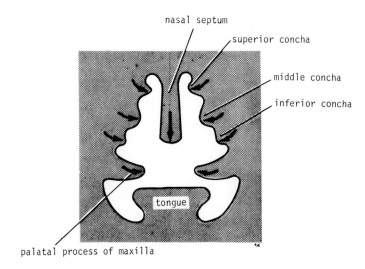

Fig. 9-5. The formation of the palate and the nasal septum (coronal section).

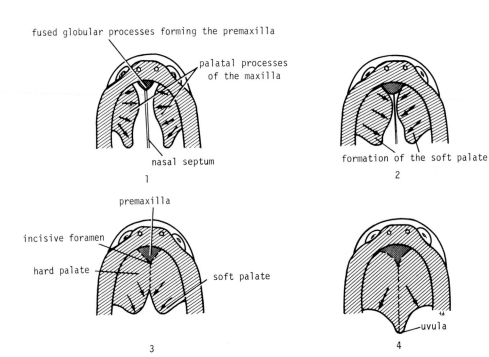

Fig. 9-6. The different stages in the formation of the palate.

sends medially a horizontal plate called the *palatal process;* these plates fuse and also unite with the premaxilla and the developing nasal septum. The fusion takes place from the anterior to the posterior region. A little later two folds grow posteriorly from the posterior edge of the palatal processes to form the *soft palate,* so that the *uvula* is the last structure to be formed (Fig. 9-6). The union of the two folds of the soft palate occurs during the eighth week. The two parts of the uvula fuse in the midline during the eleventh week. The interval between the premaxilla and the palatal processes is represented in the midline by the *incisive foramen.*

The Nose

The roof of the nose is formed from the lateral nasal processes. The lateral walls are also formed from the lateral nasal processes assisted by the maxillary processes (Figs. 9-1— 9-4). The anterior openings of the nose begin at the *olfactory pits* in the frontonasal process. Each olfactory pit is bounded medially by the median nasal process, laterally by the lateral nasal process, and inferiorly by the maxillary process (Figs. 9-1 & 9-2). As these processes fuse, the olfactory pits become deeper and form well-defined blind sacs, the opening into each of which is the *nostril* or *naris.*

The floor of the nose is at first very short and consists of the anterior part of the maxillary process on each side and the fused globular processes of the median nasal process (premaxilla). At this stage, the floors of the olfactory pits rupture so that the nasal cavities communicate with the developing mouth (Fig. 9-5). Meanwhile the *nasal septum* is forming as a downgrowth from the median nasal process (Fig. 9-5). Later the *palatal processes* of the maxilla grow medially and fuse with each other and with the nasal septum, thus completing the floor of the nose. Each nasal cavity therefore communicates anteriorly with the exterior through the nostril or naris and posteriorly through the *choana* with the nasopharynx. The external nares are closed by epithelial plugs from the second to the sixth month.

The *superior, middle,* and *inferior conchae* develop as elevations on the lateral wall of each nasal cavity (Fig. 9-5). The *olfactory cells* in the olfactory epithelium lining the upper part of the nose send their nerve fibers to the olfactory bulbs within the cranial cavity.

The *paranasal air sinuses* start to develop before birth and reach their maximum size at about puberty. At birth the *maxillary* and *sphenoidal air sinuses* are small diverticula opening off from the nasal cavities. The other sinuses at this time are merely shallow depressions of mucous membrane on the nasal wall.

In the early stages of development, the nose is a much-flattened structure and only gains its recognizable form after the facial development is complete.

The Nasolacrimal Duct

The formation of the *nasolacrimal duct* should be mentioned here, since it develops as a linear thickening of ectoderm on the developing face and extends from the medial canthus of the developing eye to the region of the developing nose (Fig. 9-4). This thickening separates the lateral nasal process from the maxillary process and forms a solid cord of cells that sinks beneath the surface and becomes embedded in the mesenchyme. The upper end of the cord becomes expanded to form the *lacrimal sac.* Further cellular proliferation results in the formation of the *lacrimal ducts,* which enter each eyelid. Ultimately the central cells of these cords degenerate so that the duct system becomes canalized and drains into the inferior meatus of the nose.

CONGENITAL ANOMALIES OF THE FACE REGION

CLEFT LIP. Cleft lip and palate are common congenital defects and they occur in one in eight hundred live births in the United States. Cleft lip most commonly involves the upper lip (Fig. 9-7).

Cleft upper lip may be confined to the lip or may be associated with a cleft palate. The anomaly is usually *unilateral cleft lip* (Figs. 9-8 & 9-9) and is caused by failure of the maxillary process to fuse with the median nasal process. The cleft may vary from a slight notch to a complete separation extending into the nostril. *Bilateral cleft lip* (Figs. 9-10 & 9-11) is caused by the failure of both maxillary processes to fuse with the median nasal process, which then remains as a central flap of tissue. *Oblique facial cleft* (Fig. 9-12) is a rare condition in which the cleft lip on one side extends to the medial margin of the orbit. This is caused by the failure of the maxillary process to fuse with the lateral and median nasal processes. *Median cleft lip* is very rare and is caused by the failure of fusion of the globular processes of the median nasal process.

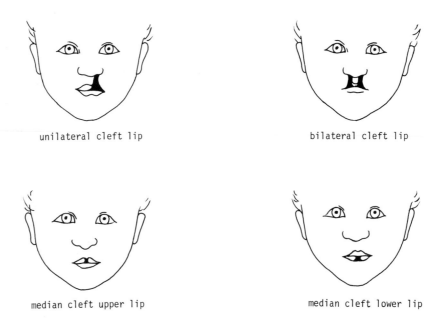

unilateral cleft lip   bilateral cleft lip

median cleft upper lip   median cleft lower lip

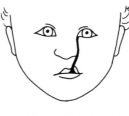

oblique facial cleft

Fig. 9-7. The various forms of cleft lip.

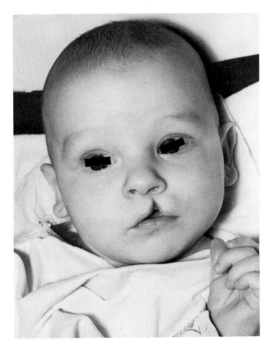

Fig. 9-8. Unilateral cleft upper lip. (Courtesy of Dr. R. Chase.)

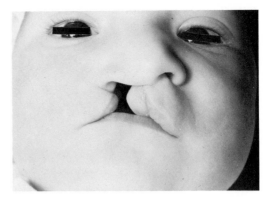

Fig. 9-9. Unilateral cleft upper lip and palate. (Courtesy of Dr. R. Chase.)

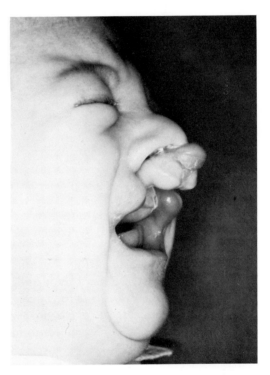

Fig. 9-11. Bilateral cleft upper lip and palate. Note the forward displacement of the premaxilla. (Courtesy of Dr. L. Thompson.)

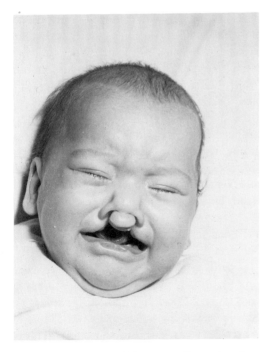

Fig. 9-10. Bilateral cleft upper lip and palate. (Courtesy of Dr. R. Chase.)

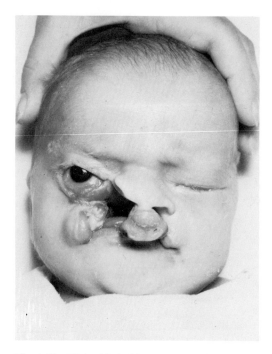

Fig. 9-12. Right-sided oblique facial cleft, and left-sided cleft upper lip; there is also total bilateral cleft palate. (Courtesy of Dr. R. Chase.)

Cleft lower lip is extremely rare. It is exactly central and is caused by incomplete fusion of the mandibular processes.

The condition of isolated cleft lip is usually treated by plastic surgery not later than 2 months after birth, provided the baby's condition permits. The surgeon strives to approximate the vermilion border and to form a normal-looking lip.

MACROSTOMA AND MICROSTOMA. The normal size of the mouth shows considerable individual variation. Rarely, there is incomplete fusion of the maxillary with the mandibular processes, producing an excessively large mouth or *macrostoma*. Very rarely, there is excessive fusion of these processes producing a small mouth or *microstoma*. These conditions can be easily corrected surgically.

CLEFT PALATE. Cleft palate is commonly associated with cleft upper lip. All degrees of cleft palate occur (Fig. 9-13) and are caused by failure of the palatal processes of the maxilla to fuse with each other in the midline and in severe cases by the failure of these processes also to fuse with the premaxilla. It will be remembered that under normal conditions this process of fusion occurs from front to back. The first degree of severity is cleft uvula, the second degree is un-united palatal processes (Figs. 9-14 & 9-15), and the third degree is un-united palatal processes and a cleft on one side of the premaxilla. Usually this type is associated with unilateral cleft lip. The fourth degree of severity is rare, and it consists of un-united palatal processes and a cleft on both sides of the premaxilla. This type is usually associated with bilateral cleft lip. A very rare form may occur in which there is a bilateral cleft lip and the premaxilla fails to fuse with palatal processes of the maxilla on each side.

A baby born with a severe cleft palate presents a difficult feeding problem, since he is unable to suck efficiently. Such a baby often receives some milk in his mouth which he frequently regurgitates through his nose or aspirates into his lungs, leading to respiratory infection. For this reason careful artificial feeding is required until the baby is strong enough to undergo surgery. Plastic surgery is usually recommended between 1 and 2 years of age, before improper speech habits have been acquired.

MEDIAN NASAL FURROW. In this condition the nasal septum is split, separating the two halves of the nose (Figs. 9-16 & 9-17).

LATERAL PROBOSCIS. This is a skin-covered process, usually with a dimple at its lower end (Fig. 9-18). It is often associated with the absence of the isolateral half of the nose.

ATRESIA OF THE NASOLACRIMAL DUCT. This is a common anomaly and is caused by failure in canalization of the developing duct. It may

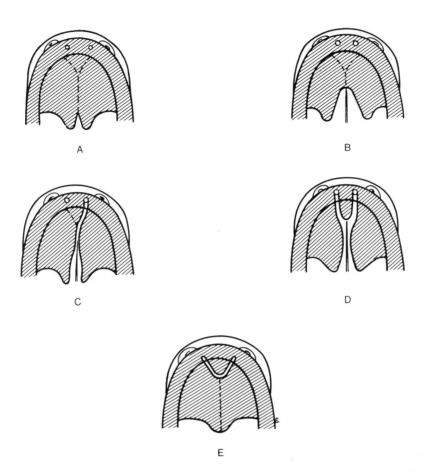

Fig. 9-13. The different forms of cleft palate: (A) cleft uvula, (B) cleft soft and hard palate, (C) total unilateral cleft palate and cleft lip, (D) total bilateral cleft palate and cleft lip, and (E) bilateral cleft lip and jaw.

Fig. 9-14. Cleft hard and soft palate. (Courtesy of Dr. R. Chase.)

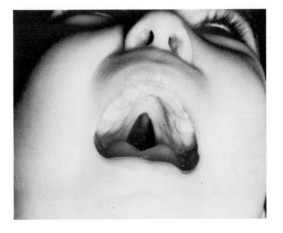

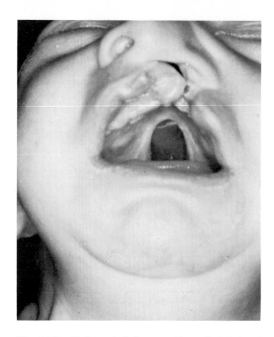

Fig. 9-15. Unilateral cleft upper lip and cleft hard and soft palate. (Courtesy of Dr. L. Thompson.)

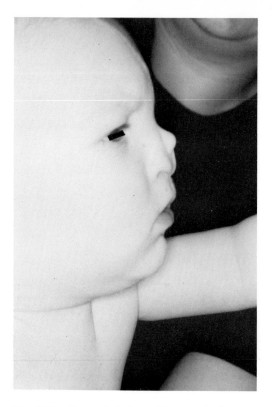

Fig. 9-16. Congenital dermoid cyst of the nose associated with median nasal furrow. In the latter anomaly the nasal septum is split anteriorly into two diverging halves. (Courtesy of Dr. L. Thompson.)

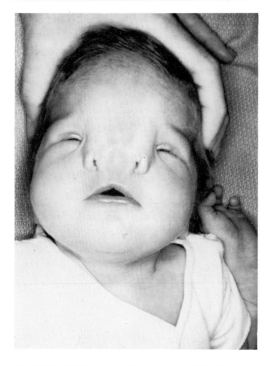

Fig. 9-17. Median nasal furrow in which the nasal septum has completely split separating the two halves of the nose. Note that the external nares are separated by a wide furrow. (Courtesy of Dr. L. Thompson.)

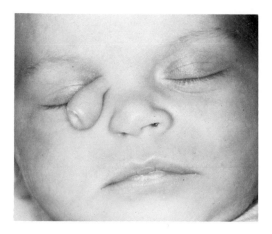

Fig. 9-18. Lateral proboscis. (Courtesy of Dr. R. Chase.)

occur at the upper end, but it usually occurs at the lower end at the entrance into the nose. Here, a flap of mucous membrane, which normally forms a valve at this site, completely covers the ostium. The obstruction is usually easily relieved by the passage of a probe.

CONGENITAL FISTULAS OF THE LACRIMAL SAC. This is a relatively rare condition, and it may occur unilaterally or bilaterally. The orifice is usually found on the side of the nose a short distance below the inner canthus of the eye. Such fistulas should be closed surgically.

Clinical Problems
Answers on page 439

1. A 1-month-old boy was examined by a pediatrician and found to have a left-sided upper cleft lip. The cleft extended from the edge of the lip up to, but not within, the left nostril of the nose. How would you explain the development of this condition? What other areas would you examine in this child? Is there a sexual or familial predisposition for this condition? At what age should this child receive treatment?

2. A 6-week-old baby boy was brought to a pediatrician because the mother felt that his mouth was too small. On examination the child was found to have a very small oral opening, and the mandible was poorly developed. What is the diagnosis? Using your knowledge of embryology, how would you explain the formation of this condition?

3. A 4-week-old baby boy was examined by a pediatrician because of failure to gain weight and difficulty with feeding. The mother said that the child was breast-fed,

eagerly accepted the milk when it was manually expressed from the breast, but was obviously having difficulty in sucking at the nipple. What congenital anomaly in the mouth do you think could be responsible for this feeding problem? How would you treat such a case?

4. A 10-week-old baby was taken to a pediatrician because the mother noticed that, when the baby cried, tears ran down his right cheek but not down his left cheek. On examination the mother's observation was confirmed; even a small amount of crying resulted in tears overflowing the lower eyelid on the right side. Gentle pressure over the lacrimal sac on the left side showed nothing abnormal. However, pressure over the lacrimal sac on the right side resulted in the appearance of mucopus in the conjunctival sac. What is the diagnosis? Could you have made the diagnosis during the first week of life?

REFERENCES

Burston, W. R. Symposium on Malformations of the Face. *Brit. Dent. J.* 116:288, 1964.

Curtis, E. J., Fraser, F. C., and Warburton, D. Congenital Cleft Lip and Palate. *Amer. J. Dis. Child.* 102:853, 1961.

Fraser, F. C. Cleft Lip and Cleft Palate. *Science* 158:1603, 1967.

Fraser Roberts, J. A. Inherited Diseases. In *Methodology in Human Genetics,* edited by W. J. Burdette. Holden-Day, San Francisco, 1962.

Grace, L. G. Frequency of Occurrence of Cleft Palate and Hare Lips. *J. Dent. Res.* 22:495, 1943.

Harris, J. W. S., and Ross, J. P. Cortisone Therapy in Early Pregnancy: Relation to Cleft Palate. *Lancet* 1:1045, 1956.

Kraus, B. S. Prenatal Growth and Morphology of the Human Bony Palate. *J. Dent. Res.* 39:1177, 1960.

MacMahon, B., and McKeown, T. The Incidence of Harelip and Cleft Palate Related to Birth Rank and Maternal Age. *Amer. J. Hum. Genet.* 5:176, 1953.

Mathews, D. N. Plastic Surgery, Cleft Lip and Palate. In *Recent Advances in Paediatric Surgery,* edited by A. W. Wilkinson. Little, Brown, Boston, 1963. P. 182.

Patten, B. M. The Normal Development of the Facial Region. In *Congenital Anomalies of the Face and Associated Structures,* edited by S. Pruzansky. Thomas, Springfield, Ill., 1961. P. 11.

Stark, R. B. The Pathogenesis of Harelip and Cleft Palate. *Plast. Reconstr. Surg.* 13:20, 1954.

Warbrick, J. G. The Early Development of the Nasal Cavity and Upper Lip in the Human Embryo. *J. Anat.* 94:351, 1960.

Warkany, J. *Congenital Malformations.* Year Book, Chicago, 1971. P. 631.

DEVELOPMENT

The Mouth

The cavity of the mouth is formed from two sources: (1) a depression from the exterior called the *stomodeum,* which is lined with ectoderm, and (2) a part immediately posterior to this, derived from the cephalic end of the foregut and lined with entoderm. These two parts are at first separated by the *buccopharyngeal membrane,* but this breaks down and disappears during the third week of development (Figs. 10-1 & 10-2). If this membrane were to persist into adult life, it would occupy an imaginary plane extending obliquely from the region of the body of the sphenoid, through the soft palate, and down to the inner surface of the mandible inferior to the teeth. This means that the structures that are situated in the mouth anterior to this plane are derived from ectoderm, and those which lie postero-inferior to it are derived from entoderm. Thus, the epithelium of the hard palate, sides of the mouth, lips, and the enamel of the teeth are ectodermal structures. Moreover, the secretory epithelium and cells lining the ducts of the *parotid salivary gland* are also derived from ectoderm. On the other hand, the epithelium of the tongue, the floor of the mouth, the palatoglossal and palatopharyngeal folds, and most of the soft palate are entodermal in origin. The secretory and duct epithelia of the *sublingual* and *submandibular salivary glands* are also believed to be of entodermal origin. Needless to say, the exact line of junction of the preexisting ectoderm and entoderm in the adult mouth is impossible to determine.

The Pharynx and Neck

The neck appears between the mouth and the heart, anterior to the hindbrain vesicle. Here the entoderm of the foregut is separated laterally from the surface ectoderm by a layer of mesenchyme. The mesenchyme on each side becomes split up into five or six vertical bars called the *pharyngeal arches.* Each arch forms a swelling on the surface of the embryo and on the wall of the foregut. As the result of this, a series of grooves or clefts are seen on the surface of the embryo between the arches, and these are known as the *pharyngeal clefts* (Fig. 10-3). Similar grooves are seen on the lateral wall of the foregut and are known as *pharyngeal pouches.* The foregut at this level is called the *pharynx.*

Fate of the Pharyngeal Arches

The mesenchymal arches grow around to the anterior aspect of the pharynx and meet and

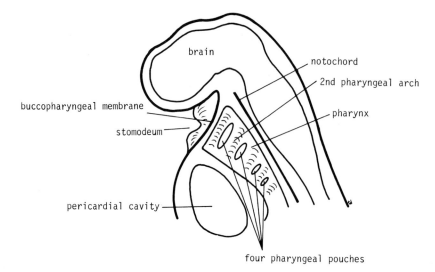

Fig. 10-1. Sagittal section of embryo showing the position of the buccopharyngeal membrane. The membrane is covered on the outside by ectoderm and on the inside by the entoderm of the foregut. Pharyngeal arches and pouches are shown.

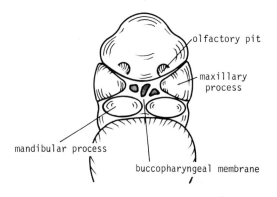

Fig. 10-2. The face of the developing embryo, showing the buccopharyngeal membrane breaking down.

fuse. The first two arches are large and overlap laterally the third and fourth arches. The fifth and sixth arches are small and cannot be seen on the surface of the embryo. The mesenchyme of each arch condenses and forms a core of cartilage and also some skeletal muscle and an artery. The musculature of each arch is supplied by a nerve which has

grown into it from the developing hindbrain. The dorsal ends of the cartilaginous part of the arches become joined to the cartilaginous part of the skull; the first two, however, are the only ones to retain this connection.

The muscles of each arch do not always confine their attachment to the bones or cartilages of their own arch but often migrate into the surrounding tissue. The developmental origin of these muscles can always be determined, since their nerve supply comes from the nerve that supplies the arch of origin.

The nerve that supplies the muscles of the first arch is the *mandibular division of the fifth cranial nerve*. The first arch also receives an additional nerve, the *chorda tympani,* a branch of the seventh cranial nerve, which is a sensory nerve to the mucous membrane of the anterior two-thirds of the tongue. The *seventh cranial nerve* supplies the muscles of the second arch. The *ninth cranial nerve* supplies the muscles of the third arch, and the *tenth* and *eleventh cranial nerves* supply the muscles of the remaining arches.

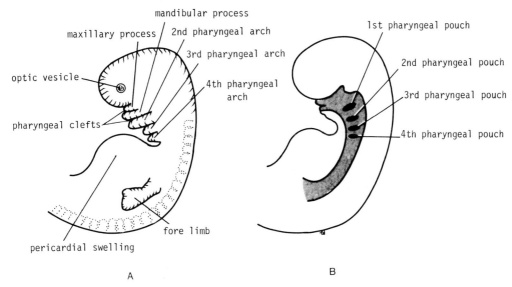

Fig. 10-3. A fetus, aged approximately 32 days, showing (A) the pharyngeal clefts on the outside of the embryo and (B) the pharyngeal pouches seen from within the pharynx.

First Pharyngeal Arch

The mesenchyme, which forms the first pharyngeal arch, divides into two processes, a short *maxillary process* and a long *mandibular process* (Fig. 10-4).

The maxillary process on each side grows anteriorly and medially beneath the developing eye into the facial region. Five areas of intramembranous bone formation become apparent and eventually give rise to the following: the *maxilla*, the *zygoma*, the *palatine*, and the *squamous temporal* bones.

The mesenchymal core of the mandibular process becomes transformed into a cartilaginous bar called *Meckel's cartilage* (Figs. 10-4 & 10-5). The dorsal end of the cartilage separates into two small fragments that later become ossified and form the ear ossicles, the *malleus* and the *incus*. The intermediate portion of the cartilage retrogresses, and its perichondrium condenses to form the *anterior ligament of the malleus* and the *sphenomandibular ligament*. The ventral end of the cartilage extends forward as a cylindrical rod,

which becomes associated with the formation of the mandible (Fig. 10-5). The body of the mandible develops as intramembranous bone lateral to Meckel's cartilage during the sixth week. The greater part of the ventral end of Meckel's cartilage now disappears without contributing to the formation of the mandible. A small portion of the anterior extremity remains and ossifies and becomes incorporated into this part of the mandible.

The muscles of the first arch are the *muscles of mastication*, the *anterior belly of the digastric*, the *mylohyoid*, the *tensor palati*, and the *tensor tympani*, and they are innervated by the mandibular division of the fifth cranial nerve.

The artery of the first arch at first connects the aortic sac to the dorsal aorta, but it later disappears (see Chap. 8).

Second Pharyngeal Arch

The mesenchymal core of this arch becomes condensed to form a cartilaginous bar. The dorsal end of this bar will eventually form an ear ossicle, the *stapes,* and the *styloid process*

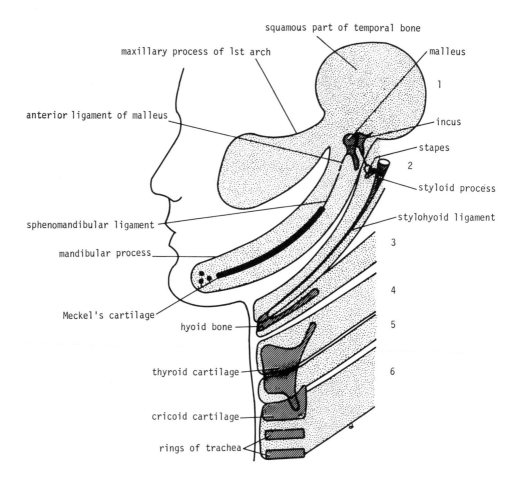

Fig. 10-4. Side of head and neck, showing the fate of the cartilages of the pharyngeal arches. The pterygo-mandibular ligament and the stylomandibular ligament are not formed from the pharyngeal arches.

of the temporal bone (Fig. 10-4). The intermediate portion will form the *stylohyoid ligament* and its ventral portion, the *lesser cornu,* and the *superior part of the body of the hyoid bone.*

The muscles of the second arch are the *stapedius,* the *stylohyoid,* and the *posterior belly of the digastric,* all of which remain attached to the arch; the *muscles of facial expression* (including the buccinator), the *auricular muscles,* the *occipitofrontalis,* and the *platysma,* all of which have migrated away from the arch. The muscles of the second arch are supplied by the seventh cranial nerve.

The artery of the second arch at first connects the aortic sac to the dorsal aorta, but it later disappears (see p. 99).

Third Pharyngeal Arch

The mesenchymal core forms a cartilaginous bar which loses its connection with the skull. The ventral portion persists as the *greater cornu of the hyoid bone* and the *inferior part of the body of the hyoid bone* (Fig. 10-4).

The muscles of the third arch are the

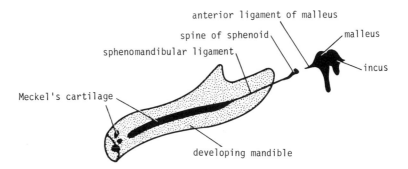

anterior ligament of malleus

spine of sphenoid

sphenomandibular ligament

malleus

incus

Meckel's cartilage

developing mandible

Fig. 10-5. The fate of the cartilage of the mandibular process of the first pharyngeal arch.

stylopharyngeus and probably some of the superior *pharyngeal muscles*. They are innervated by the ninth cranial nerve.

For the fate of the artery of the third arch, see Chapter 8.

Fourth, Fifth, and Sixth Pharyngeal Arches

As in the previous arches, the mesenchymal core becomes transformed in part into cartilage. The cartilage of the fourth and fifth arches forms the *thyroid cartilage* and that of the sixth forms the *cricoid,* the *arytenoid,* and the *rings of the trachea* (Fig. 10-4). The musculature of these arches becomes the *muscles of the larynx,* the remaining *muscles of the pharynx,* and the *soft palate.* The muscles are supplied by the tenth and eleventh cranial nerves. The *cricothyroid muscle* is supplied by the external laryngeal branch of the superior laryngeal division of the vagus, and the intrinsic muscles of the larynx are supplied by the recurrent laryngeal branch of the vagus.

For the arteries of these arches, see Chapter 8.

Fate of the Ectoderm Covering Each Pharyngeal Arch and Fate of the Pharyngeal Clefts

The ectoderm covering the first arch becomes the epidermis of the skin over the lower jaw. Superior to the first arch, the ectoderm thickens to form the *labiogingival lamina,*

which grows inferiorly on the medial aspect of the jaw invading the mesenchyme. These cells later degenerate and form a sulcus between the lip and the alveolar process (Fig. 10-9).

The *first pharyngeal cleft* forms the *external auditory meatus* and the outer epithelial covering of the *tympanic membrane* (Fig. 10-6). Around the developing meatus, the *pinna* is formed as the result of the growth and later fusion of six small surface elevations, three derived from the first arch and three from the second arch. The remaining pharyngeal clefts become buried by the second pharyngeal arch, which enlarges and grows inferiorly in the neck. As a result of this, the second, third, and fourth clefts form the floor of a cavity lined with ectoderm called the *cervical sinus.* Later the sinus becomes obliterated by apposition and fusion of its walls. These changes result in the neck's having a smooth contour.

Fate of the Pharyngeal Pouches

The lining of the pharynx is derived from the cephalic end of the foregut and is therefore entodermal in origin. It is at first smooth but later shows swellings and pouches which are caused by the appearance of the pharyngeal arches. From the five pairs of pouches, many of the neck structures will develop; some of these will remain inside the pharynx, for

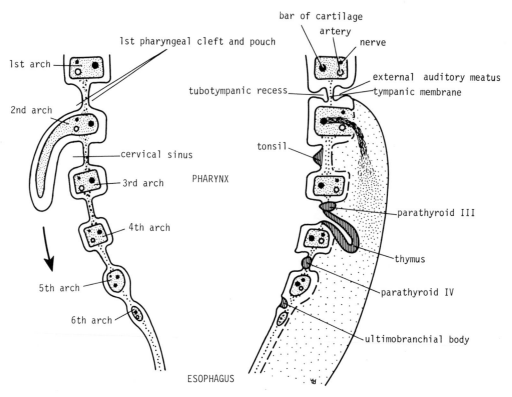

Fig. 10-6. The pharynx, showing the fate of the pharyngeal clefts and pouches. The great downgrowth of the second pharyngeal arch, burying the pharyngeal clefts, is shown.

example, the tonsil, while others will migrate into the tissues of the neck, for example, the thymus.

First Pharyngeal Pouch

A diverticulum, called the *tubotympanic recess,* grows out from the first pharyngeal pouch; this extends laterally to meet the floor of the first pharyngeal cleft (Fig. 10-6). On reaching the base of the skull, it comes into close contact with the developing internal ear and the dorsal ends of the first and second pharyngeal arches; the latter will form the bony ossicles: the *malleus,* the *incus,* and the *stapes.* The recess now wraps itself around these small bones at that level and forms the *tympanic cavity.* The neck of the recess narrows and becomes the *pharyngotympanic*

tube. The entoderm lining the tympanic cavity forms the inner epithelial covering of the tympanic membrane. The *mastoid antrum* later develops as a posterior extension of the tympanic cavity.

Second Pharyngeal Pouch

The tonsil develops from this pouch by solid buds of entoderm growing out into the mesenchyme (Fig. 10-6). The central cells of these buds break down, forming the *tonsillar crypts,* and later lymphatic tissue accumulates around the crypts. The *capsule* of the tonsil is formed from a condensation of mesenchyme.

Third Pharyngeal Pouch

The *thymus* and the *inferior parathyroid gland* develop from this pouch (Fig. 10-6).

The thymus arises as a diverticulum, which grows inferiorly into the neck to reach the superior mediastinum. Each diverticulum is at first hollow and later, as the result of cellular proliferation, becomes a solid bar. The two thymic bars become fused together in the superior mediastinum and sever their connection with the third pharyngeal pouches. The entodermal cells multiply to form solid clusters, the *corpuscles of Hassall.* By the end of the third month, the thymus becomes invaded with lymphatic tissue. For the further development of the thymus, see Chapter 17.

The inferior parathyroid, or parathyroid III, named after its pouch of origin, develops as a proliferation of entodermal cells in the third pharyngeal pouch. As the thymic diverticulum on each side grows inferiorly in the neck, it pulls the inferior parathyroid with it so that it finally comes to rest on the posterior surface of the thyroid gland, completely separated from the thymus. If the separation from the thymus is delayed, the inferior parathyroid may be pulled down into the lower part of the neck or thoracic cavity. During the descent, the inferior parathyroid is pulled past the superior parathyroid.

Fourth Pharyngeal Pouch

The *superior parathyroid gland,* or parathyroid IV, develops from this pouch as a proliferation of entodermal cells (Fig. 10-6). These sever their connection with the pharyngeal wall and take up their final position on the posterior aspect of the thyroid gland on each side.

For the further development of the superior and inferior parathyroid glands, see Chapter 18.

Fifth Pharyngeal Pouch

There is some question as to whether this pouch can be identified as a separate entity in the human embryo. Some authorities believe that entodermal cells proliferate in this region and give rise to the *ultimobranchial body.*

The cells of the ultimobranchial body may be incorporated into the thyroid gland (see Chap. 18) as the parafollicular cells.

The Tongue

At about the fourth week, a median swelling appears in the entodermal ventral wall or floor of the pharynx called the *tuberculum impar* (Fig. 10-7). A little later another, the *lateral lingual swelling,* appears on each side of the tuberculum impar, derived from the anterior end of each first pharyngeal arch. The lateral lingual swellings now enlarge and grow medially and fuse with each other, and the tuberculum impar is buried by them. The lingual swellings thus form the anterior two-thirds or body of the tongue, and since they are derived from the first pharyngeal arches, the mucous membrane on each side will be innervated by the lingual nerve, a branch of the mandibular division of the fifth cranial nerve (common sensation); the chorda tympani from the seventh cranial nerve (taste) also supplies this area.

Meanwhile a second median swelling appears in the floor of the pharynx behind the tuberculum impar called the *copula.* This extends forward on each side of the tuberculum impar and becomes V-shaped. At about this time the anterior ends of the second, third, and fourth pharyngeal arches are entering this region. The anterior ends of the third arch on each side now overgrow the other arches and extend into the copula, fusing in the midline. The copula now disappears. The mucous membrane of the posterior third of the tongue is thus formed from the third pharyngeal arches and is innervated by the ninth cranial nerves (common sensation and taste).

The anterior two-thirds of the tongue are separated from the posterior third by a groove, the *sulcus terminalis,* which represents the interval between the lingual swellings of the first pharyngeal arches and the

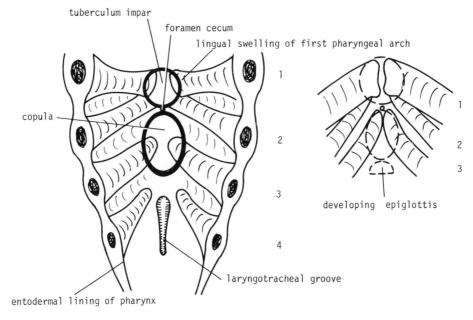

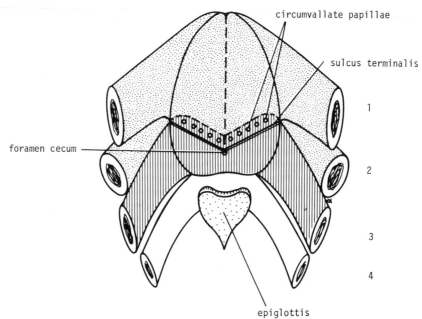

Fig. 10-7. The floor of the pharynx, showing different stages in the development of the tongue.

anterior ends of the third pharyngeal arches. Around the edge of the anterior two-thirds of the tongue, the entodermal cells proliferate and grow inferiorly into the underlying mesenchyme. Later these cells degenerate so that this part of the tongue becomes free (Fig. 10-8). Some of the entodermal cells remain in the midline and help to form the *frenulum of the tongue*.

It will be remembered that the *circumvallate papillae* are situated on the mucous membrane just anterior to the sulcus terminalis, and their taste buds are innervated by the ninth cranial nerve. It is presumed that during development the mucous membrane of the posterior third of the tongue becomes pulled anteriorly slightly so that fibers of the ninth cranial nerve cross the sulcus terminalis to supply these taste buds (Fig. 10-7).

The muscles of the tongue are derived from the *occipital myotomes*, which at first are closely related to the developing hindbrain and later migrate inferiorly and ante-

riorly around the pharynx and enter the tongue (Fig. 10-8). The migrating myotomes carry with them their innervation, the twelfth cranial nerves.

The *epiglottis* is formed by the posterior third of the copula becoming split off from the tongue by a transverse groove. The groove becomes divided into the *valleculae* by the appearance of a median *glosso-epiglottic fold*.

The thyroid gland develops as a diverticulum from the floor of the pharynx behind the tuberculum impar, the site being called the *foramen cecum* (Fig. 10-7). For the further development of the thyroid gland, see Chapter 18.

The Salivary Glands

All the salivary glands have the same plan of origin and development. They arise at about the seventh week as solid outgrowths of cells from the wall of the developing mouth; these

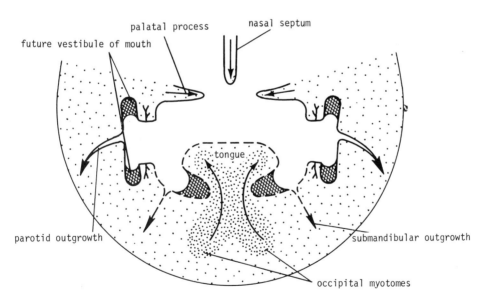

Fig. 10-8. Cross section of the developing mouth, showing the paths taken by the developing tissues as they move into position. The epithelial surface, shown as a solid line, is ectodermal in origin; the epithelial surface, shown as an interrupted line, is entodermal in origin. The epithelial area, shown crosshatched, eventually degenerates, forming the vestibule of the mouth; the anterior part of the tongue is mobilized.

cells grow into the underlying mesenchyme. The epithelial buds branch repeatedly to form solid *ducts,* the ends of which round out to form secretory *acini.* Later the solid ducts and acini become canalized. The surrounding mesenchyme condenses to form the capsule and divides each gland into lobes or lobules. The ducts and acini of the *parotid gland* are derived from ectoderm (Fig. 10-8) and those of the *submandibular* and *sublingual glands* from entoderm.

The Teeth

Deciduous Teeth

At about the sixth week the first sign of tooth development is seen. A linear thickening of ectoderm occurs along a line that represents the edge of the developing jaws and is known as the *dental lamina* (Fig. 10-9). Soon there arises from the deep margin of the lamina ten *dental buds* for the upper jaw and ten dental buds for the lower jaw, which grow into the underlying mesenchyme. Each dental bud now becomes invaginated by a condensation of mesenchyme called the *dental papilla* and becomes cap-shaped. The cells of the cap become differentiated into the *outer dental epithelium* at the convexity and an *inner dental epithelium* at the concavity. As the result of an increase in the intercellular fluid, the cells of the cap which lie between the outer and inner epithelia become loosely arranged to form the *stellate reticulum.* With further growth of the dental cap, the mesenchymal cells of the dental papilla adjacent to the inner dental epithelium enlarge and differentiate into *odontoblasts.* The odontoblasts will be responsible for the laying down of *dentine.* As more and more dentine is formed, the cell bodies of the odontoblasts recede toward the center of the dental papilla, each leaving a fine cellular process behind in the dentine, called the *ondontoblastic process.* The remaining cells in the dental papilla form the *pulp* of the tooth. Meanwhile the

mesenchyme surrounding the developing tooth becomes condensed to form the fibrous *dental sac.*

The dental cap continues to grow and the invagination by the dental papilla deepens so that the cap becomes bell-shaped. The cells of the inner dental layer now differentiate into *ameloblasts,* which will be responsible for laying down *enamel* on the outer surface of the dentine. As the enamel thickens, the ameloblasts retreat outward into the stellate reticulum. During the formation of the enamel, the layer of outer dental epithelium becomes much folded by the formation of vascular papillae from the adjacent mesenchyme of the dental sac. It is believed that this arrangement provides a rich nutritional supply for the active ameloblasts. When the enamel is completely developed, the ameloblasts, the remains of the stellate reticulum, and the outer dental epithelium become indistinguishable. These cells lay down a delicate membrane which covers the enamel called the *enamel cuticle.* Once the tooth has erupted, mastication soon wears away the cuticle on the exposed surfaces.

By the third month, the dental lamina produces further epithelial dental buds on the lingual side of each developing deciduous tooth. These will become the dental buds of the permanent teeth. For some time, the dental buds of the deciduous and permanent teeth remain attached to the epithelium of the gums by the dental lamina but ultimately it disappears completely.

Meanwhile the ectodermal cells forming the free edge of the bell-shaped dental bud proliferate and extend down around the dental papilla to form the *root sheath.* The cells of the dental papilla in contact with the sheath differentiate into odontoblasts, which start to produce dentine that is continuous with that of the crown. Later, the root sheath becomes invaded and broken down by surrounding mesenchymal cells. These mesenchymal cells differentiate into *cementoblasts,*

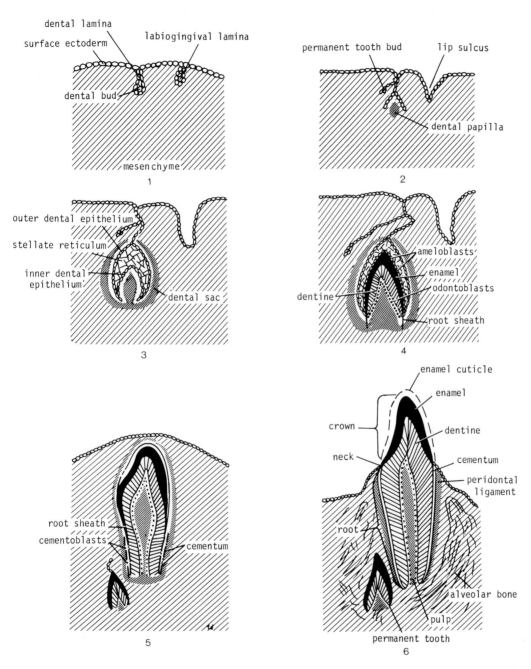

Fig. 10-9. The different stages in the development of a deciduous tooth. The dental bud of the permanent tooth is also shown.

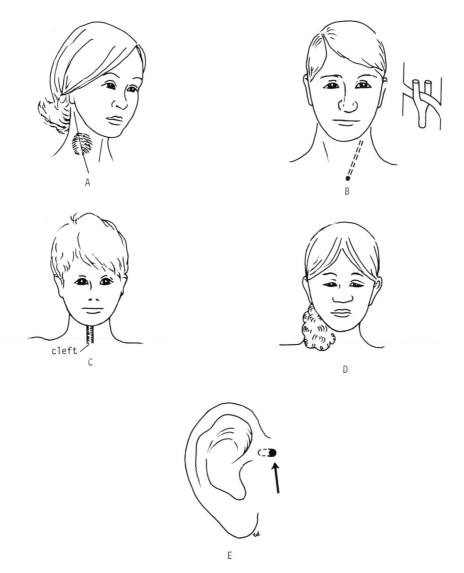

Fig. 10-10. Congenital anomalies of the neck: (A) branchial cyst in upper part of neck protruding from beneath anterior border of sternocleidomastoid muscle; (B) branchial fistula opening onto skin surface in the lower part of the neck, showing the channel extending superiorly in the neck between the internal and external carotid arteries; (C) failure of pharyngeal arches from the two sides to fuse in midline, producing a midline cleft; (D) cystic hygroma of the neck in a 2-year-old boy; and (E) preauricular sinus.

which lay down a special form of bone called *cementum*. This covers the dentine of the root and is continuous with the enamel at the neck of the tooth. Once the root is formed, the fibroblasts and fibers of the dental sac form the *peridontal ligament,* and the fibers extend from the cementum to the periosteum of the alveolar bone. The peridontal ligament thus supports and holds the tooth in position.

With continued growth of the crown and root, the deciduous teeth move toward the surface and finally erupt into the oral cavity. The eruption of deciduous teeth begins between the sixth and ninth months of postnatal life, and all should be present in a healthy child by the end of the second year or soon after. The lower central incisors are usually the first to erupt.

Permanent Teeth

During the third month of development, the dental buds for the permanent teeth arise on the lingual side of the developing deciduous teeth. In the permanent teeth, there are on both sides of each jaw three molars not represented in the deciduous set. These are formed from dental buds that arise from a posterior extension of the dental lamina. The thirty-two permanent dental buds develop in a similar manner to that described for the deciduous teeth, but they remain dormant until the sixth year, when the first molars erupt. The last permanent teeth to erupt are the third molars, and this can occur at a variable time between the seventeenth and thirtieth years.

CONGENITAL ANOMALIES OF THE NECK, TONGUE, TEETH, AND LOWER JAW

Neck

Branchial Cysts, Sinuses, and Fistulas

The burial of the second, third, and fourth pharyngeal clefts as the result of the downgrowth of the second pharyngeal arch forms

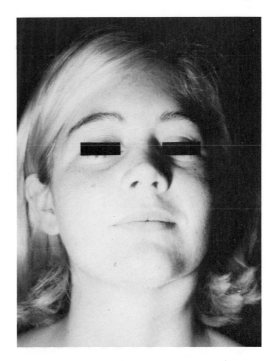

Fig. 10-11. Branchial cyst on left side of the neck in 18-year-old girl. (Courtesy of Dr. R. Chase.)

an ectodermal-lined cavity called the *cervical sinus* (Fig. 10-6). Normally this sinus becomes obliterated by apposition and fusion of its walls. Should this fail to occur, a *branchial cyst* forms. Such cysts are not apparent at birth but gradually enlarge during childhood and become conspicuous in early adult life. They are most commonly found in the superior part of the neck, protruding from beneath the anterior border of the sternocleidomastoid muscle (Figs. 10-10 & 10-11). They are lined with stratified squamous epithelium and are filled with fluid containing cholesterol crystals. It is believed that they are derived from the ectoderm lining the second pharyngeal cleft. Surgical removal is indicated, since they gradually increase in size and may become infected (Fig. 10-12).

Occasionally the second pharyngeal arch fails to bury the pharyngeal clefts completely, and the cervical sinus remains in communi-

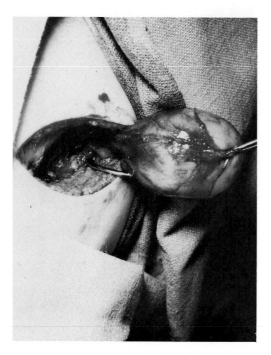

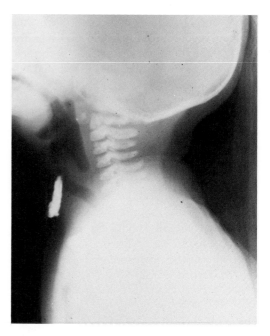

Fig. 10-12. Branchial cyst being removed from patient seen in Figure 10-11. (Courtesy of Dr. R. Chase.)

Fig. 10-13. X-ray film of branchial sinus following injection of radiopaque material into opening in the neck. (Courtesy of Dr. J. Randolph.)

cation with the surface of the neck, forming a *branchial sinus* (Fig. 10-13). A similar opening in the neck may result from infection of a branchial cyst. A branchial sinus may be found anywhere along the anterior border of the sternocleidomastoid muscle, especially in the inferior part of the neck. Such a sinus should be removed in its entirety by careful surgical dissection.

Sometimes a *branchial fistula* occurs in which the cervical sinus remains as a channel extending up the neck between the internal and external carotid arteries (Fig. 10-10) and opening into the pharynx just posterior to the tonsil. Inferiorly, it opens onto the skin of the neck at some point along the anterior border of the sternocleidomastoid muscle. It is concluded, therefore, that branchial fistulas of the neck are derived from the second pharyngeal

pouch and cleft. A branchial fistula should be removed in its entirety by careful surgical dissection.

Very rarely the pharyngeal arches from the two sides fail to fuse properly in the midline, giving rise to a *midline pharyngeal cyst* or a *cleft* (Fig. 10-10).

Branchial Cartilage

An irregular mass of cartilage, several millimeters in diameter, may be found in the subcutaneous tissues of the neck, usually just anterior to the lower third of the sternocleidomastoid muscle. It is thought that such pieces of cartilage are derived from one of the pharyngeal arches.

Preauricular and Auricular Sinuses

These open on the pinna or immediately anterior to the ear. They are thought to result from incomplete fusion of the small nodules that originate from the first and second pharyngeal arches to form the pinna. A sinus anterior to the ear is prone to infection and should be excised (Fig. 10-10).

Cystic Hygroma

At about the sixth week, primitive lymph sacs develop in the mesenchyme in the neck in association with the jugular and subclavian veins; these are called *jugular lymph sacs*. Failure of a portion of an isolated endothelial-lined sac to join with the lymphatic system results in the formation of a cystic swelling in the lower third of the neck which may be present at birth or present during early infancy (Fig. 10-10). On section, the swelling is found to consist of a large number of small cysts filled with clear lymph and lined by endothelium. A cystic hygroma should be excised.

Tongue

Aglossia

Complete or partial absence of the tongue is extremely rare.

Macroglossia

An excessively large tongue may be present at birth and is usually caused by the presence of a cystic hygroma of the lymphatics of the tongue. Congenital *neurofibromatosis,* sometimes confined to one-half of the tongue, is a rare cause of macroglossia. As in lymphangioma, the treatment is surgical reduction of the bulk of the tongue. *Congenital muscular hypertrophy* of unknown cause may result in the tongue's protruding from the mouth (Fig. 10-14). Partial glossectomy is the treatment of choice.

Bifid Tongue

A split involving the tip or anterior two-thirds of the tongue is caused by failure of

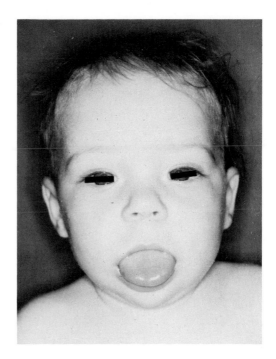

Fig. 10-14. Macroglossia due to congenital muscular hypertrophy. (Courtesy of Dr. L. Thompson.)

the lingual swellings of the first pharyngeal arches to fuse in the midline. This may require plastic closure for cosmetic reasons.

Tonguetie

This rare condition is caused by a short frenulum. No treatment is necessary unless mastication or speech is impaired.

Excessive Length of Frenulum

This condition is rare but important, since the tongue may be excessively mobile and may fall back and occlude the pharynx, causing suffocation.

Ranula

This transparent cystic swelling may be found inferior to the margin of the tongue and is caused by a failure of one of the ducts of the sublingual salivary gland to become canalized during development (Fig. 10-15).

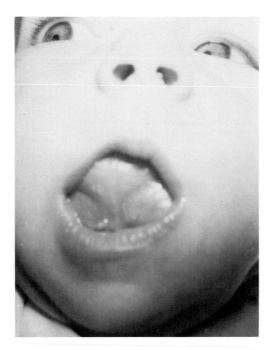

Fig. 10-15. Bilateral ranula lying inferior to the tongue. (Courtesy of Dr. G. Avery.)

Surgical removal is desirable, since the ranula is liable to become infected.

Teeth

Congenitally Absent and Supernumerary Teeth

Complete absence of teeth is very rare. Absence of single teeth, most frequently the permanent upper lateral incisors, third molars, and lower second premolars, may occur. Single or multiple supernumerary teeth resulting from the formation of additional dental buds occasionally occur.

Impaction of a Tooth

Impaction most often affects the third lower molar, which turns its crown medially and upward as it develops and only assumes the upright position in the later stages of eruption. The second molar may block the eruption of the third molar by preventing this change of position. Thus, horizontal position of the third molar may lead to impaction (impacted "wisdom" tooth) (Fig. 10-16).

Odontogenic Cysts

Aberrations of dental development cause these cysts to form, and they are found most often in the region of the third molar teeth.

PRIMORDIAL CYST. This develops as the result of degeneration of the stellate reticulum of the dental cap before any calcified tissue has been formed, causing fluid to accumulate; thus a cyst develops in place of a tooth (Fig. 10-16).

DENTIGEROUS CYST. This type of cyst occurs in an unerupted tooth after the enamel has been formed. Degeneration and accumulation of fluid occur in the remains of the stellate reticulum, and a cyst is formed, the walls of which are derived from the outer epithelial layer of the dental bud. The crown of the unerupted tooth projects into the cavity of the cyst and the root is outside the cyst (Fig. 10-16).

Odontogenic Tumors

Such tumors represent gross errors in development and arise from the ectoderm or mesenchyme of the developing tooth.

Micrognathia

This is a failure of the lower jaw to develop adequately (Figs. 10-17 & 10-18). It is thought to be caused in some cases by an excessive flexion of the cervical vertebral column pressing the developing jaw against the front of the thorax. The condition may occur in association with oligohydramnios.

Unilateral Agenesis of the Mandible

This is an asymmetry of the lower jaw; however, the muscles of mastication are usually normal. Failure of development of the first arch on one side may be the only defect or may be associated with weakness of the muscles of facial expression on the same side because of involvement of the second arch. The cause is unknown.

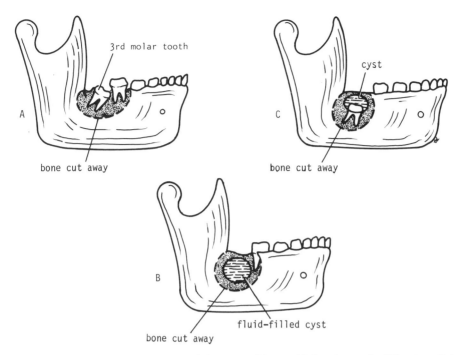

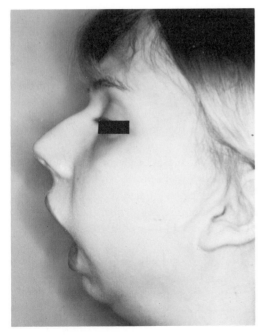

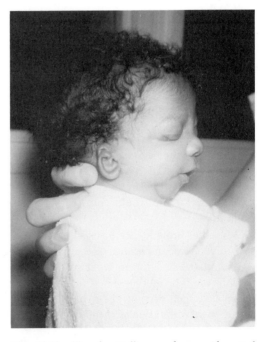

Fig. 10-16. Anomalies of tooth development: (A) impacted lower third molar tooth; (B) primordial cyst, in place of third molar tooth; (C) dentigerous cyst, crown of unerupted third molar tooth projecting into cavity of cyst.

Fig. 10-17. Micrognathia. (Courtesy of Dr. L. Thompson.)

Fig. 10-18. Treacher-Collins syndrome. Abnormal first pharyngeal arch results in micrognathia, defects in lower eyelid, and deformed auricle of ear. (Courtesy of Dr. G. Avery.)

139

1. A 25-year-old woman visited her physician because she had noticed a swelling in the front of her neck. The swelling was painless and was gradually increasing in size. On examination a swelling about 1 inch (2.5 cm) in diameter was found just beneath the upper third of the anterior border of the right sternocleidomastoid muscle. On palpation the swelling fluctuated in size and did not appear to be attached to surrounding structures. What is your diagnosis? Do you think this cyst should be removed?

2. A 40-year-old man visited his physician because he had noticed a small area of irritation in the lower part of his neck. On questioning, the patient said that a small drop of fluid sometimes exuded out onto the skin surface and stained his shirt. Three years previously he had had a painful abscess in the same area and this had been successfully treated with antibiotics. On examination a small skin opening with reddened edges was seen in the lower third of the neck, just anterior to the left sternocleidomastoid muscle. On applying gentle pressure to the neck immediately above the opening, a small drop of mucus was extruded onto the skin surface. What is the diagnosis? How would you treat this condition?

3. A mother brought her 8-year-old daughter to a pediatrician because of the presence of a lobulated swelling in front of the child's right ear. The mother stated that the swelling had been present at birth, had gradually increased in size as the child grew, and was now unsightly. On examination a sessile swelling covered with normal skin was found immediately in front of the tragus of the right ear. On palpation the swelling was found to contain a firm nodule. The opposite ear was normal, and further examination of the child revealed no other abnormality. What is the diagnosis? How would you treat this condition?

4. On examining a 3-year-old boy, a pediatrician found a pinpoint hole in a skin depression immediately anterior to the ascending limb of the helix of the right auricle of the ear. On questioning, the mother said that she had also noticed the hole, but since it did not cause her son any discomfort, she had not sought a physician's advice. What is this condition called? Is it necessary to treat it?

5. A 6-year-old boy was examined by a pediatrician for a large swelling below the jaw on the right side of the neck. The swelling extended from the parotid region down to about 2 in. (5 cm) above the clavicle. On palpation the swelling was found to be painless, soft, and fluctuant. It was not attached to the skin but appeared to extend deep, to the sternocleidomastoid muscle on the right side. The swelling had first been noticed 3 years previously and had gradually increased in size. Using your knowledge of embryology, what diagnosis would you make? How would you treat this condition?

6. A 3-month-old boy was brought to a pediatrician because the mother thought that his tongue was abnormally large. "His mouth does not seem to be large enough to hold his tongue," she said. On examination the tongue was found to be diffusely enlarged beyond normal limits. Name the common

congenital conditions responsible for diffuse enlargement of the tongue.

7. A 4-year-old girl was examined by a pediatrician and found to have a bluish cystic swelling below the left margin of the tongue. The cyst had first been noticed 1 year previously and since that time had gradually increased in size. What is your diagnosis?

8. A 30-year-old man was examined by a dentist and found to have a swelling of the body of the mandible on the right side. The swelling was situated behind the second molar tooth; the third molar tooth was unerupted. X-ray examination of the mandible revealed a cyst, and the crown of the unerupted third molar tooth could be seen projecting into the cyst. What is your diagnosis? How can you explain the presence of the cyst?

9. A boy at birth was seen to have a receding mandible. On further examination the child was found to have a cleft soft palate and a small tongue. During the first few months of life there was considerable difficulty with feeding due to the inability of the baby to get the lower lip around the nipple and thus to suck properly. What is the embryological explanation for the receding mandible and the cleft palate? What is the treatment?

REFERENCES

Alber, G. D. Branchial Anomalies. *J.A.M.A.* 183:399, 1963.

Arey, L. B. *Developmental Anatomy,* 7th ed. Saunders, Philadelphia, 1966.

Bailey, H. The Clinical Aspects of Branchial Fistulae. *Brit. J. Surg.* 21:173, 1933.

Bill, A. H., and Vadheim, J. L. Cysts, Sinuses, and Fistulas of the Neck Arising from the First and Second Branchial Clefts. *Ann. Surg.* 142:904, 1955.

Boyd, J. D. Development of the Thyroid and Parathyroid Glands and the Thymus. *Ann. Roy. Coll. Surg. Eng.* 7:455, 1950.

Brown, P. M., and Judd, E. S. Thyroglossal Cysts and Sinuses: Results of Radical (Sistrunk) Operation. *Amer. J. Surg.* 102:494, 1961.

Byers, L. T., and Anderson, R. Anomalies of the First Branchial Cleft. *Surg. Gynec. Obstet.* 93:775, 1951.

DeBord, R. A. First Branchial Cleft Sinus. *Arch. Surg.* (Chicago) 81:228, 1960.

Dennison, W. M. *Surgery in Infancy and Childhood,* 2d ed. Livingstone, Edinburgh, 1967.

Diamond, M., and Applebaum, E. The Epithelial Sheath. *J. Dent. Res.* 21:403, 1942.

Douglas, J. Branchiogenetic Cyst with Sinus Leading into Pharynx. *Ann. Surg.* 67:240, 1918.

Gilmour, J. R. The Embryology of the Parathyroid Glands, the Thymus and Certain Associated Rudiments. *J. Path. Bact.* 45:507, 1937.

Gottlieb, E., and Lenin, M. L. Congenital Midline Cervical Cysts of the Neck. *New York J. Med.* 66:712, 1966.

Henzel, J. H., Pories, W. J., and DeWeese, M. S. Etiology of Lateral Cervical Cysts. *Surg. Gynec. Obstet.* 125:87, 1967.

Johnson, P. L., and Bevelander, G. The Role of the Stratum Intermedium in Tooth Development. *Oral Surg.* 10:437, 1957.

Kingsbury, B. F. The Question of a Lateral Thyroid in Mammals, with Special Reference to Man. *Amer. J. Anat.* 65:33, 1939.

Ladd, W. E., and Gross, R. E. Congenital Branchiogenic Anomalies. *Amer. J. Surg.* 39:234, 1938.

Lincoln, J. C. R. Cervico-Auricular Fistulae. *Arch. Dis. Child.* 40:218, 1965.

Marshall, S. F., and Beeker, W. F. Thyroglossal Cysts and Sinuses. *Ann. Surg.* 129:642, 1949.

Martins, A. G. Lateral Cervical and Pre-Auricular Sinuses. *Brit. Med. J.* 5:255, 1961.

McClintock, J. C., and Mahaffey, D. E. Thyroglossal Tract Lesions. *J. Clin. Endocr.* 10:1108, 1950.

Miles, A. E. W. Malformations of the Teeth. *Proc. Roy. Soc. Med.* 47:817, 1954.

Neel, H. B., and Pemberton, J. Lateral Cervical (Branchial) Cysts and Fistulas. *Surgery* 18:267, 1945.

Norris, E. H. The Parathyroid Glands and the Lateral Thyroid in Man: Their Morphogenesis, Histogenesis, Topographic Anatomy and Prenatal Growth. *Contrib. Embryol.* 26:247, 1937.

Orban, B. Growth and Movement of the Tooth Germs and Teeth. *J. Amer. Dent. Ass.* 15:1004, 1928.

Orban's Oral Histology and Embryology, 6th ed., edited by H. Sicher. Mosby, St. Louis, 1966.

Perzik, S. L. Early Management in Extensive Cervical Cystic Hygroma and Macroglossia. *Arch. Surg.* (Chicago) 80:450, 1960.

Rickham, P. P., and Johnston, J. H. *Neonatal Surgery.* Butterworth, London, 1969.

Schour, J., and Massler, M. Studies in Tooth Development: The Growth Pattern of Human Teeth. *J. Amer. Dent. Ass.* 27:1785, 1940.

Sicher, H. Tooth Eruption: Axial Movement of Teeth with Limited Growth. *J. Dent. Res.* 21:395, 1942.

Small, A. The Surgical Removal of Branchial Sinus. *Lancet* 2:891, 1960.

Weller, G. L. Development of the Thyroid, Parathyroid, and Thymus Glands in Man. *Contrib. Embryol.* 24:93, 1933.

The digestive tube has been shown to be formed from the part of the yolk sac that lies within the body of the embryo (Chap. 3). The entoderm forms the epithelial lining, and the splanchnic mesenchyme forms the surrounding muscle and serous coats. The developing gut is divided into the foregut, midgut, and hindgut (Fig. 11-1).

DEVELOPMENT

The Esophagus

The esophagus develops from the narrow part of the foregut that succeeds the pharynx (Fig. 11-1). It is at first a short tube, but when the heart and diaphragm descend, it elongates rapidly. The entodermal lining of the esophagus proliferates and almost obliterates the lumen; later recanalization occurs. The splanchnic layer of mesenchyme forms striated muscle in the upper two-thirds of the esophagus and smooth muscle in the lower two-thirds, so that there is a mixture of the two types of muscle in the middle third. On each side of the esophagus lies the *pericardioperitoneal canal,* a part of the coelomic cavity which subsequently forms the pleural cavity.

The Stomach

The stomach commences as a fusiform dilatation of the foregut at about the fourth week (Figs. 11-1 & 11-2). At this time, it has a *ventral* and *dorsal mesentery* (see p. 188). Very active growth takes place along the dorsal border, which becomes convex and forms the *greater curvature* of the stomach. The anterior border becomes concave and forms the *lesser curvature*. The *fundus* appears as a dilatation at the upper end of the stomach. At this stage, the stomach has a right and left surface to which the right and left vagus nerves are attached, respectively. With the continued active growth of the dorsal border of the stomach, along with the great growth of the right lobe of the liver, the ventral border of the stomach gradually rotates toward the right so that the left surface becomes anterior and the right surface posterior. The ventral and dorsal mesenteries become altered in position as a result of this rotation of the stomach, and they now form the *omenta* of the stomach and various peritoneal ligaments. A pouch of peritoneum becomes located behind the stomach and is known as the *lesser sac* or *omental bursa*.

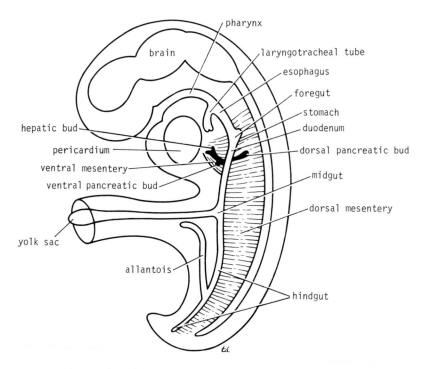

Fig. 11-1. Foregut, midgut, and hindgut, showing the ventral mesentery and dorsal mesentery, the hepatic bud, and the ventral and dorsal pancreatic buds.

The Duodenum

The duodenum is formed from the most caudal portion of the foregut and the most cephalic end of the midgut. This region of the gut rapidly grows to form a loop. At this time the duodenum has a mesentery that extends to the posterior abdominal wall and is part of the dorsal mesentery. A small part of the ventral mesentery is also attached to the ventral border of the first part of the duodenum and the upper half of the second part of the duodenum. When the stomach rotates, the duodenal loop is forced to rotate to the right, where the second, third, and fourth parts adhere to the posterior abdominal wall, and the peritoneum behind the duodenum now disappears. However, some smooth muscle and fibrous tissue that belong to the dorsal mesentery remain as the *suspensory ligament of the duodenum* (of

Treitz), and this fixes the terminal part of the duodenum and prevents it from moving inferiorly (Fig. 11-4). The liver and pancreas arise as entodermal buds from the developing duodenum.

The Liver

The liver arises as a solid bud of entodermal cells from the distal end of the foregut (Figs. 11-3 & 11-4). This site of origin lies at the apex of the loop of the developing duodenum and corresponds to a point halfway along the second part of the fully formed duodenum. The *hepatic bud* grows anteriorly into the mass of splanchnic mesoderm called the *septum transversum*. The septum transversum in this region forms the ventral mesentery. The end of the hepatic bud now divides into right and left branches, from which columns of entodermal cells grow out into the vascu-

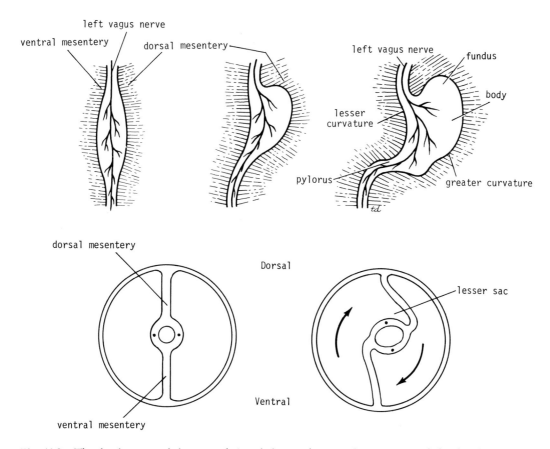

Fig. 11-2. The development of the stomach in relation to the ventral mesentery and the dorsal mesentery.

lar mesoderm. The columns of cells continue to grow and branch and anastomose with one another. The paired vitelline veins and umbilical veins that course through the septum transverum become broken up by the invading columns of liver cells to form the *liver sinusoids* (Fig. 8-6). It is thus seen that the columns of entodermal cells form the *liver cords* or parenchymatous tissue of the liver; the liver sinusoids are formed from parts of the vitelline and umbilical veins; and the fibrous capsule of the liver and the connective tissue are formed from the mesoderm of the septum transversum. Some of the cells forming the lining of the sinusoids become differentiated into large macrophages, the *Kupffer cells.* Collections of proliferating

mesenchymal cells which have a hematopoietic function are seen between the liver cells and the blood sinusoids. The newly formed erythrocytes and leukocytes enter the circulation by passing through the wall of the sinusoids.

The main hepatic bud and its right and left terminal branches now become canalized to form the *common hepatic duct* and the *right* and *left hepatic ducts.* Further canalization of the columns of cells within the liver takes place so that the duct system eventually joins the *bile capillaries.* The liver cells start to secrete bile during the fifth month of development.

The liver continues to grow rapidly in size and comes to occupy the greater part of the

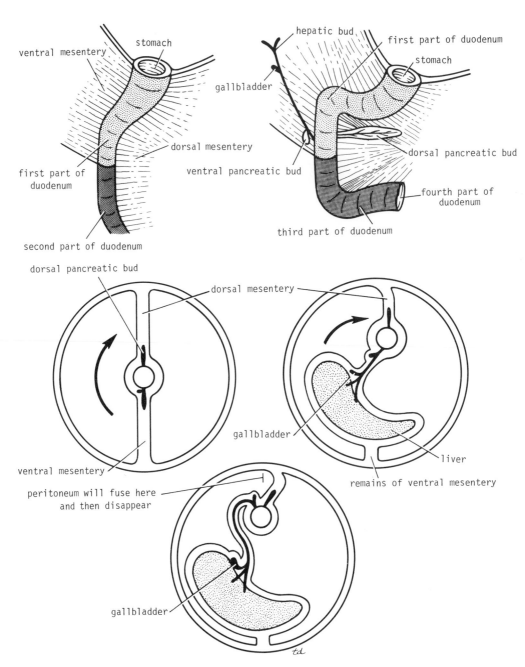

Fig. 11-3. The development of the duodenum in relation to the ventral mesentery and the dorsal mesentery. The stippled area is foregut and the crosshatched area is midgut.

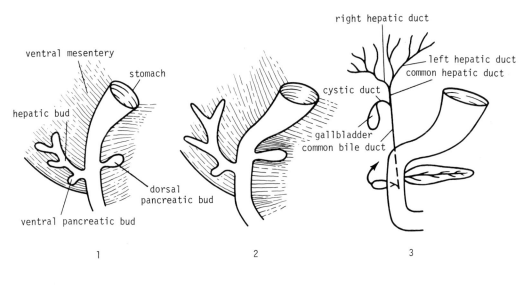

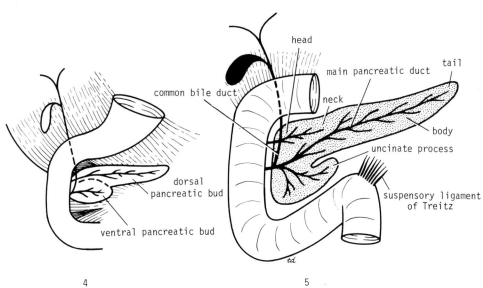

Fig. 11-4. The development of the pancreas and the extra-hepatic biliary apparatus.

abdominal cavity. In the early stage, the *right and left lobes* that correspond to the right and left branches of the hepatic bud are of equal size. Later the right lobe becomes much larger than the left lobe. The *caudate* and *quadrate lobes* develop as subdivisions of the left lobe. The development of the ligaments of the liver is discussed on page 188.

The Gallbladder and Cystic Duct

The gallbladder develops as a solid outgrowth of cells from the hepatic bud. The end of the outgrowth expands to form the *gallbladder,* while the narrow stem remains as the *cystic duct.* Later the gallbladder and cystic duct become canalized. The cystic duct now opens into the *common hepatic duct* to form the *common bile duct.*

The Pancreas

The pancreas develops from a *dorsal* and *ventral bud* of entodermal cells that arise from the foregut. The dorsal bud originates a short distance above the ventral bud and grows into the dorsal mesentery. The ventral bud arises in common with the hepatic bud close to the junction of the foregut with the midgut (Fig. 11-4). A canalized duct system now develops in each bud. The rotation of the stomach and duodenum, together with the rapid growth of the left side of the duodenum, results in the ventral bud's coming into contact with the dorsal bud, and fusion occurs (Fig. 11-5). Fusion also occurs between the ducts so that the *main pancreatic duct* is derived from the entire ventral pancreatic duct and the distal part of the dorsal pancreatic duct. The main pancreatic duct joins the common bile duct and enters the second part of the duodenum. The proximal part of the dorsal pancreatic duct may persist as an *accessory duct* that may or may not open into the duodenum about 2 cm above the opening of the main duct.

With the continued growth, the entodermal cells of the now-fused ventral and dorsal pancreatic buds extend into the surrounding mesenchyme as columns of cells. These columns give off side branches which later become canalized to form collecting ducts.

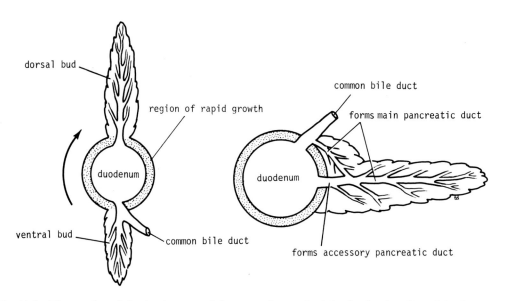

Fig. 11-5. The rotation of the duodenum and the unequal growth of the duodenal wall result in the ventral and dorsal pancreatic buds fusing together.

Secretory acini appear at the ends of the ducts.

The *pancreatic islets* arise as small buds from the developing ducts. Later these cells sever their connection with the duct system and form isolated groups of cells that start to secrete *insulin* and *glucagon* at about the fifth month (see Chap. 18).

The inferior part of the head and the uncinate process of the pancreas are formed from the ventral pancreatic bud; the superior part of the head, the neck, the body, and the tail of the pancreas are formed from the dorsal pancreatic bud (Fig. 11-4).

Entrance of Common Bile Duct and Pancreatic Duct Into the Duodenum

As would be expected from the development of these ducts, the common bile duct and the main pancreatic ducts join one another and pass obliquely through the wall of the second part of the duodenum to open on the summit of the *duodenal papilla,* which is surrounded by the *sphincter of Oddi* (Fig. 11-6). In about one-third of individuals, they pass separately through the duodenal wall, although in close contact, and open separately on the summit of the duodenal papilla. In a small number of individuals, the two ducts join and form a common dilatation, the *ampulla of Vater.* This opens on the summit of the duodenal papilla.

CONGENITAL ANOMALIES

Esophagus

Congenital Atresia of the Esophagus

Atresia with or without fistula with the trachea is considered in detail on page 179. When associated with a fistula, in the major-

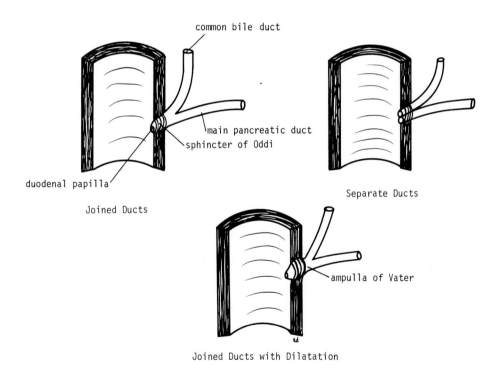

Fig. 11-6. The different ways in which the common bile duct and the main pancreatic duct open into the duodenum.

ity of cases the lower segment of the esophagus communicates with the trachea.

Esophageal Stenosis

This is a narrowing of the lumen of the esophagus and commonly occurs at the same site as atresia. It is treated by dilatation.

Congenital Short Esophagus

This condition is caused by esophageal hiatus hernia in the diaphragm. See page 198. Stomach contents flow into the esophagus, which results in esophagitis. If untreated, it results in fibrosis and shortening of the esophagus.

Esophageal Compression by an Abnormal Artery

Rarely, the right subclavian artery arises from the arch of the aorta and passes in front of or behind the esophagus, causing obstruction.

Stomach

Congenital Hypertrophic Pyloric Stenosis

This condition is a relatively common surgical emergency and presents itself between the ages of 3 and 6 weeks. The child ejects the stomach contents with considerable force called *projectile vomiting*. This is accompanied by constipation and loss of weight. There is marked hypertrophy and hyperplasia of the pyloric muscle affecting mainly the circular muscle (Fig. 11-7), which results in considerable narrowing of the pyloric canal, the mucous membrane of which is thrown into longitudinal folds.

Hereditary factors play an important part in this condition and it is three or four times more common in boys than in girls. The exact cause of pyloric stenosis is unknown, although recent research has shown that the autonomic ganglion cells in this region are fewer in number than normal. It is possible that prenatal neuromuscular incoordination produces localized muscular hypertrophy.

Mild cases of pyloric stenosis may be treated by dietetic methods and the administration of antispasmodics. The more severe cases are treated surgically by making a longitudinal incision through the hypertrophied muscle fibers.

Duodenum

Atresia and Stenosis

During the development of the duodenum, the lining cells proliferate at such a rate that the lumen becomes completely obliterated. Later, as a result of vacuolation and degeneration of these cells, the gut becomes recanalized. Failure of recanalization could produce atresia or stenosis. Atresia is the most common defect, and obstruction usually occurs in the region of the entrance of the

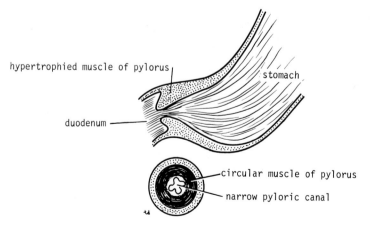

Fig. 11-7. Congenital hypertrophic pyloric stenosis. Enormous hypertrophy of the muscle in the region of the pylorus and its abrupt termination at the gastroduodenal junction are shown.

hypertrophied muscle of pylorus

stomach

duodenum

circular muscle of pylorus

narrow pyloric canal

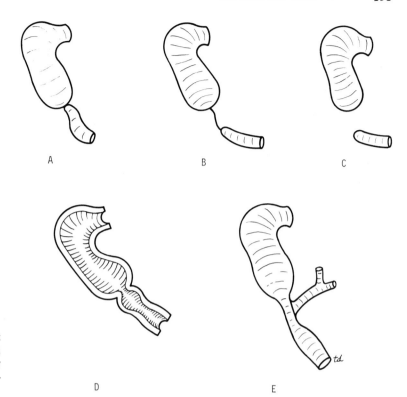

Fig. 11-8. The different types of duodenal atresia; it occurs most commonly at the junction of the foregut and midgut.

common bile and pancreatic ducts, although it may occur at any level in the duodenum. Figure 11-8 shows the different forms of duodenal atresia and stenosis. These conditions are often associated with other malformations, especially mongolism.

Vomiting is the most common presenting symptom, and the vomitus is usually bile-stained. Surgical treatment during the first few days of life is essential.

Duplication of the Duodenum

The embryological factors involved in the formation of duplications of the alimentary tract are considered in Chapter 12.

Pancreas

Annular Pancreas

It is generally believed that in this condition the ventral pancreatic bud becomes fixed so that, when the stomach and duodenum rotate, the ventral bud is pulled around the right side of the duodenum to fuse with the dorsal bud of the pancreas, thus encircling the duodenum (Fig. 11-9). In this manner, the duodenum may be obstructed, and vomiting usually starts a few hours after birth. Early surgical relief of the obstruction is necessary.

Ectopic Pancreas

This may be found in the submucosa of the stomach, duodenum, or small intestine (including Meckel's diverticulum) and gallbladder, and in the spleen. Its importance lies in the fact that it may protrude into the lumen of the gut and be responsible for causing intussusception (Fig. 11-10).

Congenital Fibrocystic Disease

Basically this condition in the pancreas is caused by an abnormality in the secretion of mucus. The mucus produced is excessively

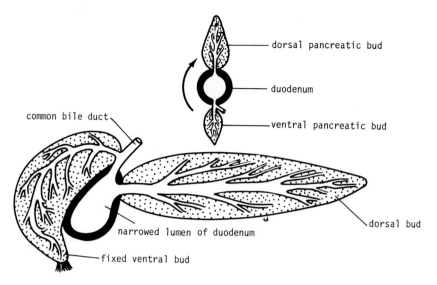

Fig. 11-9. The formation of annular pancreas producing duodenal obstruction.

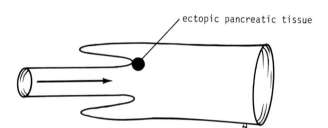

Fig. 11-10. An ectopic piece of pancreas causing an intussusception.

viscid and obstructs the pancreatic ducts, which leads to pancreatitis with subsequent fibrosis. The condition also involves the lungs, the kidneys, and the liver.

Bile Passages

Biliary Atresia

This is thought to be a result of a failure of the bile ducts to canalize during development. The various forms that occur are shown in Fig. 11-11. Jaundice appears soon after birth; clay-colored stools and very dark-colored urine are also present. Surgical cor-

rection of the atresia should be attempted where possible. Where the atresia cannot be corrected, the child will ultimately die of liver failure.

Absence of the Gallbladder

Occasionally the outgrowth of cells from the hepatic bud fails to develop. In these cases there is no gallbladder and no cystic duct (Fig. 11-12).

Double Gallbladder

Rarely the outgrowth of cells from the hepatic bud bifurcates so that two gallbladders are formed (Fig. 11-12).

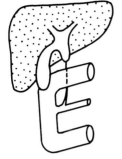

Atresia of common bile duct

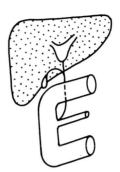

Atresia of common hepatic duct

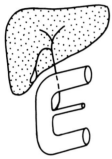

Atresia of entire extra-hepatic apparatus

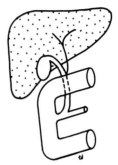

Atresia of hepatic ducts

Fig. 11-11. The different forms of biliary atresia.

Absence of the Cystic Duct

In this condition the gallbladder drains directly into the common bile duct. The entire outgrowth of cells from the hepatic bud has developed into the gallbladder and has failed to leave the narrow stem that would normally form the cystic duct. The condition may not be recognized when performing a cholecystectomy, and the common bile duct may be seriously damaged by the surgeon (Fig. 11-12).

Abnormally Long Cystic Duct

The cystic duct may open into the common bile duct near its entrance into the duodenum. A portion of the duct may be left behind following cholecystectomy (Fig. 11-12).

Accessory Bile Duct

A small bile duct may open directly from the liver into the gallbladder, which may cause leakage of bile into the peritoneal cavity following cholecystectomy if not recognized at operation (Fig. 11-12).

Congenital Choledochal Cyst

This is a rare condition caused by an area of weakness in the wall of the common bile duct. The cyst may contain as much as 1 to 2 liters of bile. Its importance lies in the fact that it may press on the common bile duct and cause obstructive jaundice (Fig. 11-12).

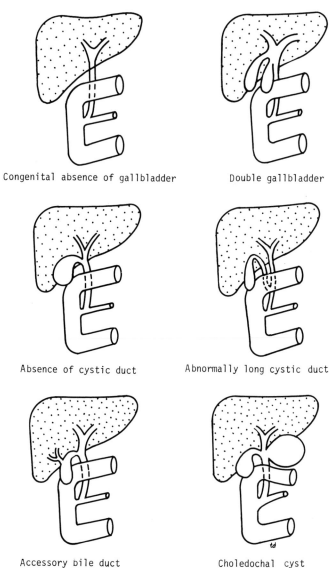

Congenital absence of gallbladder

Double gallbladder

Absence of cystic duct

Abnormally long cystic duct

Accessory bile duct

Choledochal cyst

Fig. 11-12. Some congenital anomalies of the gallbladder and biliary ducts.

Clinical Problems

Answers on page 441

1. A mother took her 20-day-old baby boy to a pediatrician because he had started to vomit after his feeds. The baby was breast-fed. On careful questioning, the mother said that for the first 15 days after birth the baby had taken his feeds very well and had slept contentedly in his crib following the normal after-feed burp. However, in the previous 5 days the baby had begun to feed hungrily and then, toward the end of

each feed, would vomit violently, shooting the milk out of his mouth for a distance of 1 to 2 feet. On several occasions the feed was completed, only to be followed in a few minutes by the same type of projectile vomiting. Once the milk had been vomited, the child would immediately feed again, only to repeat the same performance. On examination, the baby was noted to be restless, with dry skin and a depressed anterior fontanelle. On gentle palpation of the anterior abdominal wall a small, firm swelling could be felt just below and medial to the tip of the right ninth costal cartilage. On observation of the anterior abdominal wall in a good light, an occasional wave of gastric peristalsis could be seen traveling across the epigastrium from left to right. What is your diagnosis? How would you treat this infant? What is now believed to be the underlying cause of this condition?

2. A pediatric resident was called to the intensive care unit to examine a day-old baby girl. The nurse in charge of the case said that the infant had repeatedly vomited her food since birth. The vomiting was projectile in nature and the vomit was bile-stained. Only a small amount of pale-yellow meconium had been passed since birth. On examination the baby was found to be dehydrated, with dry skin, dry tongue, and a depressed anterior fontanelle. On palpation of the anterior abdominal wall, no swelling could be detected in the epigastrium or below the right costal margin. However, visible gastric peristalsis could be seen through the abdominal wall if the baby was given a bottle of glucose water to suck on. An anteroposterior x-ray film of the abdomen revealed no air in the gut. What is the most likely diagnosis? How would you treat this child? What is your embryological explanation for the condition?

3. A 20-year-old male with mongolism (Down's syndrome) was operated on for acute intestinal obstruction. At laparotomy a ring of tissue was found to encircle the second part of the duodenum. Can you explain the presence of this ring of tissue embryologically? How would you treat this patient?

4. A 3-month-old baby boy was examined by a pediatrician because he was jaundiced. The mother said that the jaundice had been present at birth, but since that time had become progressively deeper in color. The baby's stools were pale yellow in color and were of a putty-like consistency. On examination the child was found to be severely jaundiced and to have an enlarged liver and spleen. What is the diagnosis? Using your knowledge of embryology, can you explain the condition? How can you explain the color of the stools? Why are the liver and spleen enlarged? How would you treat this infant?

REFERENCES

Ahrens, E. H., Harris, R. C., and MacMahan, M. E. Atresia of the Intrahepatic Bile Ducts. *Pediatrics* 8:628, 1951.

Aitken, J. Congenital Intrinsic Duodenal Obstruction in Infancy. *J. Pediat. Surg.* 1:546, 1966.

Barbosa, J., Dockerty, M. B., and Waugh, J. Pancreatic Heterotopia. *Surg. Gynec. Obstet.* 82:527, 1946.

Boyden, E. A. The Problem of the Pancreatic Bladder. *Amer. J. Anat.* 36:151, 1925.

Burmeister, R. E., and Stanley-Brown, E. G. Congenital Hypertrophic Pyloric Stenosis. *Surg. Gynec. Obstet.* 115:405, 1962.

Cameron, R., and Bunton, G. L. Congenital Biliary Atresia. *Brit. Med. J.* 2:528, 1960.

Cozzi, F., and Wilkinson, A. W. Oesophageal Atresia. *Lancet* 2:1222, 1967.

Dawson, W., and Langman, J. An Anatomical-Radiological Study on the Pancreatic Duct Pattern in Man. *Anat. Rec.* 139:59, 1961.

Dennison, W. M. *Surgery in Infancy and Childhood,* 2d ed. Livingstone, Edinburgh, 1967.

Gross, R. E., and Chisholm, J. C. Annular Pancreas Producing Duodenal Obstruction. *Ann. Surg.* 119:759, 1944.

Haas, L., and Sturridge, M. F. Congenital Tracheo-Oesophageal Fistula. *Proc. Roy. Soc. Med.* 54: 329, 1961.

Houle, M. P., and Hill, P. S. Congenital Absence of the Gallbladder. *J. Maine Med. Ass.* 51:108, 1960.

Jacoby, N. M. Pyloric Stenosis. *Lancet* 1:119, 1962.

Kiesewetter, W. B., and Koop, C. E. Annular Pancreas in Infancy. *Surgery* 36:145, 1954.

Ladd, W. E. Congenital Obstruction of the Duodenum in Children. *New Eng. J. Med.* 206: 277, 1932.

Langman, J. Oesophageal Atresia Accompanied by a Remarkable Vessel Anomaly. *Arch. Chir. Neerl.* 4:39, 1952.

Lee, E. T. C., and Rickham, P. P. Neonatal Jaundice. *Clin. Pediat.* (Phila.) 3:197, 1964.

Lister, J. The Blood Supply of the Oesophagus in Relation to Oesophageal Atresia. *Arch. Dis. Child.* 39:131, 1964.

McKeown, T. Infantile Hypertrophic Pyloric Stenosis. *Proc. Roy. Soc. Med.* 54:453, 1961.

Myers, R. L., Baggenstoss, A. F., Logan, G. B., and

Hallenbeck, G. A. Congenital Extrahepatic Atresia of Extrahepatic Biliary Tract. *Pediatrics* 18:767, 1956.

Popper, H., and Shaffner, F. *Liver: Structure and Function.* McGraw-Hill, New York, 1957.

Rains, A. J. H., and Capper, W. M. *Bailey and Love's Short Practice of Surgery,* 14th ed. Lippincott, Philadelphia, 1968.

Rickham, P. P., and Johnston, J. H. *Neonatal Surgery.* Butterworth, London, 1969.

Rintoul, J. R., and Kirkman, N. F. The Myenteric Plexus in Infantile Pyloric Stenosis. *Arch. Dis. Child.* 36:474, 1961.

Salebury, A. M., and Collins, R. E. Congenital Pyloric Atresia. *A.M.A. Arch. Surg.* 80:501, 1960.

Saunders, J. B., and Lindner, H. H. Congenital Anomalies of the Duodenum. *Ann. Surg.* 112: 321, 1940.

Sterling, J. A. *Experiences with Congenital Biliary Atresia.* Thomas, Springfield, Ill., 1960.

Weatherill, D., Forgrave, E. G., and Carpenter, W. S. Annular Pancreas Producing Duodenal Obstruction in the Newborn. *A.M.A. Amer. J. Dis. Child.* 95:202, 1958.

Wilkinson, A. W., Hughes, E. A., and Stevens, C. H. Neonatal Duodenal Obstruction. *Brit. J. Surg.* 52:410, 1965.

DEVELOPMENT

The Jejunum, Ileum, Cecum, Appendix, Ascending Colon, and Proximal Two-Thirds of the Transverse Colon

In Chapter 11 the distal half of the duodenum was shown to be developed from the midgut. The succeeding part of the small bowel and the large bowel as far as the distal one-third of the transverse colon also develop from the midgut. The midgut increases rapidly in length and forms a loop to the apex of which is attached the *vitelline duct,* the latter passing through the widely open umbilicus (Fig. 12-1). At the same time the dorsal mesentery elongates, and passing through it from the aorta to the yolk sac are the *vitelline arteries.* These arteries now fuse to form the *superior mesenteric artery,* which supplies the midgut and its derivatives.

At this time the rapidly growing liver and the enlargement of the developing kidneys so encroach on the abdominal cavity that the intestinal loop is forced out of the abdominal cavity through the umbilicus into the remains of the extra-embryonic coelom in the umbilical cord. This physiological herniation of the midgut takes place during the sixth week of development.

Just before the herniation occurs, a diverticulum appears at the caudal end of the bowel loop, and this is the beginning of the formation of the cecum. At first the diverticulum is conical; later the upper part expands and forms the *cecum,* while the lower part remains rudimentary and forms the *appendix* (Fig. 12-2). After birth the wall of the cecum grows unequally and the appendix comes to lie on its medial side.

While the loop of gut is in the umbilical cord, its cephalic limb becomes greatly elongated and coiled and forms the future jejunum and greater part of the ileum. The caudal limb of the loop also increases in length, but it remains uncoiled and forms the future distal part of the ileum, the cecum and the appendix, the ascending colon, and the proximal two-thirds of the transverse colon.

Rotation of the Midgut Loop in the Umbilical Cord

While in the extra-embryonic coelom in the umbilical cord, the midgut loop rotates around an axis formed by the superior

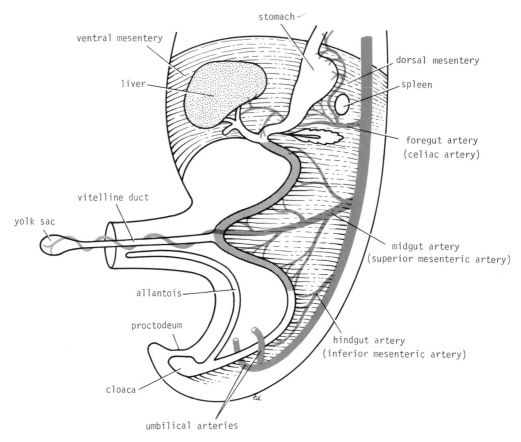

Fig. 12-1. The formation of the midgut loop (*hatched*), showing how the superior mesenteric artery and vitelline duct form an axis for the future rotation of the midgut loop.

mesenteric artery and the vitelline duct. As one views the embryo from the anterior aspect, a counterclockwise rotation occurs of approximately 90 degrees (Fig. 12-3).

Return of the Midgut to the Abdominal Cavity and Further Rotation of the Loop

During the third month, the abdominal cavity is large enough to hold the whole bowel and the midgut loop is rapidly withdrawn into the abdomen. The cephalic limb of the loop returns first, possibly because the cecum impedes the return of the caudal limb. The jejunum is the first part of the gut to reenter

the abdominal cavity, and it comes to lie high up on the left side. Succeeding loops of the ileum then return gradually, filling the left side of the abdomen. The caudal limb of the loop finally returns, and it comes to lie superiorly and ventral to the cephalic loop derivatives. During this process of return to the abdominal cavity, the midgut loop rotates counterclockwise a further 180 degrees as seen from the anterior aspect of the embryo (Fig. 12-4). Thus the loop rotates through a total of 270 degrees counterclockwise. In this manner, the cecum and appendix come into close contact with the right lobe of the liver. Later the cecum and appendix descend into

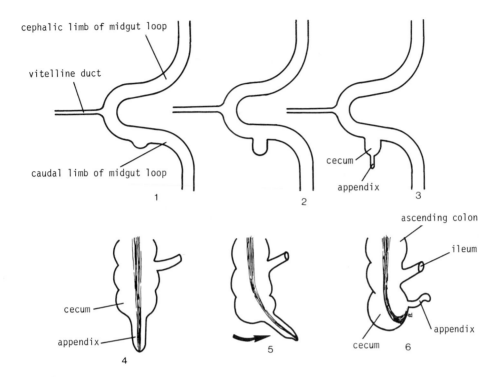

cephalic limb of midgut loop

vitelline duct

caudal limb of midgut loop

cecum

appendix

1   2   3

ascending colon

ileum

cecum

appendix

cecum

appendix

4   5   6

Fig. 12-2. The different stages in the development of the cecum and appendix. The final stages of development (stages 4, 5, and 6) take place after birth.

the right iliac fossa so that the *ascending colon* and *hepatic flexure* of the colon are formed (Fig. 12-4).

The Final Position of the Gut and Its Relation to the Peritoneum

During the rotation of the stomach and duodenum, the duodenal loop moves to the right and comes into contact with the posterior abdominal wall. The dorsal mesentery of the duodenum now fuses with the peritoneum on the posterior abdominal wall, and the peritoneum covering the posterior surface of the duodenum largely disappears (Fig. 12-5). Most of the duodenum thus becomes retroperitoneal. The duodenojejunal flexure is drawn superiorly and to the left and fixed to the posterior abdominal wall by the *suspensory ligament of Treitz.*

The dorsal mesentery from the duodenojejunal flexure to the ileocecal junction remains as the *mesentery of the small intestine.* Following the descent of the cecum into the right iliac fossa, the cecum remains surrounded by peritoneum. However, when the ascending colon comes into contact with the posterior abdominal wall, the dorsal mesentery in this region fuses with the peritoneum covering the posterior abdominal wall and the peritoneum posterior to the ascending colon disappears. In this way, the ascending colon becomes retroperitoneal. The dorsal mesentery of the transverse colon remains as the *transverse mesocolon,* but its attachment to the posterior abdominal wall changes so that it no longer remains as a longitudinal midline structure but becomes transversely oriented and is attached to the anterior surface of the pancreas.

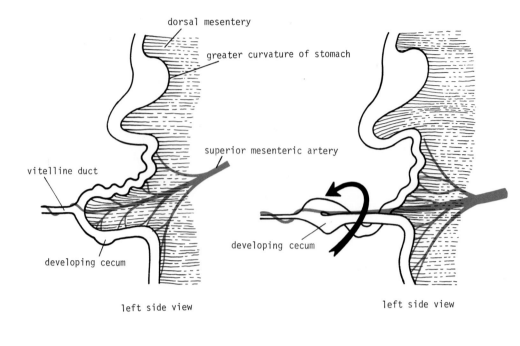

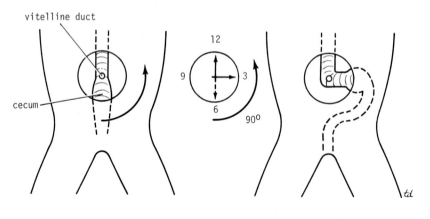

Fig. 12-3. Counterclockwise 90-degree rotation of midgut loop while it is in the extra-embryonic coelom in the umbilical cord.

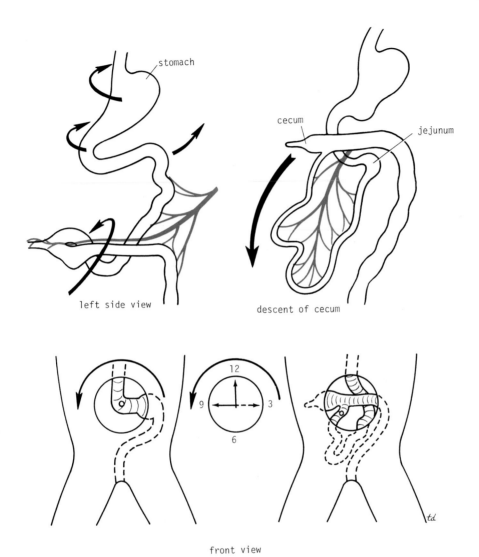

Fig. 12-4. Counterclockwise 180-degree rotation of midgut loop as it is withdrawn into the abdominal cavity. The descent of the cecum takes place later.

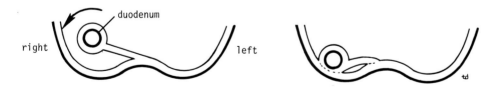

Fig. 12-5. How the dorsal mesentery of the duodenum comes to fuse with the peritoneum on the posterior abdominal wall. The peritoneum behind the duodenum disappears so that the duodenum becomes retroperitoneal.

The Fate of the Vitelline Duct

The midgut is at first connected with the yolk sac by the vitelline duct. When the midgut loop lies within the extra-embryonic coelom in the umbilical cord, the duct becomes greatly narrowed and the yolk sac much smaller. By the time the gut returns to the abdominal cavity, the vitelline duct is normally obliterated and severs its connection with the gut.

Development of the Left Colic Flexure, Descending Colon, Pelvic Colon, Rectum, and the Upper Half of the Anal Canal

These structures are developed from the hindgut. Distally this terminates as a blind

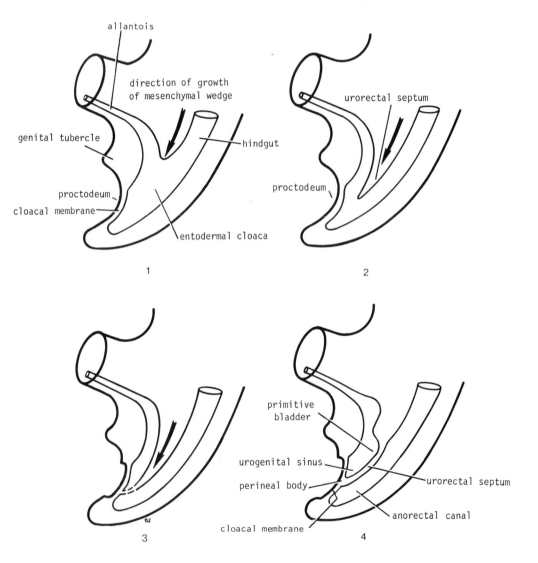

Fig. 12-6. The formation of the urorectal septum which divides the cloaca into an anterior part, the primitive bladder and the urogenital sinus, and a posterior part, the anorectal canal. The numbers indicate the progressive stages in development.

sac of entoderm which is in contact with a shallow ectodermal depression called the *proctodeum.* The apposed layers of ectoderm and entoderm form the *cloacal membrane,* which separates the cavity of the hindgut from the surface (Fig. 12-6). It has already been pointed out that the hindgut sends off a diverticulum called the *allantois,* which passes into the umbilical cord. Distal to the allantois, the hindgut dilates to form the *entodermal cloaca* (Fig. 12-6). In the interval between the allantois and the hindgut, a wedge of mesenchyme invaginates the entoderm. With continued proliferation of the mesenchyme, a septum is formed that grows inferiorly and divides the cloaca into anterior and posterior parts. The septum is called the *urorectal septum,* the anterior part of the cloaca becomes the *primitive bladder* and the *urogenital sinus,* and the posterior part of the cloaca forms the *anorectal canal.* On reaching

the cloacal membrane, the urorectal septum fuses with it and forms the future *perineal body* (Fig. 12-6).

The fate of the primitive bladder and of the urogenital sinus in both sexes is considered in detail in Chapters 15 and 16.

The anorectal canal forms the rectum and the superior half of the anal canal. The lining of the inferior half of the anal canal is formed from the ectoderm of the proctodeum (Fig. 12-7). The posterior part of the cloacal membrane soon breaks down so that the gut opens onto the surface of the embryo.

Blood Supply to the Derivatives of the Foregut, Midgut, and Hindgut

Foregut Arteries

The cephalic end of the foregut, which includes the pharynx, and the cervical and thoracic portions of the esophagus are sup-

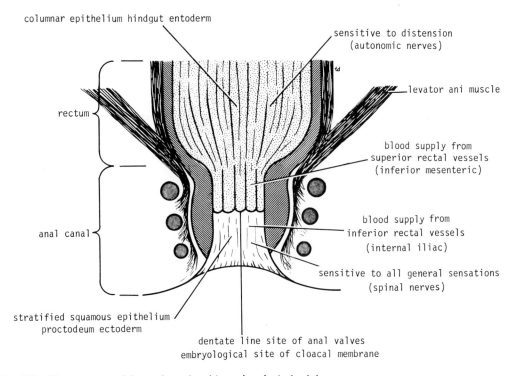

Fig. 12-7.   The structure of the anal canal and its embryological origin.

plied by the *ascending pharyngeal arteries, palantine arteries, superior and inferior thyroid arteries, bronchial arteries,* and the *esophageal branches from the aorta.* This extensive blood supply is acquired when the foregut greatly elongates into the developing neck. The caudal end of the foregut, which includes the distal third of the esophagus, the stomach, and the proximal half of the duodenum, is supplied by a number of vessels that fuse to form a single trunk, the *celiac artery* (Fig. 12-1). It is interesting to note that this artery also supplies the liver and pancreas, which are glandular derivatives of this part of the gut. The spleen is supplied by the same artery, and this is not surprising since this organ develops in the dorsal mesentery of the foregut; the artery to the spleen runs in the lienorenal ligament.

Midgut Artery

The midgut, which extends from halfway along the second part of the duodenum to the left colic flexure, is supplied by the *superior mesenteric artery,* which represents the fused pair of vitelline arteries (Fig. 12-1).

Hindgut Artery

The hindgut, which extends from the left colic flexure to halfway down the anal canal, is supplied by the *inferior mesenteric artery* (Fig. 12-1). This represents a number of ventral branches of the aorta which fuse to form a single artery.

Meconium

At full term, the large intestine is filled with a mixture of intestinal gland secretions, bile, and amniotic fluid. This substance is dark green in color and is called *meconium.* It starts to accumulate at 4 months and reaches the rectum at the fifth month.

CONGENITAL ANOMALIES

Diverticula of the Intestine

All coats of the bowel are found in the wall of a congenital diverticulum. In the duodenum, they are found on the medial wall of the second and third parts (Fig. 12-8). Usually they are symptomless. Jejunal diverticula occasionally occur and usually give rise to no symptoms. Meckel's diverticulum of the ileum is considered under congenital anomalies of the vitelline duct, below. Diverticulum of the cecum is commonly situated on the medial side of the cecum close to the ileocecal valve. It may be subject to acute inflammation and is then confused with appendicitis. Diverticula of the colon are acquired and not congenital.

Atresia and Stenosis of the Intestine

The commonest site of the obstruction is in the duodenum (see p. 150). The next most common site is the ileum and then the

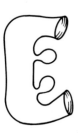

duodenum

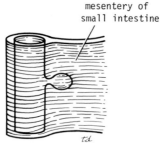

mesentery of small intestine

jejunum

Fig. 12-8. Congenital diverticula of the duodenum and jejunum. Those of the jejunum occur on the mesenteric border.

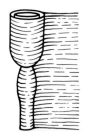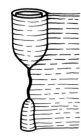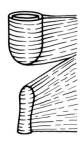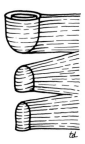

Fig. 12-9. Different types of atresia and stenosis of the small intestine.

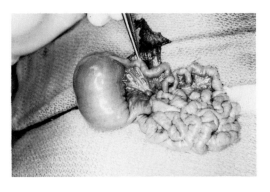

Fig. 12-10. Atresia of the jejunum. (Courtesy of Dr. J. Randolph.)

jejunum (Figs. 12-9 & 12-10). Frequently the obstruction occurs at multiple sites. For many years the explanation given as to its origin was a failure of the lumen to become recanalized after epithelial proliferation of the cells of the mucous membrane had completely blocked the lumen. While this may be the cause in some cases, it is now generally believed that atresia and stenosis occurring below the duodenum are caused by damage to the bowel during intrauterine life. Such damage may be caused by peritonitis followed by adhesions; it may also be caused by strangulation and vascular damage following twisting or volvulus of the intestine. Persistent bile-stained vomiting occurs from birth. Surgical relief of the obstruction should be carried out as soon as possible.

Duplication of the Digestive System

This may occur anywhere from the mouth to the anus and may be spherical or tubular in shape (Fig. 12-11). Duplication may occur when excessive proliferation of the mucous membrane cells takes place during development. Normally vacuolation and degeneration of these cells occur, and a single lumen is established. It is possible that degeneration of these central cells could occur at two sites simultaneously, so that two lumina are formed instead of one. The additional segment of bowel should be removed as soon as possible, since it may cause obstruction or be the site of hemorrhage or perforation.

Arrested Rotation of the Midgut Loop

Complete Absence of Rotation

This condition is rare. *Incomplete rotation* means no further rotation occurs after the initial counterclockwise rotation of 90 degrees in the umbilical cord. In these cases the duodenum, jejunum, and ileum remain on the right side of the abdomen, and the cecum and colon are on the left side of the abdomen (Fig. 12-12). In other cases, a counterclockwise rotation of 180 degrees occurs, and although the duodenum may take up its correct position posterior to the superior mesenteric artery, the cecum comes to lie anterior and to the left of the duodenum. Abnormal adhesions form which run across the anterior surface of the duodenum and cause obstruction to its second part.

Malrotation of the Midgut Loop

Counterclockwise rotation of 90 degrees, followed by clockwise rotation of 90 or 180 degrees, may occur. In these cases, the duo-

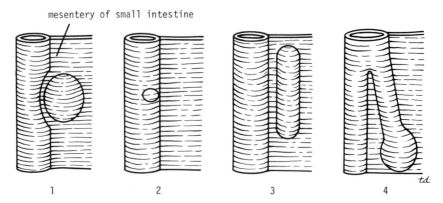

mesentery of small intestine

1   2   3   4

Fig. 12-11. Examples of duplications of the jejunum and ileum. Types 1 & 2 are in the form of cysts and types 3 & 4 are tubular. Only in type 4 does the lumen of the tube communicate with the gut; in these cases, the distal end becomes greatly dilated.

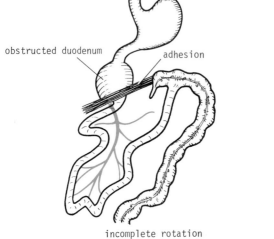

obstructed duodenum   adhesion

incomplete rotation

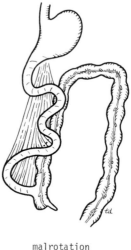

malrotation

Fig. 12-12. Two forms of anomalous rotation of the gut.

denum comes to lie anterior to the superior mesenteric artery, and the colon may come to lie anterior to the mesentery of the small intestines (Fig. 12-12).

In the majority of cases, repeated vomiting, which is usually caused by duodenal obstruction, is the presenting symptom. Surgical correction of the incomplete rotation or malrotation of the gut is performed, and all adhesions are divided.

The Vitelline Duct (Vitello-Intestinal Duct)

This may persist and give rise to one of the following conditions (Fig. 12-13):

1. FISTULA. In this condition, the terminal part of the ileum communicates with the abdominal wall skin at the umbilicus (Figs. 12-14 & 12-15). The fistula may discharge mucus or feces.

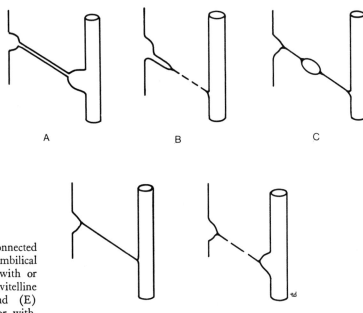

Fig. 12-13. The anomalies connected with the vitelline duct: (A) umbilical fistula, (B) umbilical sinus (with or without a fibrous band), (C) vitelline cyst, (D) fibrous band, and (E) Meckel's diverticulum (with or without a fibrous band).

2. SINUS. A small portion of the duct may remain and open onto the skin at the umbilicus. The sinus may discharge mucus.

3. CYST. Both ends of the duct may close, leaving an intermediate portion patent. The mucous membrane will produce mucus which will accumulate in the intermediate segment and form a cyst.

4. FIBROUS BAND. The entire lumen of the duct may become obliterated, but the duct fails to degenerate and persists as a fibrous band that extends from the ileum to the umbilicus. A coil of bowel may become twisted around the band and cause intestinal obstruction.

5. MECKEL'S DIVERTICULUM. This is caused by a persistence of a short length of the vitelline duct that remains attached to the antimesenteric border of the ileum (Fig. 12-16). It occurs in about 2 percent of people, about 2 feet from the ileocecal valve, and may be as much as 2 inches long. In 20 percent there is present ectopic gastric mucosa or pancreatic tissue. The diverticulum may become in-

fected, cause intussusception, or may be the site of peptic ulcer. If connected to the umbilicus by a fibrous band which is a remnant of a further portion of the vitelline duct, it may cause obstruction of the bowel (see above). Anomalies of the vitelline duct should be treated surgically if they are causing symptoms.

Meconium Ileus

This is a manifestation of fibrocystic disease of the pancreas. During the later months of fetal life, the ileum becomes filled with viscid mucus mixed with meconium, which causes intestinal obstruction. The ileal loop containing the material is opened surgically and the contents removed.

Undescended Cecum and Appendix

An inflammation of the appendix would give rise to tenderness in the right hypochondrium, which may lead to a mistaken diag-

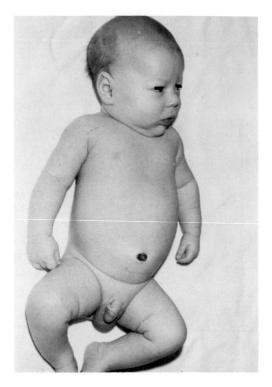

Fig. 12-14. Persistent vitelline duct in 3-month-old infant. (Courtesy of Dr. H. Miller.)

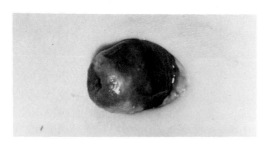

Fig. 12-15. Umbilical region of infant in Figure 12-14. Shows opening of fistula of persistent vitelline duct. (Courtesy of Dr. H. Miller.)

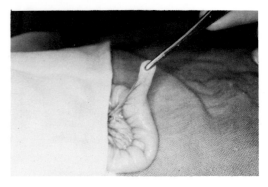

Fig. 12-16. Meckel's diverticulum. (Courtesy of Dr. J. Randolph.)

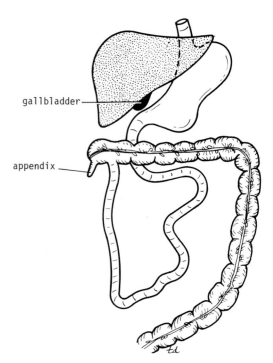

Fig. 12-17. Undescended cecum and appendix, showing the close relation of the appendix to the gallbladder.

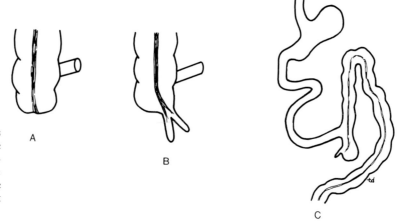

Fig. 12-18. (A) Agenesis of appendix, (B) double appendix, and (C) appendix in the left iliac fossa resulting from the nonrotation of the midgut loop.

nosis of inflammation of the gallbladder (Fig. 12-17).

Anomalies of the Appendix

Agenesis, or failure of the appendix to develop, is extremely rare; however, a few examples of *double appendix* have been reported (Fig. 12-18). The possibility of *left-sided appendix* in individuals with transposition of thoracic and abdominal viscera or in

cases of arrested rotation of the midgut should always be remembered.

Primary Megacolon (Hirschsprung's Disease)

This disease shows a familial tendency and is more common in males than in females. Symptoms usually appear during the first few days after birth. The child fails to pass meconium and the abdomen becomes enor-

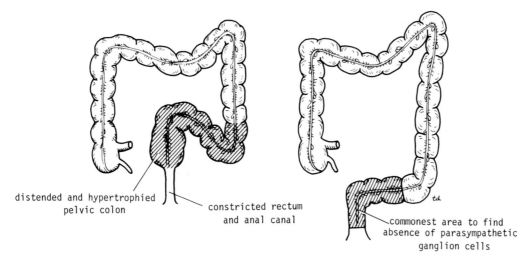

distended and hypertrophied pelvic colon

constricted rectum and anal canal

commonest area to find absence of parasympathetic ganglion cells

Fig. 12-19. Hirschsprung's disease.

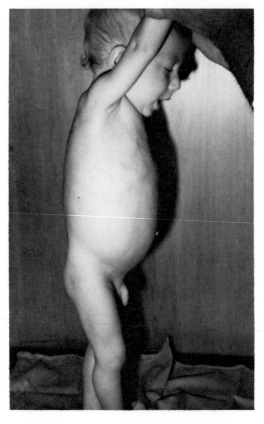

Fig. 12-20. A case of Hirschsprung's disease. (Courtesy of Dr. J. Randolph.)

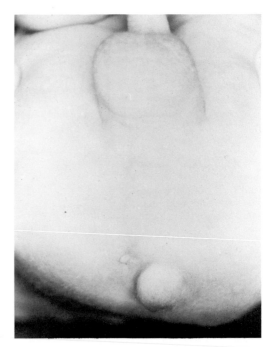

Fig. 12-21. Imperforate anus. In this case the proctodeum failed to develop. (Courtesy of Dr. G. Avery.)

mously distended. The pelvic colon is greatly distended and hypertrophied, while the rectum and anal canal are constricted (Figs. 12-19 & 12-20). It is the constricted segment of the bowel that causes the obstruction, and histological examination reveals a complete failure of development of the parasympathetic ganglion cells in this region. The treatment is operative excision of the aganglionic segment of the bowel.

Anorectal Anomalies

About 1 child in 4,000 is born with *imperforate anus* (Fig. 12-21), or imperfect fusion of the entodermal cloaca with the proctodeum. The condition may be divided into two main types, the low and the high (Figs. 12-22 & 12-23).

Low Anomalies

1. THE COVERED ANUS. The anus is absent. The anal canal communicates with the surface and opens onto the skin in the midline at any point between the prepuce and the perineal body. This condition is probably caused by the genital swellings (see p. 228) extending posteriorly and fusing in the midline to cover the proctodeum.

2. ECTOPIC ANUS. The anus is situated anteriorly and may open in the female into the posterior part of the vulva or vagina. In the male, this type of anus opens in the perineum (Fig. 12-24). This anomaly may be caused by a failure in the complete development of the urorectal septum.

3. STENOSED ANUS. The anus is in a normal position, but the opening is microscopic in size (Fig. 12-25). This condition may result

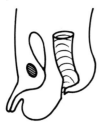

covered anus

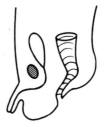

ectopic anus

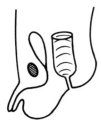

stenosed anus

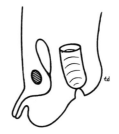

anal membrane stenosis

Fig. 12-22. The different forms of low anorectal anomalies.

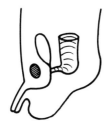

anorectal agenesis
with rectourethral fistula

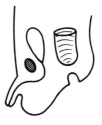

rectal atresia

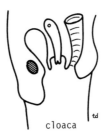

cloaca

Fig. 12-23. The different forms of high anorectal anomalies.

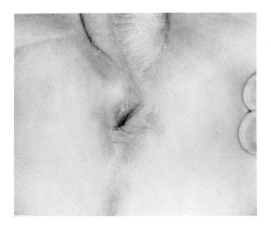

Fig. 12-24. Ectopic anus. The anus is situated anteriorly, just behind the scrotum. (Courtesy of Dr. G. Avery.)

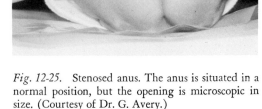

Fig. 12-25. Stenosed anus. The anus is situated in a normal position, but the opening is microscopic in size. (Courtesy of Dr. G. Avery.)

from failure of the cloacal membrane to rupture adequately and poor development of the proctodeum.

4. ANAL MEMBRANE STENOSIS. The anus is at the normal site, but the cloacal membrane has persisted at the level of the anal valves.

High Anomalies

1. ANORECTAL AGENESIS. The anus, anal canal, and inferior part of the rectum are absent. The rectum ends as a blind pouch superior to the pelvic floor. In the male, there is often a fistula between the rectal pouch and the bladder or urethra. In the female, a similar fistula extends between the rectum and vagina. This condition is probably caused by a failure in the growth of the proctodeum and the urorectal septum.

2. RECTAL ATRESIA. The anus and anal canal are normal. The rectum ends blindly superior to the pelvic floor, and there is no fistula present. This is an uncommon anomaly and is difficult to explain on embryological grounds. A local interference in the blood supply of the developing rectum may account for its failure to develop.

3. CLOACA. This occurs only in the female. The vagina, the bladder, and the rectum open into a single wide cavity. This anomaly could be explained on the basis that the urorectal septum failed to develop.

While the low anomalies are relatively simple to treat surgically, the high anomalies require prolonged surgical care, often involving a number of plastic operations, extending over many years.

Clinical Problems

Answers on page 442

1. A surgical resident was called to the neonatal ward to examine a 36-hour-old boy. The child was vomiting bile-stained fluid. The vomit was not great in volume and the vomiting was not forceful. On examination the abdomen showed generalized

distension with ballooning forward of the anterior abdominal wall. The skin covering the abdominal wall was tightly stretched and shiny. Only a small amount of grayish meconium had been passed since birth. Peristalsis was not visible through the abdominal wall. Rectal examination with the little finger revealed nothing abnormal. X-ray examination showed the presence of air in the distended small intestine, together with fluid levels. However, the air and fluid levels were limited to the upper part of the intestine; no air was seen in the distal part of the ileum or the colon. What is your diagnosis? What are the possible embryological explanations for this condition? How would you treat this patient?

2. A 5-year-old boy died of large bowel obstruction. On postmortem examination he was found to have a duplicated descending colon. How would you explain this condition embryologically?

3. A 3-day-old girl vomited some bile-stained fluid on the first day. During the second day the child vomited three times and on the third day vomited six times. The vomiting was projectile in character and the vomit was green-stained with bile. During this period a little normal-looking meconium was passed per rectum. During the third day some blood was passed per rectum. To begin with there was no abdominal distension, but during the third day the abdomen became generally distended. The child was found to be dehydrated. A diagnosis of high intestinal obstruction was made. At operation the child was found to have malrotation of the gut; the duodenum was situated anterior to the superior mesenteric artery, and the colon was lying posterior to the mesentery of the small intestine. In addition, a volvulus of the small intestine was present. Can you explain the condition of malrotation of the gut? Why has volvulus of the small intestine occurred?

4. A 6-year-old boy was examined by a pediatrician because of a history of recurrent pain in the region of the umbilicus. The pain was dull and aching in nature and lasted for about a week. It had recurred on four occasions in the previous 2 years. Two days before the examination the child had had severe rectal bleeding and had fainted. On examination, some tenderness of the anterior abdominal wall was noted in the region of the right iliac fossa, and the child was obviously anemic. Examination of the stools showed them to be streaked with dark-red blood. Has the patient an appendicitis or a Meckel's diverticulum? How would you treat this patient?

5. A 3-month-old girl was brought to a pediatrician because the mother had noticed an extrusion of fecal material through the umbilicus. The child was otherwise perfectly normal. What is the diagnosis? How can you explain the embryology of this condition? How would you treat this child?

6. A 75-year-old man visited his physician because he had noticed a watery discharge from his umbilicus. On questioning, it was found that he had the symptoms of an enlarged prostate with urethral obstruction. With your knowledge of embryology, can you explain the umbilical discharge?

7. A 4-day-old girl was operated on for low intestinal obstruction. The clinical picture was a history of bile-stained vomiting with general abdominal distension. On examination distended loops of intestine could be visualized through the anterior abdominal wall, and visible intestinal peristalsis was present. On palpation the intestine was felt to be filled with dough-like material which indented on pressure. At no time had the child passed meconium rectally. Rectal examination revealed an empty rectum. What is your diagnosis? Is this condition a part of a

more general disease? How would you treat this condition?

8. A 40-year-old woman was thought to have chronic cholecystitis. It was decided to perform a cholecystectomy to relieve her of her symptoms. At operation the cecum and a chronically inflamed appendix were found high up beneath the right lobe of the liver. The gallbladder was found to be perfectly normal. Can you explain the abnormal position of the cecum and appendix?

9. A 3-week-old boy was taken to a pediatrician because of repeated vomiting and reluctance to feed. On questioning, the mother said the child had started to vomit on the first day of life and had vomited at least once a day since then. To begin with the mother had been reassured and told that the baby was taking its feeds too quickly and that the vomiting would eventually cease. While initially accepting this reassurance, the mother had now noticed that the child did not seem hungry at feeding time; moreover, she had noticed that the abdomen was becoming distended. She added that the child was definitely constipated; very occasionally, hard meconium was passed.

On examination the abdomen was found to be greatly distended. A rectal examination with the gloved little finger resulted in the passage of a large amount of flatus, and the abdominal distension became visibly less. A low barium enema followed by an x-ray examination showed

a normal rectum; above it, a narrowed part of the colon led to a funnel-shaped expansion, which in turn led to a greatly dilated descending colon and transverse colon. What is your diagnosis? Using your knowledge of embryology, can you explain the nature of the disease? How would you treat this patient?

10. A 3-day-old baby girl was examined because the nurse had failed to identify the anus. The diaper was stained with meconium, but the anal orifice could not be seen. On careful examination of the posterior vaginal wall, a minute opening could be identified through which meconium was exuding. Pricking the skin just in front of the coccygeal region caused contraction of the external anal sphincter and showed where the normal anal orifice should have been. An x-ray film of the perineal region was then made. For this purpose the infant was carefully inverted for 3 minutes prior to taking the film, so that air in the rectum could rise past the meconium and lie in the anal canal close to the skin. The skin covering the anal sphincter was marked by placing a quarter on the skin surface. The radiogram showed that the air-filled anal canal was situated very close to the skin surface. However, a small diverticulum extended forward to the region of the posterior vaginal wall. What is the diagnosis? How would you explain this anomaly?

REFERENCES

Abrami, G., and Denison, W. M. Duplications of the Stomach. *Surgery* 49:794, 1961.

Aschner, P. W., and Karelitz, S. Peptic Ulcer of Meckel's Diverticulum and Ileum. *Ann. Surg.* 91:583, 1930.

Basu, R., Forshall, I., and Rickham, P. P. Duplications of Alimentary Tract. *Brit. J. Surg.* 47:477, 1960.

Beach, P. D., Brascho, D. J., Hein, W. R., Nichol, W. W., and Geppert, L. J. Duplication of the Primitive Hindgut of the Human Being. *Surgery* 49:779, 1961.

Bentley, J. F. R. Some New Observations on Hirschsprung's Disease in Infancy and Childhood. *Dis. Colon Rectum* 7:462, 1964.

Bentley, J. F. R., and O'Donnell, M. B. Mesenteric

Cyst with Malrotated Intestine. *Brit. Med. J.* 2:223, 1959.

Bill, A. H., and Johnson, R. J. Failure of Migration of the Rectal Opening as the Cause for Most Cases of Imperforate Anus. *Surg. Gynec. Obstet.* 106:643, 1958.

Bremer, J. L. Diverticula and Duplications of the Intestinal Tract. *Arch. Path.* (Chicago) 38:326, 1944.

Brookes, V. B. Meckel's Diverticulum in Children. *Brit. J. Surg.* 42:57, 1954.

Brown, J. J. M. Small Intestinal Obstruction in the Newborn. *Ann. Roy. Coll. Surg. Eng.* 20:280, 1957.

Chester, S. T., and Robinson, W. T. Congenital Atresia of the Transverse Colon. *Ann. Surg.* 146:824, 1957.

Christensen, E. R. Duplications in the Gastro-Intestinal Tract in Children. *Danish Med. Bull.* 6:281, 1959.

Custer, B. S., Kellner, A, and Escue, H. M. Enterogenous Cysts. *Ann. Surg.* 124:508, 1946.

Daudet, M., Chappnis, J. P., and Daudet, N. Duplications Intestinales. *Ann. Chir. Infant* 8:5, 1967.

Davis, D. L., and Poynter, C. W. M. Congenital Occlusions of the Intestines. *Surg. Gynec. Obstet.* 34:35, 1922.

Dennison, W. M. *Surgery in Infancy and Childhood.* Livingstone, Edinburgh, 1967.

Dott, N. M. Anomalies of Intestinal Rotation. *Brit. J. Surg.* 11:251, 1923.

Dott, N. M. Volvulus Neonatorum. *Brit. Med. J.* 1:250, 1927.

Edelman, S., Strauss, L., Becker, J. M., and Arnheim, E. Visceral Aganglionosis of the Colon. *Surgery* 47:557, 1960.

Ellis, D. G., and Clatworthy, H. W. The Meconium Plug Syndrome Revisited. *J. Pediat. Surg.* 1:54, 1966.

Emery, J. C. Abnormalities in Meconium of the Foetus and Newborn. *Arch. Dis. Child.* 32:17, 1957.

Estrada, R. L. *Anomalies of Intestinal Rotation and Fixation.* Thomas, Springfield, Ill., 1958.

Feggetter, S. Congenital Intestinal Atresia. *Brit. J. Surg.* 42:378, 1955.

Fisher, J. H., DeLuca, F. G., and Swenson, O. Rectal Biopsy in Hirschsprung's Disease. *Z. Kinderchir.* 2:67, 1965.

Fock, G., and Kostia, J. Familial Occurrence of Hirschsprung's Disease. *Clin. Pediat.* 2:371, 1963.

Forshall, I. Duplication of Intestinal Tract. *Postgrad. Med. J.* 37:570, 1961.

Fraser, G. C., and Berry, C. L. Neonatal Mortality in Hirschsprung's Disease. *J. Pediat. Surg.* 2:205, 1967.

Frazer, J. E., and Robbins, R. H. On Facts Concerned in Causing Rotation of Intestine in Man. *J. Anat.* 50:75, 1915.

Gardner, C. E., and Hart, D. Anomalies of Intestinal Rotation as a Cause of Intestinal Obstruction. *Arch. Surg.* (Chicago) 29:942, 1934.

Gillis, D. A., and Grantmyre, E. B. The Meconium Plug Syndrome and Hirschsprung's Disease. *Canad. Med. Ass. J.* 92:225, 1965.

Grob, M. Intestinal Obstruction in the Newborn. *Arch. Dis. Child.* 35:40, 1960.

Gross, R. E., Holcomb, G. W., and Farber, S. Duplications of the Alimentary Tract. *Pediatrics* 9:449, 1952.

Hardin, C. A., and Friesen, S. R. Congenital Atresia of the Colon. *Arch. Surg.* (Chicago) 80:616, 1960.

Hiatt, R. B., and Santulli, T. V. Important Factors Influencing the Treatment of Imperforate Anus. *Dis. Colon Rectum* 5:110, 1962.

Holshaw, D. S., Eckstein, H. B., and Nixon, H. H. Meconium Ileus. *Amer. J. Dis. Child.* 100:113, 1965.

Howard, S., Moss, P. D., and O'Domhnaill, S. Patent Vitello-Intestinal Duct with Associated Fistula and Prolapse. *Lancet* 2:968, 1953.

Howell, L. M. Meckel's Diverticulum. *Amer. J. Dis. Child.* 71:365, 1946.

Johnston, J. H., and Penn, I. A. Extrophy of the Cloaca. *Brit J. Urol.* 38:302, 1966.

Kiesewetter, W. B., Sukarochona, K., and Sieber, W. K. The Frequency of Aganglionosis Associated with Imperforate Anus. *Surgery* 58:877, 1965.

Kiesewetter, W. B., Turner, R. C., and Sieber, W. K. Imperforate Anus. *Amer. J. Surg.* 107:412, 1964.

Knutrud, O., and Eek, S. Combined Intrinsic Duodenal Obstruction and Malrotation. *Acta Chir. Scand.* 119:506, 1960.

LeDuc, E. Congenital Recto-Urethral Fistula: Report of Case Without Rectal Anomaly. *J. Urol.* 93:272, 1965.

Louw, J. H. Investigation into the Etiology of Congenital Atresia of the Colon. *Dis. Colon Rectum* 7:471, 1964.

Louw, J. H. Congenital Abnormalities of the Anus and Rectum. *Curr. Probl. Surg.* 3:5, 1965.

Louw, J. H. Jejunoileal Atresia and Stenosis. *J. Pediat. Surg.* 1:8, 1966.

McIntosh, R., and Donovan, E. J. Disturbances of Rotation. *Amer. J. Dis. Child.* 57:116, 1939.

McLetchie, N. G. B., Purvis, J. K., and Saunders,

R. C. The Genesis of Gastric and Certain Intestinal Diverticula and Enterogenous Cysts. *Surg. Gynec. Obstet.* 99:135, 1954.

Nixon, H. H. Hirschsprung's Disease. *Arch. Dis. Child.* 39:109, 1964.

Okamoto, E., and Ueda, T. Embryogenesis of Intramural Ganglia of the Gut and Its Relations to Hirschsprung's Disease. *J. Pediat. Surg.* 2:437, 1967.

Pegum, J. M., Loly, P. C. M., and Falkiner, N. Mcl. Development and Classification of Ano-Rectal Anomalies. *Arch. Surg.* (Chicago) 89:481, 1964.

Ravitch, M. M. Duplications of the Alimentary Canal. In *Pediatric Surgery*. Year Book, Chicago, 1962.

Santulli, T. V. Meconium Ileus. In *Pediatric Surgery*. Year Book, Chicago, 1962.

Santulli, T. V., Shullinger, J. N., and Amoury, R. A. Malformations of Anus and Rectum. *Surg. Clin. N. Amer.* 70:1253, 1966.

Schultz, L. R., Lasher, E. P., and Bill, A. H. Abnormalities of Rotation of the Bowel. *Amer. J. Surg.* 101:128, 1961.

Shim, W. K. T., and Swenson, O. Treatment of Congenital Megacolon in 50 Infants. *Pediatrics* 38:145, 1966.

Snyder, W. H., and Chaffin, L. Malrotation of the Intestine. In *Pediatric Surgery*. Year Book, Chicago, 1962.

Suruga, K., Tsunoda, A., Fukuda, A., and Masatake, Y. Some Problems of Congenital Intestinal Atresia. *Z Kinderchir.* 3:29, 1966.

Tench, E. M. Development of the Anus in the Human Embryo. *Amer. J. Anat.* 59:333, 1936.

Walker, A. W., Kempson, R. L., and Ternberg, J. L. Aganglionosis of the Small Intestine. *Surgery* 60:449, 1966.

DEVELOPMENT

At about the fourth week of development, a median longitudinal groove, the *laryngotracheal groove,* develops in the pharyngeal floor caudal to the copula. The entodermal lining of this groove will give origin to the lining epithelium and glands of the larynx, trachea, and bronchi, and to the epithelium of the alveoli.

The margins of the laryngotracheal groove now fuse. This process starts caudally and extends cranially so that the *laryngotracheal tube* is formed and its lumen becomes separated from the foregut (Fig. 13-1). A small opening persists just behind the copula, and this will become the permanent opening into the larynx. At about the same time, the foregut lengthens rapidly and its lumen becomes narrowed so that the *esophagus* is formed. The laryngotracheal tube now grows caudally into the splanchnic mesoderm on the ventral surface of the foregut and divides into right and left *lung buds.* Cartilage develops in the mesenchyme of the tube, and the upper part of the tube becomes the *larynx* and the lower part the *trachea.*

Each lung bud consists of an entodermal tube surrounded by splanchnic mesoderm, and from this, all the tissues of the corresponding lung will be derived. Each bud grows laterally and projects into the pleural part of the intra-embryonic coelom. The right lung bud divides into three lobes and the left into two, corresponding to the number of *main bronchi* and *lobes* found in the fully developed lung. Each main bronchus then divides repeatedly in a dichotomous manner until eventually the terminal bronchioles and alveoli are formed. It is interesting to note that division of the terminal bronchioles, with the formation of additional bronchioles and alveoli, continues for some time after birth.

As the lungs grow, they migrate inferiorly and further invaginate the intra-embryonic coelom (Fig. 13-1). This part of the coelom will form the *pleural sacs.* Each lung will receive a covering of *visceral pleura* derived from splanchnic mesoderm. The *parietal pleura* will be derived from somatic mesoderm. The mesenchyme surrounding the entodermal bronchial tree will differentiate into connective tissue, cartilage, muscle, and pulmonary and bronchial blood vessels. By the seventh month, the capillary loops connected with the pulmonary circulation have become closely related to the alveoli and are

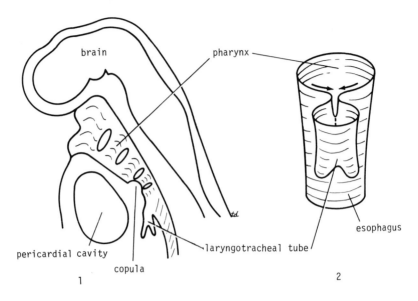

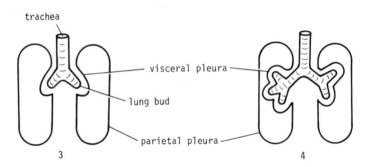

Fig. 13-1. The development of the lungs: 1. The laryngotracheal groove and tube have been formed. 2. The margins of the laryngotracheal groove fuse to form the laryngotracheal tube. 3. The lung buds invaginate the wall of the intra-embryonic coelom. 4. The lung buds divide to form the main bronchi.

sufficiently well developed to support life, should premature birth take place.

In the earliest stage, the opening into the larynx is a median slit. Later this becomes T-shaped with the development of the arytenoid cartilages. The opening then becomes temporarily closed by the fusion of its walls until the third month.

Although it is possible under experimental conditions to elicit respiratory movements in the fetus at the end of the third month,

normally these do not occur until birth. With the onset of respiration at birth, the lungs expand and the alveoli become dilated. However, it is only after 3 to 4 days of postnatal life that the alveoli in the periphery of each lung become fully expanded. It is now generally agreed that aeration of the lung at birth is not the inflation of a collapsed empty organ but the replacement of fluid within the alveoli by air. The fluid found in the bronchial tree just before birth is probably a mixture of amniotic fluid and glandular secretions produced by the gland cells of the lining mucous membrane. The fluid in the lung is rapidly removed at birth almost certainly through the pulmonary blood capillaries or lymphatics.

In recent years it has been shown that there is present within the lungs a substance which has remarkable surface-acting properties. It is the presence of this substance called *surfactant* which allows the surface-tension forces within the alveoli to be overcome so that effective ventilation can be established at birth. Surfactant is thought to be produced by cells lining the alveoli and appears at about the thirtieth week of intra-uterine life.

During labor, the baby is subjected to considerable compression as he passes down the birth canal. As he emerges into the cold dry environment, he leaves behind the warm moist uterine cavity. He is usually a little anoxic on delivery, and even more so when his umbilical cord is tied. It is as a result of these various stimuli that the first breath is taken, and this is normally followed by rhythmic respiration.

CONGENITAL ANOMALIES

Esophageal Atresia and Tracheo-Esophageal Fistula

If the margins of the laryngotracheal groove fail to fuse adequately, an abnormal opening may be left between the laryngotracheal tube and the esophagus. If the tracheo-esophageal septum formed by the fusion of the margins of the laryngotracheal groove should be deviated posteriorly, the lumen of the esophagus would be much reduced in diameter. The different types of atresia with and without fistula are shown in Figure 13-2. Obstruction of the esophagus (Fig. 13-2A, B, & C) prevents the child from swallowing saliva and milk, and this leads to aspiration into the larynx and trachea, which usually results in pneumonia. A communication between the trachea and esophagus (Fig. 13-2A, B, D, & F) results in air being forced into the stomach when the child cries. The stomach dilates and elevates the diaphragm with consequent embarrassment of respiration. Acid gastric contents may be forced up the esophagus through the fistula into the trachea and down into the bronchial tree, producing severe chemical pneumonitis.

With early diagnosis and careful preoperative preparation, it is possible in many cases to correct this serious anomaly with surgery.

Neonatal Lobar Emphysema

This condition occurs shortly after birth and is an overdistension of one or more lobes of the lung. It is a result, in many cases, of a failure of development of bronchial cartilage, which causes the bronchi to collapse. Air is inspired through the collapsed bronchi, but it is trapped during expiration.

Congenital Cysts of the Lungs

The cysts may be solitary or form multiple honeycomb-like masses. They are believed to be caused by sequestration of lung tissue occurring during development. Prompt surgical removal of the cysts is necessary to prevent compression and collapse of surrounding lung and infectious complications.

Respiratory Distress Syndrome (Hyaline Membrane Disease)

This disease accounts for 30 percent of all neonatal deaths and 50 to 70 percent of deaths in premature infants. Basically, the disease is a failure of the alveoli to ventilate adequately, resulting in a gross hypoxemia. It has been shown that the lungs of infants dying from this condition do not contain *surfactant*. This

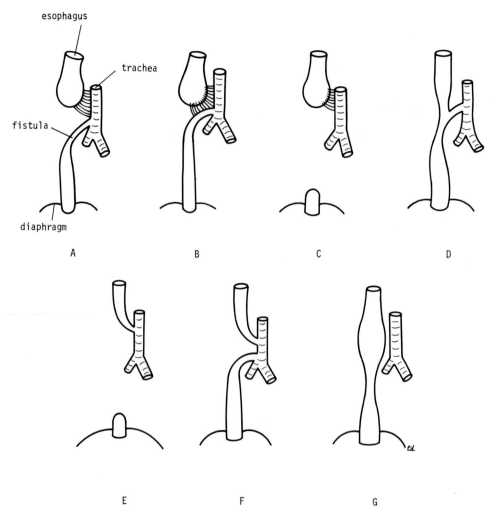

Fig. 13-2. The different types of esophageal atresia and tracheo-esophageal fistula. In the majority of cases the lower esophageal segment communicates with the trachea, and types A and B occur more commonly.

substance is necessary to overcome the surface-tension forces in the alveoli when the lungs are inflated.

Agenesis of One or Both Lungs

These conditions are extremely rare and are a result of the failure of the lung bud or buds to develop at the caudal end of the laryngo-tracheal tube.

Accessory Lung Lobes

Additional branching of the stem bronchi sometimes occurs, leading to the formation of accessory bronchi and lobes.

Clinical Problems

Answers on page 444

1. A 30-year-old pregnant woman with hydramnios gave birth to what appeared to be a perfectly normal male child. Once the child had taken his first breath and normal respiration had become established, it was noticed that bubbling saliva started to flow from his mouth. The pediatrician quickly wiped the mouth dry, whereupon the saliva started to reaccumulate and the child began to choke and cough and become cyanotic. Feeding the child with a little sterile water made the choking and breathlessness worse. Examination of the abdomen showed distension. Passage of a radiopaque catheter through the nose and down the esophagus, followed by x-ray, revealed a complete blockage of the esophagus. The presence of gas in the stomach and intestine showed the existence of a tracheo-esophageal fistula. On embryological grounds, how would you explain this congenital anomaly? How would you treat this infant?

2. A 10-month-old baby boy was examined by a pediatrician because he had had attacks of dyspnea and cyanosis. Radiography revealed displacement of the mediastinum and evidence of emphysema. A diagnosis of congenital lobar emphysema was made. How would you explain this rare condition embryologically?

3. A 2-year-old boy had a routine chest x-ray following the visit of an aunt who was found to have active pulmonary tuberculosis. On examination of the boy's chest radiograph there was no evidence of pulmonary tuberculosis, but it was noted that the upper lobe of the right lung had a honeycomb appearance. Nothing else abnormal was seen. What congenital anomaly of the lung could give this radiographic appearance? What is the embryological explanation for this condition?

4. One hour after the birth of what appeared to be a normal girl, the attending nurse noticed that the child's respiratory rate was gradually rising and had reached a rate of 70 per minute. The breathing was now obviously labored, with rib retraction and expiratory grunting. Auscultation of the chest revealed that there was diminished air entry and some fine moist sounds over the lung bases posteriorly. Within 2 hours the child became cyanotic and was obviously exhausted from excessive respiratory effort; 3 hours later the child died. At postmortem the lungs were noted to be dull red in color, fleshy in consistency, and airless. Microscopically the alveoli were collapsed and lined by an eosinophilic membrane. What is your diagnosis? What is the possible underlying defect in this condition?

REFERENCES

Barnard, W., and Day, T. D. The Development of the Terminal Air Passages of the Human Lung. *J. Path. Bact.* 45:67, 1937.

Birdsell, P., Wentworth, P., Reilly, B. J. and Donohue, W. L. Congenital Cystic Adenomatous Malformation of the Lung. *Canad. J. Surg.* 9: 350, 1966.

Bucher, U., and Reid, L. Development of the Intrasegmental Bronchial Tree. *Thorax* 16:207, 1961.

Clements, J. A. *The Alveolar Lining Layer: Development of the Lung.* Ciba Foundation Symposium. Edited by A. V. S. de Reuck and R. Porter. Churchill, London, 1967. P. 202.

Cross, K., Klaus, M., Tooley, W. H., Weisser, K. H., and Clements, J. A. The Response of the New-Born Baby to Inflation of the Lungs. *J. Physiol.* 151:551, 1960.

Davis, J. A. The First Breath and Development of Lung Tissue. In *Scientific Foundations of Obstetrics and Gynaecology,* edited by E. E. Philipp, J. Barnes, and M. Newton. Davis, Philadelphia, 1970. P. 401.

Davis, M., and Potter, E. Intra-Uterine Respiration of the Human Fetus. *J.A.M.A.* 131:1194, 1946.

Dawes, G. S. *Foetal and Neonatal Physiology.* Year Book, Chicago, 1968.

Dunnill, M. S. Postnatal Growth of the Lung. *Thorax* 17:329, 1962.

Engel, S. *The Prenatal Lung.* Pergamon, New York, 1966.

Fawcitt, J., Lind, J., and Wegelius, C. The First Breath: A Preliminary Communication Describing Some Methods of Investigation of the First Breath of a Baby and the Results Obtained from Them. *Acta Paediat.* (Stockholm) 49 (Suppl. 123):5, 1960.

Fischer, C. C., Tropear, F., and Bailey, C. P. Congenital Pulmonary Cysts. *J. Pediat.* 23:219, 1943.

Fluzz, Z., and Poppen, K. J. Embryogenesis of Tracheo-Oesophageal Atresia. *A.M.A. Arch. Path.* 52:1968, 1951.

Gruenwald, P. A. A Case of Atresia of the Esophagus Combined with Tracheo-Esophageal Fistula in a 9 mm Human Embryo, and Its Embryological Explanation. *Anat. Rec.* 78:293, 1940.

Haas, L., and Sturridge, M. F. Congenital Tracheo-Oesophageal Fistula. *Proc. Roy. Soc. Med.* 54:329, 1961.

Ham, A. W., and Baldwin, K. W. Histological Study of Development of Lung with Particular Reference to Nature of Alveoli. *Anat. Rec.* 8:363, 1941.

Holder, T. M., and Ashcroft, T. W. Esophageal Atresia and Tracheo-Esophageal Fistula. In *Current Problems in Surgery.* Year Book, Chicago, 1966.

Johnston, P. W., and Hastings, N. Congenital Tracheo-Esophageal Fistula Without Esophageal Atresia. *Amer. J. Surg.* 112:233, 1966.

Levine, R. M. Congenital Cystic Disease of the Lung. *Canad. Med. Ass. J.* 62:181, 1950.

Low, F. N. The Pulmonary Alveolar Epithelium of Laboratory Mammals and Man. *Anat. Rec.* 117:241, 1951.

Lynn, H. B. J., and Davies, L. A. Tracheo-Esophageal Fistula Without Atresia of the Esophagus. *Surg. Clin. N. Amer.* 41:871, 1961.

Palmer, D. M. The Lung of a Human Fetus at 170 mm. *Amer. J. Anat.* 158:59, 1935.

Pattle, R. E. Properties, Function and Origin of the Alveolar Lining Layer. *Proc. Roy. Soc.* [Biol.] 148:217, 1958.

Plank, J. *A Morphological Contribution to the Development of the Human Lung: Observations in the Non-Retracted Lung: Development of the Lung.* Ciba Foundation Symposium. Edited by A. V. S. de Reuck and R. Porter. Churchill, London, 1967. P. 156.

Purves, M. *Initiation of Respiration: Development of the Lung.* Ciba Foundation Symposium. Edited by A. V. S. de Reuck and R. Porter. Churchill, London, 1967. P. 317.

Reid, L. *The Embryology of the Lung: Development of the Lung.* Ciba Foundation Symposium. Edited by A. V. S. de Reuck and R. Porter. Churchill, London, 1967. P. 109.

Reynolds, E. O. R., Roberton, N. R. C., and Wigglesworth, J. S. Hyaline Membrane Disease, Respiratory Distress and Surfactant Deficiency. *Pediatrics* 42:758, 1968.

Smith, E. I. The Early Development of the Trachea and Oesophagus in Relation to Atresia of the Oesophagus and Tracheo-Oesophageal Fistula. *Contr. Embryol.* 245:36, 1957.

Sorokin, S. Histochemical Events in Developing Human Lungs. *Acta Anat.* (Basel) 40:105, 1960.

Thomas, L. B., and Boyden, E. A. Agenesis of the Right Lung. *Surgery* 31:429, 1952.

Waterston, D. J., Bonham-Carter, R. E., and Aberdeen, E. Oesophageal Atresia: Tracheo-Oesophageal Fistula. *Lancet* 2:819, 1962.

Weibel, E. R. *Post-Natal Growth of the Lung and Pulmonary Gas Exchange Capacity: Development of the Lung.* Ciba Foundation Symposium. Edited by A. V. S. de Reuck and R. Porter. Churchill, London, 1967. P. 137.

Wells, L. J. Development of the Human Diaphragm and Pleural Sacs. *Contrib. Embryol.* 35:107, 1954.

Wells, L. J., and Boyden, E. A. Development of Bronchopulmonary Segments in Human Embryos and Horizons XVII–XIX. *Amer. J. Anat.* 95:163, 1954.

Willis, R. A. *The Borderland of Embryology and Pathology.* Butterworth, London, 1962.

Zatzkin, H. R., Cole, P. M., and Bronsther, B. Congenital Hypertrophic Lobar Emphysema. *Surgery* 52:505, 1962.

The Pericardial Cavity, the Pleural Cavities, the Diaphragm, the Peritoneal Cavity, and the Umbilicus

14

DEVELOPMENT

Pericardial Cavity

The development of the pericardial cavity from the cranial portion of the intra-embryonic coelom has been described in Chapter 7. In the earliest stages, it lies in the midline of the embryo cranial to the buccopharyngeal membrane. With the formation of the head fold, the pericardium and the endocardial heart tube rotate so that the pericardial cavity comes to lie ventral to the pharynx. At this stage, the pericardial cavity is in free communication with the peritoneal cavity through the *pericardioperitoneal canals* (Fig. 14-1). The formation of the serous pericardium, the oblique and transverse sinuses, and the fibrous pericardium is described in Chapter 7.

Pleural Cavities

With the development of the lung buds, the splanchnopleuric mesoderm covering them is invaginated into the pericardioperitoneal canals. This portion of the pericardioperitoneal canals becomes the pleural cavity on each side (Fig. 14-1). The primitive pleural cavities now greatly enlarge. The developing heart and pericardial cavity, which are situated anterior to the pharynx, descend into the thorax. The pleural cavities remain continu-

ous with the pericardial and peritoneal cavities by way of the *pleuropericardial* and *pleuroperitoneal* canals, respectively. As the lungs and pleural cavities undergo further development, the pleuropericardial canals become closed off by the appearance of *pleuropericardial membranes* (Fig. 14-1). Continued expansion of the pleural cavity leads to the formation of the *pleuroperitoneal membrane* on each side. This projects into the pleuroperitoneal canal from the lateral side and eventually fuses with the septum transversum and the dorsal mesentery to form the diaphragm. In this manner the pleural and peritoneal cavities become separated.

Diaphragm

The diaphragm forms between the eighth and tenth weeks of intra-uterine life. It is derived from the following structures: (1) the septum transversum, which forms the muscle and central tendon; (2) the two pleuroperitoneal membranes, which are largely responsible for the peripheral areas of diaphragmatic pleura and peritoneum, which cover its upper and lower surfaces, respectively; and (3) the dorsal mesentery of the esophagus, in which the crura develop (Fig. 14-2).

183

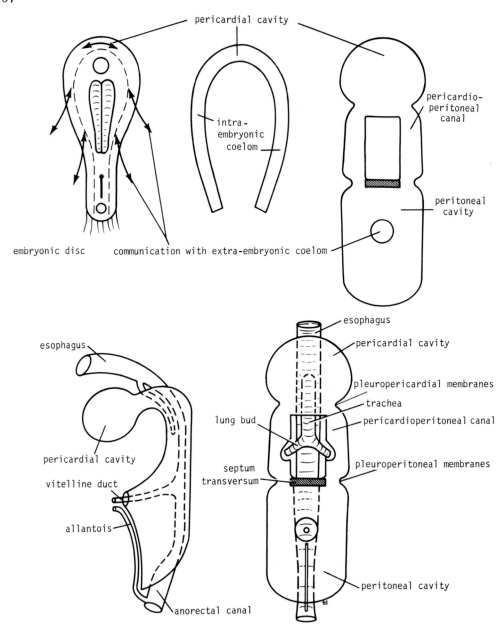

Fig. 14-1. The formation of the pericardial, pleural, and peritoneal cavities from the intra-embryonic coelom.

The septum transversum is a mass of mesoderm that lies between the pericardial cavity and the vitelline duct. It is, however, an incomplete septum, since the pleuroperitoneal canals lie posterolaterally on each side. The septum transversum is formed in the neck region by the fusion of the myotomes of the third, fourth, and fifth cervical segments. With the descent of the heart from the neck to the thorax, the septum is pushed caudally, pulling its nerve supply with it; thus its motor nerve supply is derived from the third, fourth, and fifth cervical nerves, which are contained within the phrenic nerve.

Meanwhile the pleuroperitoneal membrane on each side starts growing medially from the body wall and encroaches on the pleuroperitoneal canal until it finally fuses with the septum transversum anterior to the esophagus and the dorsal mesentery posterior to the esophagus. During the process of fusion, the mesoderm of the septum transversum extends into and pervades the other parts, thus forming the entire muscle of the diaphragm. The *motor nerve supply to the entire muscle of the diaphragm is the phrenic nerve.* The *sensory nerve supply* to the central pleura and peritoneum covering the central parts of

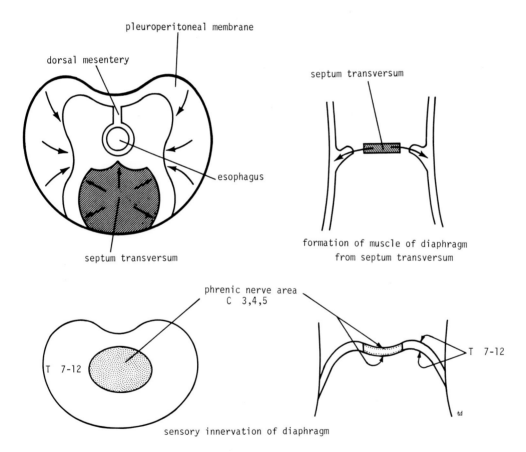

Fig. 14-2. The formation of the diaphragm from the septum transversum, the pleuroperitoneal membranes, and the dorsal mesentery. The muscle is formed from the septum transversum and is innervated by the phrenic nerve. The sensory innervation of the diaphragm is from cervical segments 3, 4, and 5 and thoracic segments 7–12 as shown.

the upper and lower surfaces of the diaphragm is also the phrenic nerve. The sensory innervation of the peripheral parts of the pleura and peritoneum covering the peripheral areas of the upper and lower surfaces of the diaphragm is from the lower six thoracic nerves (Fig. 14-2). This is understandable, since the peripheral pleura and peritoneum are derived from the pleuroperitoneal membranes from the body wall.

The Fate of the Septum Transversum

The septum transversum is formed in the neck by the fusion of the myotomes of the third, fourth, and fifth cervical segments and lies between the pericardial cavity and the vitelline duct. Within this mesodermal mass are the vitelline veins and the common cardinal veins prior to their entrance into the sinus venosus of the heart. Following the descent of the septum with the heart into the thorax, it comes to project horizontally posteriorly from the anterior or ventral body wall to meet the dorsal mesentery. The septum

transversum now becomes separated into three layers (Fig. 14-3): (1) a superior layer, which helps to form the fibrous pericardium; (2) a middle layer, which forms all the muscle of the diaphragm, the central tendon of the diaphragm, and the central areas of the pleura and peritoneum covering the diaphragm; and (3) an inferior layer, which forms the fibrous capsule and connective tissue of the liver and the ventral mesentery of the developing gut.

The enlarging pleural cavities tend to separate the fibrous pericardium from the diaphragm around the periphery, but in the center the fibrous pericardium remains fused with the central tendon. The enlarging peritoneal cavity tends to separate the fibrous capsule of the liver from the diaphragm, but it remains attached by areas of mesenchyme, which become the *falciform ligament,* the *right* and *left triangular ligaments,* and the *coronary ligament.* These ligaments are in fact two-layered folds of peritoneum, and in places the layers separate so that the liver

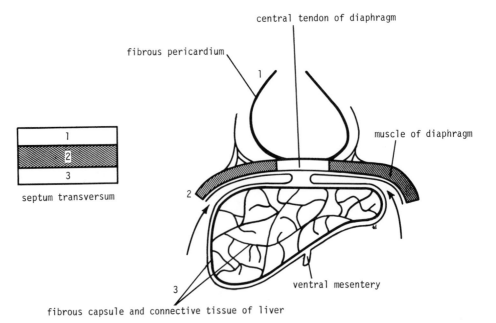

Fig. 14-3. The fate of the septum transversum.

capsule is in direct contact with the diaphragm, the so-called *bare areas.* The separation of the fibrous capsule of the liver from the diaphragm allows the contracting diaphragm freedom of movement.

Peritoneal Cavity

The peritoneal cavity is formed from that part of the intra-embryonic coelom situated caudal to the septum transversum. In the earliest stages, the peritoneal cavity is in free communication with the extra-embryonic coelom on each side. Later, with the development of the head, tail, and lateral folds of the embryo, this wide area of communication becomes restricted to the small area within the umbilical cord. Early in development, the peritoneal cavity is divided into right and left halves by a central partition formed by the *dorsal mesentery,* the gut, and a small *ventral mesentery* (Fig. 14-4). However, the ventral mesentery only extends for a short distance along the gut (see below), so that below this level the right and left halves of the peritoneal cavity are in free communication. As a result of the enormous growth of the liver and the enlargement of the developing kidneys, the capacity of the abdominal cavity becomes greatly reduced at about the sixth week of development. It is at this time that the small remaining communication between the peritoneal cavity and the extra-embryonic coelom becomes important. This enables physiological herniation of the rapidly developing midgut loop to take place, and this

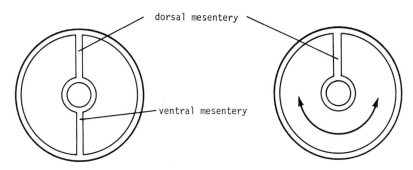

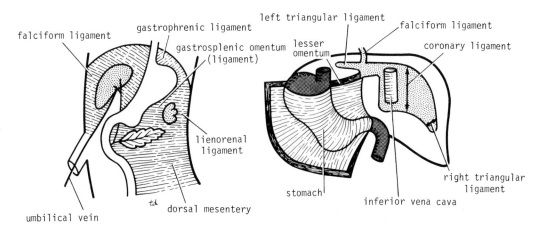

Fig. 14-4. The ventral and dorsal mesenteries.

phenomenon has received special consideration on page 157.

Origin and Fate of the Ventral Mesentery

The ventral mesentery is formed from the mesoderm of the septum transversum. In fact it may be regarded as that portion of the septum transversum which lies caudal to the diaphragm. That being the case the hepatic bud, an outgrowth of entoderm from the foregut, grows into the ventral mesentery (the septum transversum), and the latter will form the fibrous capsule and connective tissue of the liver. The remainder of the ventral mesentery will form the following peritoneal ligaments: (1) The *falciform ligament* extends from the anterior abdominal wall to the anterior surface of the liver. The free margin of the falciform ligament contains the umbilical vein, which after birth becomes obliterated and forms a fibrous cord, the *ligamentum teres* (Figs. 14-4 & 14-10). (2) The *lesser omentum* extends from the liver (porta hepatis and fissure of the ligamentum venosum) to the lesser curvature of the stomach and border of the first and second parts of the duodenum (Fig. 14-4). The free margin of the lesser omentum contains the common bile duct, hepatic artery, and portal vein. (3) The *coronary* and *triangular ligaments* extend from the liver to the undersurface of the diaphragm (Fig. 14-4).

Origin and Fate of the Dorsal Mesentery

The dorsal mesentery is formed from a fusion of the splanchnopleuric mesoderm of the two sides of the embryo and extends from the dorsal or posterior abdominal wall to the dorsal border of the abdominal part of the gut. The spleen (derived from mesenchyme) and the dorsal bud of the pancreas (derived from entoderm) develop between the layers of the dorsal mesentery. The fate of the different parts of the mesentery is as follows: (1) The *gastrophrenic ligament* extends between the abdominal part of the esophagus and the adjacent part of the stomach to the diaphragm (Fig. 14-4). (2) The *gastrosplenic omentum* or *ligament* extends between the upper part of the greater curvature of the stomach and the hilum of the spleen (Fig. 14-4). (3) The *lienorenal ligament* extends between the hilum of the spleen and the left kidney (Fig. 14-4). (4) The *greater omentum* extends between the extensive lower part of the greater curvature of the stomach and eventually fuses with the transverse colon (Fig. 14-5). (5) The mesenteries of the small intestine and large intestine extend between the gut and the posterior abdominal wall (Figs. 14-5—14-8).

Formation of the Lesser and Greater Peritoneal Sacs

The superior part of the lesser sac develops as a recess in the mesenchyme on the right side of the esophagus. This at first extends superiorly into the right side of the thorax, but later this extension becomes cut off by the development of the diaphragm. Meanwhile the extensive growth of the right lobe of the liver pulls the ventral mesentery to the right and causes rotation of the stomach and duodenum (Fig. 14-5). In this manner the upper right part of the peritoneal cavity becomes incorporated in the lesser sac. The right free border of the lesser omentum, i.e., the ventral mesentery, becomes the anterior boundary of the *epiploic foramen* (Fig. 14-7). The *superior recess of the lesser sac* is that part which lies posterior to the lesser omentum and extends superiorly behind the caudate lobe of the liver as far as the diaphragm. The *inferior recess* is that part which lies posterior to the stomach and runs for a variable distance in the greater omentum (Fig. 14-7).

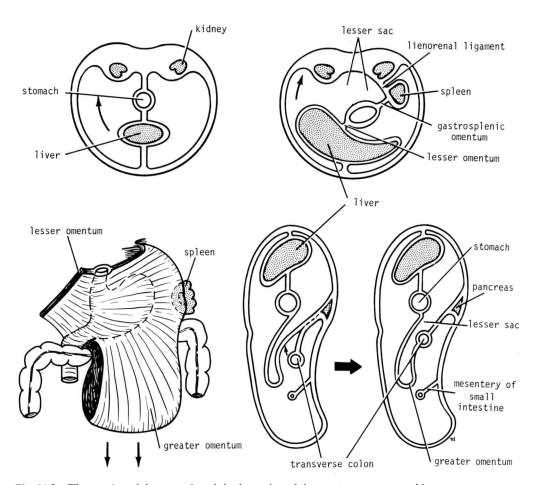

Fig. 14-5. The rotation of the stomach and the formation of the greater omentum and lesser sac.

The *lienal recess* is that part which lies in the concavity of the dorsal mesentery.

The remaining part of the peritoneal cavity, which is not included in the lesser sac, is now called the greater sac, and the two sacs are in communication through the epiploic foramen (Fig. 14-7).

Greater Omentum

The greater omentum is formed as a result of the rapid and extensive growth of the dorsal mesentery caudal to the spleen. It extends from the greater curvature of the stomach and, to begin with, is attached to the pos-terior abdominal wall superior to the transverse mesocolon. With continued growth, it reaches inferiorly as an apron-like double fold of peritoneum anterior to the transverse colon. Later the posterior layer of the omentum fuses with the transverse mesocolon, and as a result the greater omentum becomes attached to the anterior surface of the transverse colon (Fig. 14-5). As development proceeds, the omentum becomes laden with fat. The inferior recess of the lesser sac extends inferiorly between the anterior and posterior layers of the fold of the greater omentum.

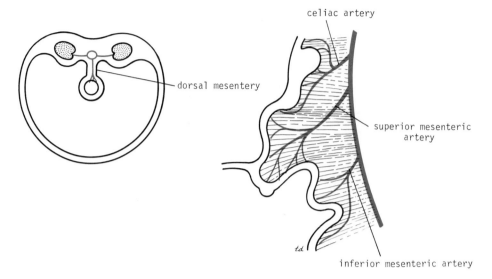

Fig. 14-6. The dorsal mesentery forming the mesenteries of the small and large intestines.

Mesenteries of the Small and Large Intestines

Duodenum

Following the rotation of the stomach and duodenum and the fusion of the ventral and dorsal pancreatic buds, the greater part of the ventral mesentery in this region disappears. A small part remains attached to the superior border of the beginning of the first part of the duodenum as the free border of the lesser omentum (Fig. 14-7). The dorsal mesentery in this region, the *mesoduodenum,* fuses with the peritoneum on the posterior abdominal wall and disappears. The peritoneum covering the posterior surface of the duodenum

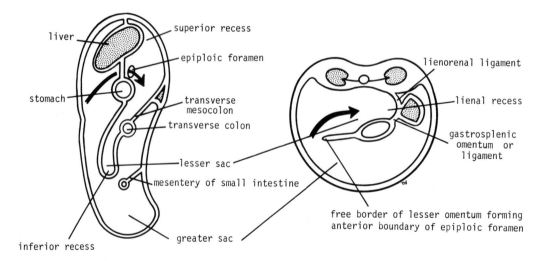

Fig. 14-7. The different parts of the lesser sac.

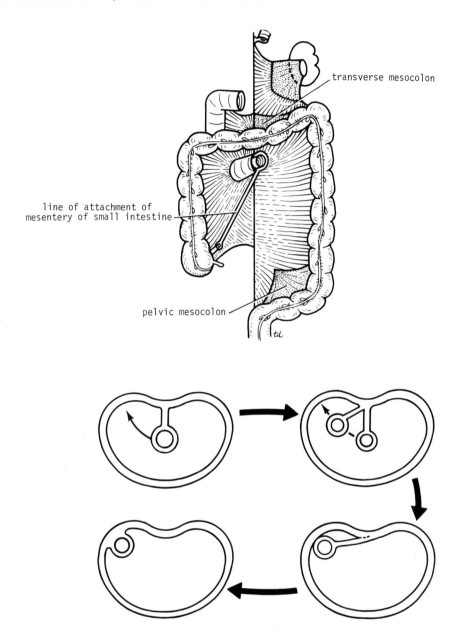

Fig 14-8. Fusion of parts of the dorsal mesentery with the peritoneum on the posterior abdominal wall (stippled areas indicate where fusion has not taken place).

now disappears so that this part of the gut becomes retroperitoneal (Fig. 14-8).

Jejunum and Ileum

The dorsal mesentery becomes the *mesentery of the small intestine*. Originally it is attached to the posterior abdominal wall in the midline. Later, with the rotation of the midgut loop, the mesentery twists around the origin of the superior mesenteric artery. After the ascending mesocolon (see below) has fused with the peritoneum on the posterior abdominal wall, the mesentery of the small intestine obtains a new attachment that extends from the duodenojejunal junction inferiorly and to the right to the ileocecal junction (Fig. 14-8).

Cecum and Appendix

The cecum has no mesentery, since it originates as a diverticulum from the antimesenteric border of the midgut and is therefore covered on all surfaces with peritoneum. Later, when the mesocolon of the ascending colon fuses with the peritoneum on the posterior abdominal wall, some fusion of the peritoneum on the posterior surface of the cecum with that of the posterior abdominal wall may take place. This may result in the formation of one or more *retrocecal recesses* or *fossae*. The appendix does not possess a true mesentery, but there is a peritoneal fold, which contains the *appendicular artery,* a branch of the posterior cecal artery, which extends from the mesentery of the ileum to the appendix (Fig. 14-9).

Colon

Following the descent of the cecum into the right iliac fossa, the part of the dorsal mesentery that is attached to the ascending colon, the *ascending mesocolon,* fuses with the peri-

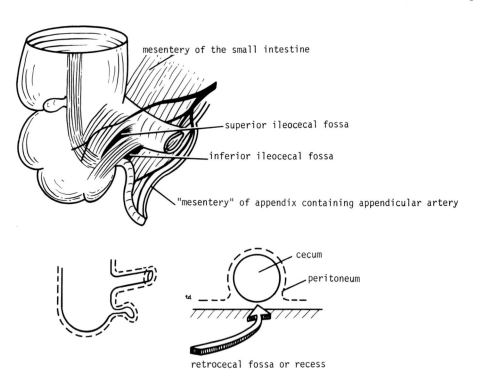

mesentery of the small intestine

superior ileocecal fossa

inferior ileocecal fossa

"mesentery" of appendix containing appendicular artery

cecum

peritoneum

retrocecal fossa or recess

Fig. 14-9. The peritoneal relations of the cecum and appendix.

toneum on the posterior abdominal wall and disappears (Fig. 14-8). The peritoneum on the posterior surface of the ascending colon also disappears so that this structure becomes retroperitoneal.

The dorsal mesentery, which attaches the transverse colon to the posterior abdominal wall, becomes attached to the anterior surface of the pancreas and fuses with the greater omentum; it is known as the *transverse mesocolon* (Fig. 14-7).

The part of the dorsal mesentery that attaches the descending colon to the posterior abdominal wall, the *descending mesocolon,* fuses with the peritoneum on the posterior abdominal wall and disappears (Fig. 14-8). The peritoneum on the posterior surface of the descending colon also disappears, so that this part of the gut becomes retroperitoneal.

The dorsal mesentery of the pelvic colon remains as the *pelvic mesocolon.* The attachment of the pelvic mesocolon to the posterior abdominal wall changes from a midline linear attachment to an inverted "V" attachment in the left iliac fossa (Fig. 14-8).

Rectum and Anal Canal

The dorsal mesentery of the rectum and upper half of the anal canal disappears, and this part of the gut becomes applied to the anterior surface of the sacrum.

Umbilicus

The umbilicus may be defined as the part of the anterior abdominal wall that was attached to the umbilical cord (Fig. 14-10). At birth, with the separation of the umbilical cord, it becomes a fibrous scar which gradually sinks beneath the surface to form an obvious landmark in the midline of the anterior abdominal wall. In fetal life it transmits the following structures: (1) The *right* and *left umbilical arteries,* which after birth be-

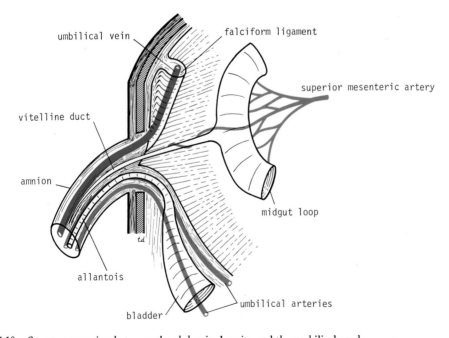

Fig. 14-10. Structures passing between the abdominal cavity and the umbilical cord.

come obliterated and fibrosed and form the *lateral umbilical ligaments.* (2) The *umbilical vein* (the left umbilical vein), which after birth forms a fibrous cord which runs in the free margin of the falciform ligament and is called the *ligamentum teres.* (3) The *vitelline duct,* which connects the midgut to the yolk sac. With the return of the midgut loop to the abdominal cavity following physiological herniation, it becomes obliterated and disappears. (4) The *allantois,* which is a diverticulum from the anterior part of the hindgut, passes into the umbilical cord for a variable distance (Fig. 14-10). After birth this becomes obliterated and remains as a fibrous cord extending from the umbilicus to the apex of the bladder forming the *urachus* or *median umbilical ligament.* (5) The *extra-embryonic coelom,* which communicates with the intra-embryonic coelom (peritoneal cavity) through the umbilicus. From the sixth to the twelfth week, the midgut loop herniates out of the peritoneal cavity into the extra-embryonic coelom contained within the umbilical cord. Once the gut has returned to the peritoneal cavity, the remnants of the extra-embryonic coelom disappear.

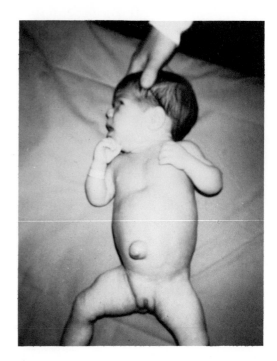

Fig. 14-11. Small umbilical hernia. (Courtesy of Dr. G. Avery.)

CONGENITAL ANOMALIES

Umbilicus

Infantile Umbilical Hernia

This is a small hernia that sometimes occurs in children and is due to a weakness in the scar of the umbilicus (Fig. 14-11). The majority become smaller and disappear without treatment as the abdominal cavity enlarges.

Exomphalos (Omphalocele)

This is the herniation of some of the intra-abdominal contents through the open umbilicus. The protrusion is covered by a translucent membrane consisting of peritoneum inside and amnion outside, separated by Wharton's jelly (Figs. 14-12 & 14-13). The

umbilical cord is attached to the apex of the protrusion and the umbilical arteries and vein run within its walls. Sometimes a large hernial sac ruptures in utero, during labor, or after birth. The size of the abdominal wall defect varies from a small opening, which allows only a loop or part of a loop of small intestine to pass through, to a very large defect with the liver, the spleen, and the greater part of the gut outside the abdominal cavity.

The anterior abdominal wall is closed by a process of folding of the embryonic disc (see Chap. 3). Failure of the formation of adequate lateral folds causes a defect in the umbilical region, which is filled in by amnion only.

Surgical excision of the amniotic sac, and the return of the protruding viscera into the abdominal cavity followed by closure of the abdominal wall defect, is the treatment of choice. In some cases the abdominal cavity is

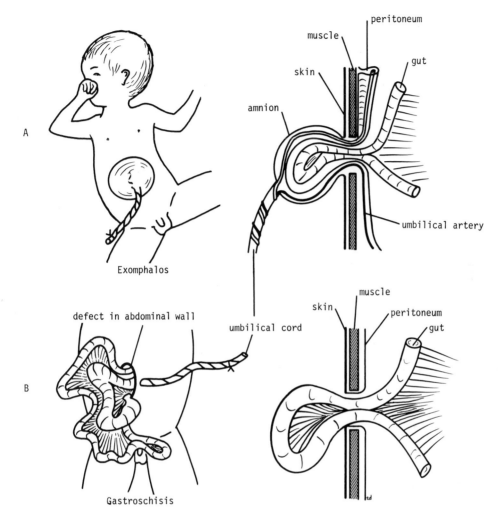

Fig. 14-12. The conditions of (A) exomphalos and (B) gastroschisis. In exomphalos, the umbilical cord is attached at the apex of the swelling and the umbilical vessels can be seen through the translucent wall of the exomphalos sac. In gastroschisis, there is a full-thickness abdominal wall defect and no hernial sac.

too small to hold the viscera, and a plastic skin flap must be constructed to cover the exomphalos.

Gastroschisis

In this condition the abdominal contents herniate through a defect in the anterior abdominal wall *adjacent* to the umbilicus (Figs. 14-12 & 14-14). It is caused by a defect in the development of one of the lateral folds of the embryo, resulting in a full-thickness defect of the abdominal wall. The umbilical cord is attached to the abdominal wall in a normal manner.

The condition is more serious than exomphalos, but the treatment is similar. The mortality is high. Both exomphalos and gastroschisis are frequently associated with other congenital abnormalities.

Fistula of Vitelline Duct

This is considered in detail in Chapter 12.

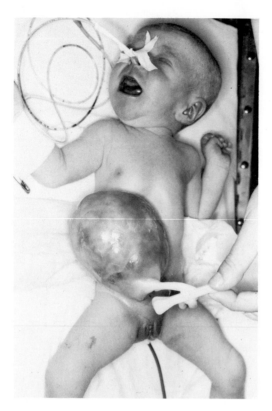

Fig. 14-13. Exomphalos (omphalocele). Note that the umbilical cord is attached to the apex of the protrusion. (Courtesy of Dr. G. Avery.)

Patent Urachus

This is considered with the development of the urinary bladder in Chapter 15.

Diaphragm

Diaphragmatic Hernia and Eventration of the Diaphragm

Congenital herniation of an abdominal viscus through the diaphragm into the thorax is caused by a failure of fusion of the various elements that form the diaphragm (Fig. 14-15).

1. HERNIA THROUGH THE PLEUROPERITONEAL CANAL. In many of these cases, the canal remains open and there is free communication between the abdominal and pleural cavities (Fig. 14-16). The peritoneum and pleura are continuous so that there is no hernial sac. In a few cases the canal is closed by a layer of peritoneum and pleura, the muscle having failed to develop adequately. In these circumstances there is a hernial sac formed by the layers of peritoneum and pleura. The condition is found much more commonly on the

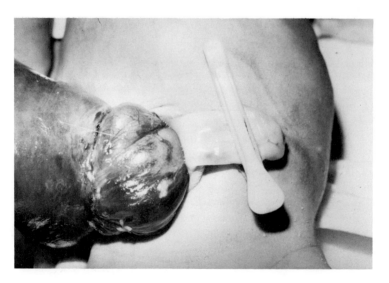

Fig. 14-14. Gastroschisis. Note the full-thickness abdominal wall defect and absence of the amniotic sac. Coils of intestine are stuck together. (Courtesy of Dr. J. Randolph.)

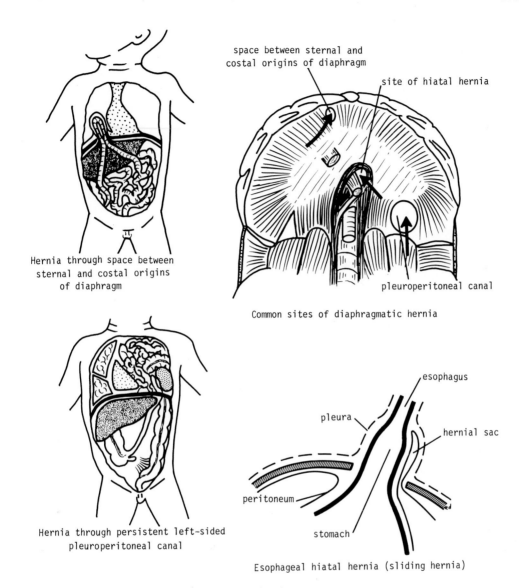

space between sternal and
costal origins of diaphragm

site of hiatal hernia

Hernia through space between
sternal and costal origins
of diaphragm

pleuroperitoneal canal

Common sites of diaphragmatic hernia

Hernia through persistent left-sided
pleuroperitoneal canal

esophagus

pleura

hernial sac

peritoneum

stomach

Esophageal hiatal hernia (sliding hernia)

Fig. 14-15. Three types of congenital diaphragmatic hernia.

left, presumably because the large right lobe of the liver blocks the defect if it should occur on the right (Fig. 14-15). The treatment is surgical reduction of the hernia and repair of the defect.

2. HERNIA THROUGH THE SPACE BETWEEN THE STERNAL AND COSTAL ORIGINS OF THE MUSCLE OF THE DIAPHRAGM. Normally these spaces are small and allow the superior epigastric vessels to enter the anterior abdominal wall. In this condition a small part of the muscle presumably fails to develop from the septum transversum and a defect occurs. A small hernial sac of peritoneum and pleura protrudes up into the thorax and may contain loops of intestine (Fig. 14-15). The treatment is surgi-

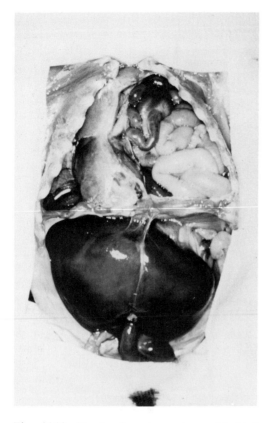

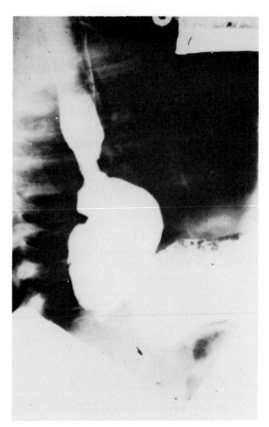

Fig. 14-16. Hernia through persistent left-sided pleuroperitoneal canal. (Courtesy of Dr. J. Randolph.)

Fig. 14-17. An esophageal hiatal hernia. Radiograph of thorax and abdomen following a barium meal. Note the presence of part of the stomach in the thoracic cavity. (Courtesy of Dr. J. Randolph.)

cal reduction of the hernia and repair of the defect.

3. ESOPHAGEAL HIATAL HERNIA. In hiatal hernia a part of the stomach protrudes through the esophageal hiatus of the diaphragm into the thorax (Figs. 14-15 & 14-17). There is a widening of the esophageal hiatus and a weakness of muscle of the right crus of the diaphragm. The combined effects of a positive intra-abdominal pressure and a negative intrathoracic pressure cause the cardia of the stomach to be pushed upward. A small peritoneal hernial sac is present on the left side of the stomach. (There is no sac on the right side, since this is a bare area.) The result of herniation is that the cardio-esopha-

geal junction becomes incompetent and the stomach contents flow into the esophagus, which results in *esophagitis*. The latter condition if untreated may lead to esophageal stricture and shortening of the esophagus.

In the newborn, the presenting symptom is vomiting of stomach contents, which is often projectile (similar to the type of vomiting seen in congenital hypertrophic pyloric stenosis). Typically, the child vomits when laid on its back, as the stomach contents then drain up the esophagus. The treatment is medical. The child always is nursed in an upright position. Surgery is not used in the treatment of this condition.

4. EVENTRATION OF THE DIAPHRAGM. This is caused by a defective development of the whole or part of the muscle of the diaphragm, which is represented by a sheet of fibrous tissue covered on the superior surface with pleura and on the inferior surface with peritoneum. The immobile diaphragm is pushed up into the thorax and is found at a higher level than normal. Symptoms are uncommon, although in severe cases cyanosis may occur, especially after feeding, because of respiratory embarrassment.

Accessory Phrenic Nerve

The muscle of the diaphragm is innervated by the phrenic nerves (the third, fourth, and fifth cervical nerves). As the septum transversum descends into the thorax, it draws the phrenic nerve behind it. It is important to remember that in some individuals the contribution from the fifth segment of the cervical spinal cord enters the phrenic nerve in the thorax via the nerve to subclavius; this contribution is referred to as the *accessory phrenic nerve*. In these cases the operation of phrenic nerve crush in the neck to paralyze the diaphragm for the treatment of lung tuberculosis would not be effective unless the accessory phrenic nerve was also crushed.

Paraduodenal Fossae

As a result of fusion of the various layers of peritoneum on the posterior abdominal wall in the region of the duodenojejunal junction, an occasional fossa or pocket of peritoneum may be formed (Fig. 14-18). The importance of the fossa or fossae lies in the fact that a loop of small intestine may become imprisoned in one of them and cause intestinal obstruction.

Fossae in the Region of the Cecum and Appendix

The *superior and inferior ileocecal fossae* are

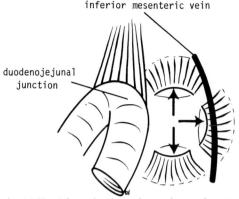

Fig. 14-18.   Three duodenal fossae (*arrows*), which may be the site of internal hernia of a loop of small intestine.

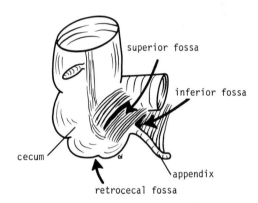

Fig. 14-19. Sites where loops of small intestine may become imprisoned and cause intestinal obstruction.

formed as the result of the appearance of folds of peritoneum during development (Fig. 14-19). If the folds are excessively developed, the fossae may be deep and a loop of small intestine may become trapped. A deep *retrocecal fossa* may form because of excessive fusion of peritoneum behind the cecum. Here again a loop of small bowel may become imprisoned.

Mobile Cecum and Ascending Colon

Incomplete fusion of the ascending mesocolon with the peritoneum on the posterior abdominal wall may lead to twisting or volvulus of the ascending colon with intestinal obstruction. Surgical correction of the twisted large bowel, followed by fixation of the ascending colon to the posterior abdominal wall, is the treatment.

Defects in the Mesentery of the Small Intestine, Transverse Mesocolon, or Pelvic Mesocolon

These may snare a loop of small bowel and cause intestinal obstruction.

Clinical Problems
Answers on page 445

1. Immediately following delivery it was noted that a 7½ lb. male child had a large swelling on the anterior abdominal wall. The swelling consisted of a large sac, the walls of which were translucent and soft. The umbilical cord was attached to the apex of the sac, and the umbilical arteries and vein ran within its walls. On closer examination it was possible to see (within the sac) coils of small intestine and the lower margin of the liver. As the baby cried and started to swallow air, the sac became larger. What is the diagnosis? How can you explain the formation of this sac? What would happen to the sac if you did not treat this condition? How would you treat this patient? Is this condition frequently associated with other congenital anomalies?

2. Following delivery of a female child it was noted that coils of small intestine protruded through a large defect in the child's anterior abdominal wall. The umbilical cord was seen to be attached normally to the anterior abdominal wall on the right side of the defect. On close examination the wall of the intestine was seen to be thickened and edematous. Some of the coils of intestine were stuck together by a gelatinous material. What is the diagnosis? How would you treat this patient? What is the prognosis?

3. A 10-day-old baby boy was taken to a pediatrician because his mother had noticed that he was breathless and on three occasions had become blue in color. On one occasion when the child was very breathless and blue, the mother had noticed that his condition was greatly improved by altering his position. On physical examination the left side of the thorax was seen to move less on breathing than did the right side. The apex beat of the heart was pushed over toward the right. Percussion of the left side of the thorax revealed excessive resonance in the lower areas. Auscultation revealed absent breath sounds over the lower part of the left side of the thorax. An anteroposterior x-ray film of the chest and abdomen showed coils of gas-filled loops of intestine on the left side of the thorax. The mediastinal shadow was displaced to the right. What is your diagnosis? How would you treat this patient?

4. A pediatrician examined a day-old baby girl with a history of repeated vomiting since birth. The child was breast-fed and was obviously hungry at each feed. On laying the child down in the cot after each feed, it was noted that she immediately vomited in a projectile manner. On examination the child was seen to be restless and dehydrated. X-ray examination following a barium swallow revealed a small piece of stomach above the diaphragm. What is the diagnosis? What is the underlying embryological explanation for this condition? How would you treat this infant?

REFERENCES

Aitken, J. Exomphalos. *Arch. Dis. Child.* 38:126, 1963.

Allen, M. S., and Thomson, S. A. Congenital Diaphragmatic Hernia in Children Under One Year of Age. *J. Pediat. Surg.* 1:157, 1966.

Allison, P. R. Reflux Oesophagitis, Hiatus Hernia and the Anatomy of Repair. *Surg. Gynec. Obstet.* 92:419, 1951.

Arey, L. B. *Developmental Anatomy,* 7th ed. Saunders, Philadelphia, 1966.

Bay Nielsen, H., and Larsen, E. Omphalocele. *Dan. Med. Bull.* 10:75, 1963.

Belsey, R. H. R. The Surgery of the Diaphragm. In *Surgery of Childhood,* edited by J. J. Mason Brown. Edward Arnold, London, 1962.

Bernstein, R. Gastroschisis. *Arch. Pediat.* 57:505, 1940.

Bonham-Carter, R. E., Waterston, D. J., and Aberdeen, E. Hernia and Eventration of the Diaphragm in Childhood. *Lancet* 1:656, 1962.

Bremer, J. L. The Diaphragm and Diaphragmatic Hernia. *Arch. Path.* (Chicago) 36:539, 1943.

Butler, N., and Claireaux, A. E. Congenital Diaphragmatic Hernia. *Lancet* 1:659, 1962.

Coupland, G. A. E., and Rickham, P. P. Vagotomy and Pyloroplasty in the Surgical Treatment of Hiatus Hernia in Children. *Aust. New Zeal. J. Surg.* 37:1, 1968.

Duhamel, B. Embryology of Exomphalos and Allied Malformations. *Arch. Dis. Child.* 38:142, 1963.

Eckstein, H. B. Exomphalos. *Brit. J. Surg.* 50:405, 1963.

Findley, C., and Kelly, A. B. Congenital Shortening of the Oesophagus and the Thoracic Stomach Resulting Therefrom. *J. Laryng.* 46:797, 1931.

Fitchett, C. N., and Tavarez, V. Bilateral Congenital Diaphragmatic Herniation. *Surgery* 57:305, 1965.

Hamilton, W. J., Boyd, J. D., and Mossman, H. W. *Human Embryology,* 3d ed. Williams & Wilkins, Baltimore, 1962.

Hutchin, P. Gastroschisis with Antenatal Evisceration of the Entire Gastro-Intestinal Tract. *Surgery* 57:297, 1965.

Hutchin, P. Somatic Anomalies of the Umbilicus and Anterior Abdominal Wall. *Surg. Gynec. Obstet.* 120:1075, 1965.

Jones, P. G. Exomphalos. *Arch. Dis. Child.* 38:180, 1963.

Kanagasuntheram, R. Development of the Human Lesser Sac. *J. Anat.* 91:188, 1957.

Kiesewetter, W. B., Gutierrez, I. Z., and Sieber, W. K. Diaphragmatic Hernia in Infants Under One Year of Age. *Arch. Surg.* (Chicago) 83:560, 1961.

Michelson, E. Eventration of the Diaphragm. *Surgery* 49:410, 1961.

Rickham, P. P. Rupture of Exomphalos and Gastroschisis. *Arch. Dis. Child.* 38:138, 1963.

Simpson, R. L., and Gaylor, H. D. Gastroschisis. *Amer. J. Surg.* 96:675, 1966.

Snyder, W. H., and Greanly, E. M. Congenital Diaphragmatic Hernia. *Surgery* 57:576, 1965.

Waterston, D. Hiatus Hernia. In *Pediatric Surgery.* Year Book, Chicago, 1962.

Wells, L. J. Observations on the Development of the Diaphragm in the Human Embryo. *Anat. Rec.* 100:778, 1948.

Wells, L. J. Development of the Human Diaphragm and Pleural Sacs. *Contrib. Embryol.* 35:107, 1954.

The greater part of the urinary system is formed from the mesoderm of the intermediate cell mass.

DEVELOPMENT

Kidneys and Ureters

Three sets of structures appear successively, called the *pronephros,* the *mesonephros,* and the *metanephros.*

Pronephros

The pronephros of each side is rudimentary in the human subject and consists of several tubules formed from mesodermal cells of the intermediate cell mass in the cervical region (Fig. 15-1). Glomeruli do not develop and the tubules do not open into an excretory duct. The first formed tubules regress before the more caudally placed last ones are formed, and the entire pronephros disappears by the end of the fourth week.

Mesonephros

The mesonephros, like the pronephros, consists of a number of tubules and is formed from the mesodermal cells of the intermediate cell mass in the thoracic and lumbar regions (Fig. 15-1). The medial end of each tubule enlarges and becomes pear-shaped, and its wall is invaginated by a cluster of capillaries which form a *glomerulus.* The capillaries are connected to a branch of the aorta. The lateral end of each tubule opens into a longitudinal collecting duct called the *mesonephric* (or *Wolffian*) *duct.* The mesonephric duct develops as a solid rod of cells in the intermediate cell mass. This canalizes and its caudal end grows to reach the lateral wall of the cloaca, which it perforates (Fig. 15-1). Meanwhile each mesonephric tubule undergoes further development. With the formation of the glomerulus, the indented medial end of the tubule forms the *glomerular capsule* (*Bowman's capsule*). The glomerular capsule and the glomerulus together are known as the *mesonephric corpuscle.* The increase in the length of the tubule causes it to become bent and S-shaped, and the equivalent of the *proximal* and *distal convoluted tubules* and the *collecting tubule* are formed.

As the mesonephric tubules continue to form and grow, the mesonephros forms a spindle-shaped ridge, which projects into the coelomic cavity on each side of the midline. Later it becomes an ovoid body, which is suspended from the posterior abdominal wall by a thick *mesonephric mesentery.* During the second month, the mesonephros reaches

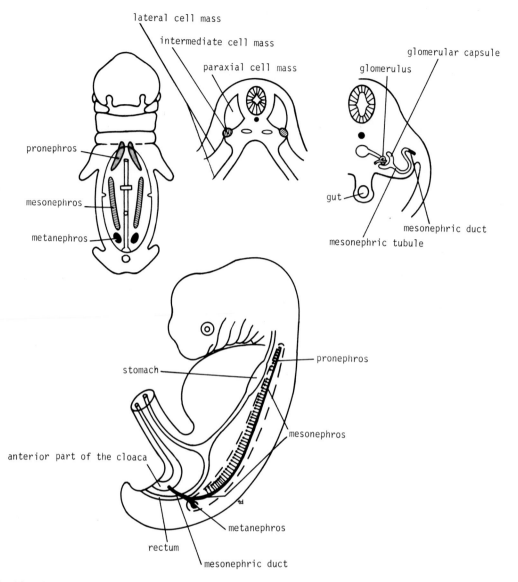

Fig. 15-1. The origin and positions of the pronephros, mesonephros, and metanephros.

its maximum degree of development and extends on each side from the region of the septum transversum down to the third lumbar segment. After functioning for a short period, the tubules start to degenerate, and this proceeds in a craniocaudal direction. By the beginning of the third month, the majority of the mesonephric tubules and glomeruli

have disappeared. However, a few caudal mesonephric tubules remain and become associated with the genital system in both sexes.

FATE OF THE MESONEPHRIC TUBULES IN THE MALE. The majority disappear, but a few remain and form the functional *efferent ductules of the testis,* the nonfunctional *superior and inferior aberrant ductules,* and the *appendix of the epididymis* (Fig. 16-2).

FATE OF THE MESONEPHRIC TUBULES IN THE FEMALE. Here again, the majority of the tubules disappear, but a few remain to form nonfunctioning *tubules of the epoophoron,* a vestigial structure, which lies in the broad ligament superior to the attachment of the mesovarium. They also form nonfunctioning *tubules of the paroophoron,* another vestigial structure which lies medial to the ovary between the layers of the broad ligament (Fig. 16-3).

Metanephros

The metanephros, or permanent kidney, develops from two sources: (1) the ureteric bud from the mesonephric duct and (2) the metanephrogenic cap from the intermediate cell mass of the lower lumbar and sacral regions.

The *ureteric bud* arises as an outgrowth of the mesonephric duct near the opening of the latter into the anterior part of the cloaca (Figs. 15-1 & 15-2). The bud grows dorsocranially into the mesoderm of the intermediate cell mass, which condenses around it to form the metanephrogenic cap (Fig. 15-2). The ureteric bud forms the *ureter,* which dilates at its upper end to form the *pelvis of the ureter.* Later the pelvis gives off branches that form the *major calyces,* and these in turn divide and branch to form the *minor calyces* and *collecting tubules.* New collecting tubules continue to be formed until the end of the fifth month of fetal life.

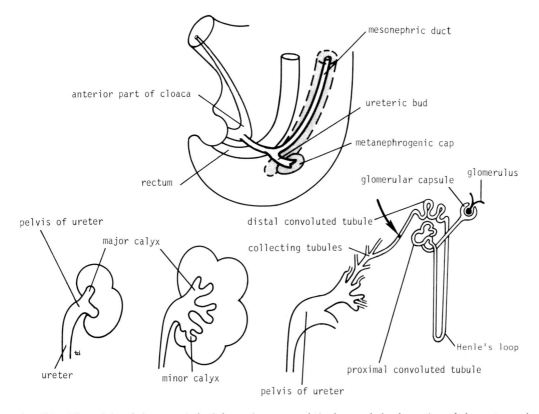

Fig. 15-2. The origin of the ureteric bud from the mesonephric duct and the formation of the major and minor calyces and the collecting tubules. The point of union between the collecting tubules and the convoluted tubules is shown by an *arrow.*

The mesodermal cells of the *metanephrogenic cap* form the glomerular capsules (*Bowman's capsules*), the *proximal and distal convoluted tubules,* and the *loops of Henle.* The glomerular capsule becomes invaginated by a cluster of capillaries that form the glomerulus. Each tubule elongates in a manner similar to that seen in the development of the mesonephric tubule (see above). It is important to realize that the metanephrogenic tissue proliferates and divides with the ureteric bud, so that each new tubule has its own cap of mesoderm. Each distal convoluted tubule formed from the metanephrogenic cap tissue becomes joined to a collecting tubule derived from the ureteric bud. The surface of the kidney is at first lobulated, but after birth this lobulation usually soon disappears.

The metanephros is at first a pelvic organ. It is found at the level of the upper sacral segments and receives its arterial supply from the pelvic continuation of the aorta, the middle sacral artery (Fig. 15-3). As development proceeds, the kidneys change their position and gradually "ascend" up the posterior abdominal wall. This so-called ascent of the kidney is largely apparent and is caused mainly by the growth of the body in the lumbar and sacral regions and by the straightening of its curvature. The ureter elongates as the "ascent" continues. The kidney is vascularized at successively higher levels by successively higher *lateral splanchnic arteries,* branches of the aorta. The kidneys ultimately reach their final position opposite the second lumbar vertebra. Because of the large size of the right lobe of the liver, the right kidney lies at a slightly lower level than the left kidney.

It is generally believed that the mesonephric and metanephric kidneys produce urine before birth. This is passed via the cloaca into the amniotic cavity and contributes to the liquor amnii. It should be pointed out, however, that the placenta functions as the kidney in the fetus, and it is only at birth

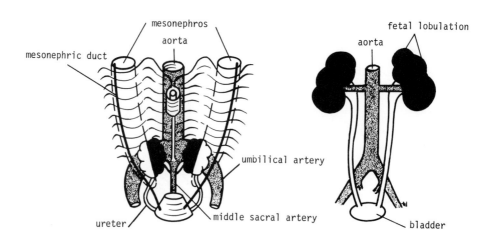

Kidneys rising out of the pelvis

Kidneys at final position opposite second lumbar vertebra

Fig. 15-3. The "ascent" of the kidneys from the pelvis. The mesonephric ducts cross in front of the ureters on each side, and the kidneys initially receive their blood supply from the middle sacral artery.

that the kidneys assume their important function.

The Bladder

In Chapter 12 the division of the cloaca by the development of the *urorectal septum* into anterior and posterior parts was described. The posterior portion forms the *anorectal canal* (Fig. 15-4). The entrance of the distal ends of the mesonephric ducts into the anterior part of the cloaca on each side enables one, for purposes of description, to divide the anterior part of the cloaca into an area above the duct entrances called the *primitive bladder* and another area below called the *urogenital sinus*.

The caudal ends of the mesonephric ducts

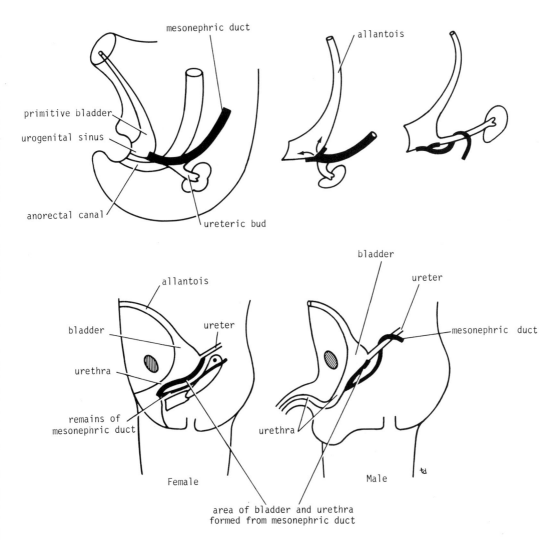

Fig. 15-4. The formation of the urinary bladder from the anterior part of the cloaca and the terminal parts of the mesonephric ducts in both sexes. The mesonephric ducts and the ureteric buds are drawn into the developing bladder.

now become absorbed into the lower part of the bladder so that the ureters and ducts have individual openings in its dorsal wall (Fig. 15-4). With differential growth of the dorsal bladder wall, the ureters come to open through the lateral angles of the bladder, and the mesonephric ducts open close together in what will be the future urethra. That part of the dorsal bladder wall marked off by the openings of these four ducts forms the *trigone* of the bladder (Fig. 15-5). It is thus seen that in the earliest stages the lining of the bladder over the trigone is mesodermal in origin; later this mesodermal tissue is thought to be replaced by epithelium of entodermal origin. The smooth muscle of the bladder wall is derived from the splanchnopleuric mesoderm.

The primitive bladder may now be divided into an upper dilated portion, the *bladder,* and a lower narrow portion, the *urethra* (Fig. 15-4). The apex of the bladder is continuous with the *allantois,* which now becomes obliterated and forms a fibrous cord, the *urachus.* The urachus persists throughout life as a ligament which runs from the apex

of the bladder to the umbilicus, and is called the *median umbilical ligament.*

Fate of the Mesonephric Duct, or Wolffian Duct

In both sexes this duct gives origin on each side to the *ureteric bud,* which forms the *ureter,* the *pelvis of the ureter,* the *major and minor calyces,* and the *collecting tubules of the kidney.* Its inferior end is absorbed into the developing bladder and forms the trigone and part of the urethra.

In the male, its upper or cranial end is joined to the developing testis by the efferent ductules of the testis and so it becomes the *duct of the epididymis,* the *vas deferens,* and the *ejaculatory duct.* From the latter, a small diverticulum arises which forms the *seminal vesicle* (Fig. 16-2).

In the female, the mesonephric duct largely disappears. Only small remnants persist, as the *duct of the epoophoron* and the *duct of the paroophoron.* The caudal end may persist and extend from the epoophoron to the hymen as *Gartner's duct* (Fig. 16-3).

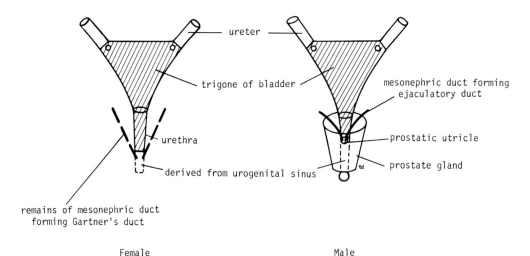

Female Male

Fig. 15-5. The parts of the bladder and urethra derived from the mesonephric ducts, in both sexes (*hatched lines*). The lower end of the urethra in the female and the lower part of the prostatic urethra in the male are formed from the urogenital sinus.

The Urethra

In the male, the *prostatic urethra* is formed from two sources. The proximal part as far as the openings of the ejaculatory ducts is derived from the mesonephric ducts. The distal part of the prostatic urethra is formed from the urogenital sinus (Fig. 15-5). The *membranous urethra* and the greater part of the *penile urethra* are also formed from the urogenital sinus. The distal end of the penile urethra is derived from an ingrowth of ectodermal cells on the glans penis. (For details on the formation of the penile urethra, see Chap. 16.)

In the female, the upper two-thirds of the urethra are derived from the mesonephric ducts. The lower end of the urethra is formed from the urogenital sinus (Fig. 15-5).

CONGENITAL ANOMALIES

Kidney

Renal Agenesis

An absent or congenitally atrophic kidney is present in about 1 in 1,400 individuals. An absent kidney is caused by a failure of the ureteric bud to develop as an outgrowth of the mesonephric duct on one side. For obvious reasons, it is important to recognize that a patient has a solitary kidney before embarking on surgical treatment of kidney disease. Children born with bilateral renal agenesis survive only a few days.

Renal Cysts

These occur in two main forms: (1) polycystic kidney and (2) solitary cyst of the kidney (Fig. 15-6).

POLYCYSTIC KIDNEY. This is a hereditary disease and can be transmitted by either parent. It may be associated with congenital cysts of the liver, pancreas, and lung. Both kidneys are enormously enlarged and riddled with cysts of varying size (Figs. 15-6 & 15-7). The kidneys may even be so large as to obstruct labor. The condition is most commonly diagnosed in early adult life as the result of pain caused by the weight of the organ or as the result of rupture of one of the cysts, causing hematuria. The failing renal tissue produces symptoms of uremia. Polycystic kidney is possibly a result of a failure of union between the convoluted tubules derived from the metanephrogenic cap and the collecting tubules derived from the metanephric or ureteric bud. The accumulation of

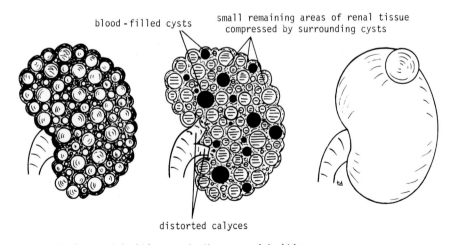

blood-filled cysts

small remaining areas of renal tissue compressed by surrounding cysts

distorted calyces

Fig. 15-6. Polycystic disease of the kidneys and solitary cyst of the kidney.

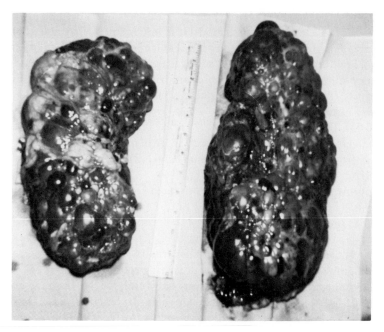

Fig. 15-7. Polycystic kidneys. (Courtesy of Dr. H. Miller.)

urine in the proximal tubules results in the formation of retention cysts. Other possible causes are sequestration of tubules during early kidney development or an abnormal development of the collecting tubules. The treatment should be surgical incision of the cysts, which relieves the pressure on the remaining renal tissue, though the disease is almost invariably fatal.

MULTICYSTIC KIDNEY. This is a rare condition and may be unilateral or bilateral. The kidney is vestigial, and in its place are several large cysts which usually communicate with the pelvis. It is thought to arise through renal hypoplasia with dysgenesis. Nephrectomy may be necessary.

SOLITARY CYST OF THE KIDNEY. This is a misnomer, since not infrequently more than one cyst is found in the kidney. However, the cysts are usually larger and much fewer in number than those found in polycystic disease (Fig. 15-6). The cause of a solitary cyst is thought to be the same as that in the polycystic kidney. Since it is likely to cause pain eventually, and may become infected, it should be removed surgically by partial nephrectomy.

Pelvic Kidney

The kidney is arrested in some part of its normal ascent; it is usually found at the brim of the pelvis (Figs. 15-8 & 15-9). Such a kidney may give rise to no signs or symptoms and may function normally. However, should an ectopic kidney become inflamed, it may, because of its unusual position, give rise to a mistaken diagnosis.

Horseshoe Kidney

This is caused by a fusion of the most medial subdivisions of the ureteric bud, resulting in a union of the caudal ends of both kidneys (Figs. 15-8, 15-10, & 15-11). Both kidneys commence to ascend from the pelvis, but the interconnecting bridge becomes trapped behind the inferior mesenteric artery so that the kidneys come to rest in the low lumbar region. The suprarenal glands, being developed separately, are found in their normal positions. Both ureters are kinked as they

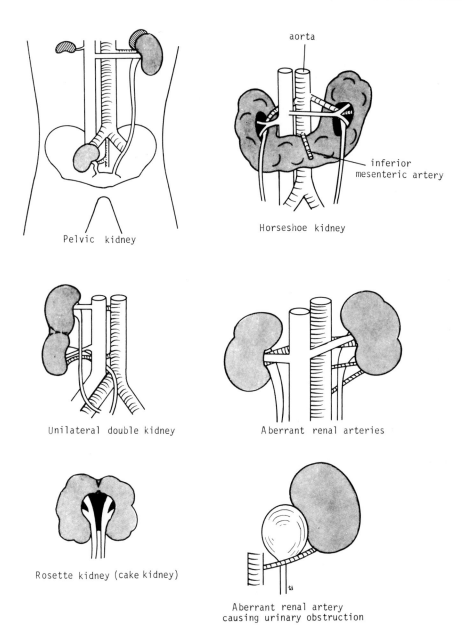

Fig. 15-8. The different forms of anomalous development of the kidney.

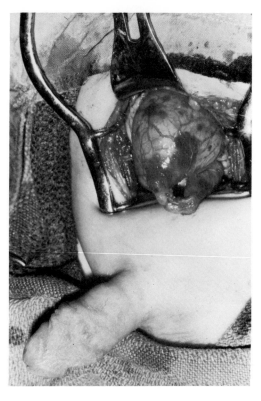

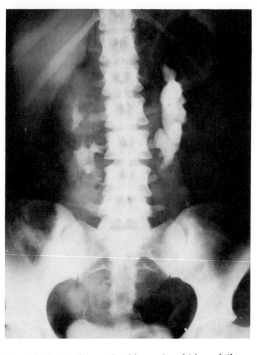

Fig. 15-10. Radiograph of horseshoe kidney following intravenous injection of iodine-containing compound, which is excreted by kidney. The ureters are not visualized. (Courtesy of Dr. H. Miller.)

Fig. 15-9. Operation for removal of right-sided pelvic kidney. (Courtesy of Dr. H. Miller.)

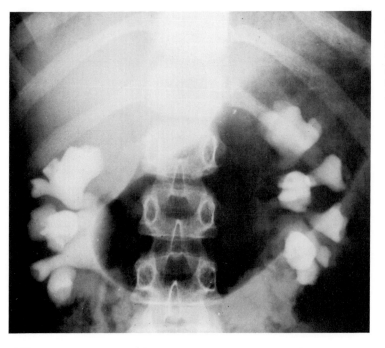

Fig. 15-11. Radiograph of horseshoe kidney following intravenous injection of iodine-containing compound. Major and minor calyces are shown. (Courtesy of Dr. H. Miller.)

pass inferiorly over the connecting bridge of renal tissue, and this produces urinary stasis; consequently infection and stone formation are frequent complications. Surgical division of the isthmus corrects the condition.

Unilateral Double Kidney

The kidney on one side may be double, with separate ureters and blood vessels. In this condition the ureteric bud on one side crosses the midline as it ascends and its upper pole fuses with the lower pole of the normally placed kidney (Fig. 15-8). Here again, angulation of the ureter may result in stasis of the urine and may require surgical treatment.

Rosette Kidney (Cake Kidney)

Both kidneys fuse together at their hila, and they usually remain in the pelvis. The two

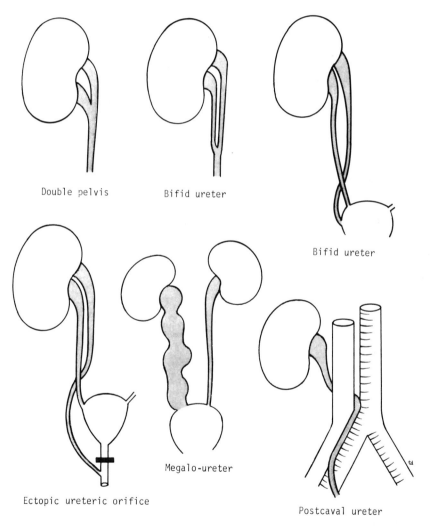

Double pelvis

Bifid ureter

Bifid ureter

Ectopic ureteric orifice

Megalo-ureter

Postcaval ureter

Fig. 15-12. The different forms of anomalous development of the ureter.

kidneys together form a rosette or cake (Fig. 15-8). This is a result of the early fusion of the two ureteric buds in the pelvis.

Aberrant Renal Vessels

These may occur on one or both sides (Fig. 15-8). If they occur at the lower pole of the kidney, they often cross in front of the ureter and produce renal stasis and even obstruction. An aberrant renal artery represents a persistent lateral splanchnic artery, a branch of the aorta. Normally, once the ascending kidney reaches its final position in the abdomen and acquires its permanent renal arteries, the lower lateral splanchnic vessels disappear. Occasionally one of these aberrant arteries may be large and supply a large segment of the kidney. Division of such a vessel would produce infarction of a portion of the renal tissue.

Ureter

Double Pelvis of the Ureter

This is usually unilateral (Fig. 15-12). The upper pelvis is small and drains the upper group of calyces; the larger lower pelvis drains the middle and lower groups of calyces. The cause is a premature division of the ureteric bud near its termination.

Bifid Ureter

Double ureters and double pelves are present. The ureters may join in the lower third of their course (Figs. 15-12 & 15-13); they may open through a common orifice into the bladder; or they may open independently into the bladder (Fig. 15-12), in which case the ureter draining the upper pelvis opens into the bladder below the orifice of the other ureter. In the latter case, one ureter crosses its fellow and may produce urinary obstruction. The cause of bifid ureter is a premature division of the ureteric bud.

Cases of double pelves and double ureters may be found by chance on radiological investigation of the urinary tract. They are

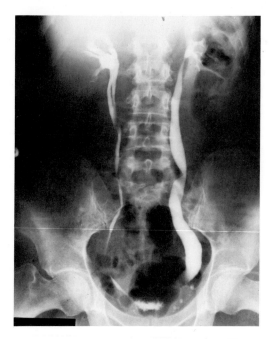

Fig. 15-13. Radiograph of right-sided bifid ureter following intravenous injection of iodine-containing compound; the left ureter is also moderately dilated. (Courtesy of Dr. H. Miller.)

more liable to become infected or be the seat of calculus formation than a normal ureter.

Ectopic Ureteric Orifice

This condition is the result of a second ureteric bud arising from a single mesonephric duct. In the male, the additional ureter may open into the lower part of the trigone, the prostatic urethra, the ejaculatory duct, or even the seminal vesicle. Since the opening is above the sphincter urethrae, the patient is continent. In the female, the additional ureter may open into the urethra below the sphincter urethrae or even into the vagina (Fig. 15-12). The patient is incontinent. Fortunately this condition is a rare anomaly. For treatment, the ureter, if normal, is implanted into the bladder.

Megalo-Ureter

This condition may be unilateral or bilateral and shows complete absence of motility

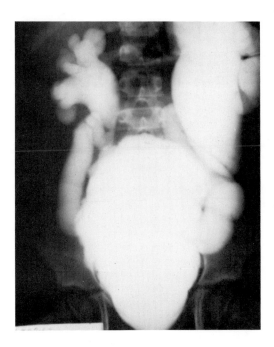

Fig. 15-14. Radiograph of bilateral megalo-ureter following intravenous injection of iodine-containing compound. (Courtesy of Dr. H. Miller.)

(Figs. 15-12 & 15-14). The cause is unknown. The ureter is prone to infection because of urinary stasis; therefore some form of plastic surgical procedure is required in order to improve the rate of drainage from the ureter.

Postcaval Ureter

The right ureter ascends posterior to the inferior vena cava and may be obstructed by it (Fig. 15-12). If necessary, surgical division of the ureter near the bladder, with reimplantation into the bladder so that the ureter has a normal relationship to the vena cava, is the treatment of choice.

Atresia of the Ureter

This occurs at the ureteric orifice of the bladder. The atresia may cause back pressure effects on the kidney (Fig. 15-15), a tendency to stone formation, and urinary infection. If the atresia is producing symptoms, surgical enlargement of the orifice is required.

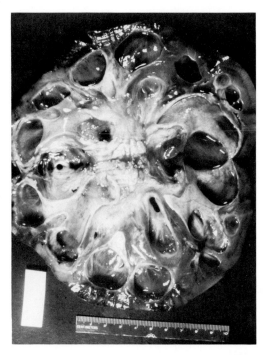

Fig. 15-15. Specimen of hydronephrotic kidney caused by congenital obstruction of lower end of ureter. Shows enlarged kidney with grossly dilated calyces. The renal cortex is thinned and atrophic. (Courtesy of Dr. H. Miller.)

Bladder

Exstrophy of the Bladder (Ectopia Vesicae)

This occurs three times more commonly in males than females. The posterior bladder wall protrudes through a defect in the anterior abdominal wall below the umbilicus (Figs. 15-16 & 15-17). The ureteric orifices are clearly discernible. In the male, there is complete epispadias (see Chap. 16), the scrotum is wide and shallow, and unilateral or bilateral undescended testes are common. In the female, the clitoris is bifid and the labia are widely separated anteriorly. In both sexes, there is separation of both pubic bones at the symphysis.

The condition is caused by a failure of the embryonic mesenchyme to invade the embry-

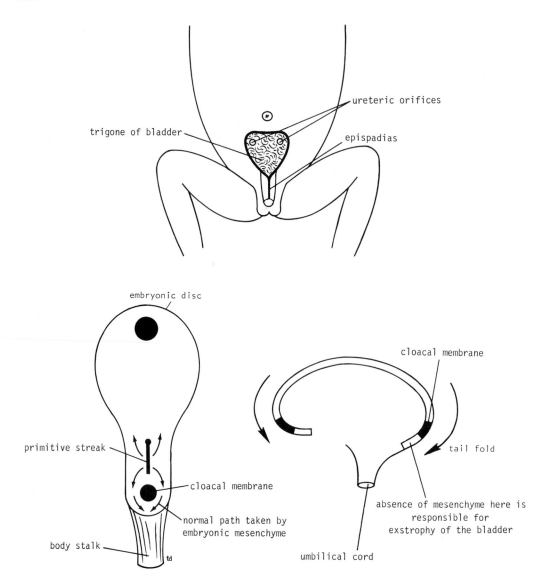

Fig. 15-16. Exstrophy of the bladder and the basis for its occurrence.

onic disc caudal to the cloacal membrane (Fig. 15-16). It will be remembered that this area bends forward with the tail fold and ultimately forms the anterior abdominal wall between the umbilicus and the cloacal membrane. The absence of intervening mesenchyme between the ectoderm and entoderm produces an unstable state which is followed by breakdown of this area in the same way as

occurs normally in the cloacal membrane. On each side of the ventral defect, the somatopleuric mesoderm from the thoracic somites grows in normally. The disorganization of the growth processes in this region leads to separation of the pubes and anomalies of development of the penis and clitoris.

Because of the urinary incontinence and the almost certain occurrence of ascending

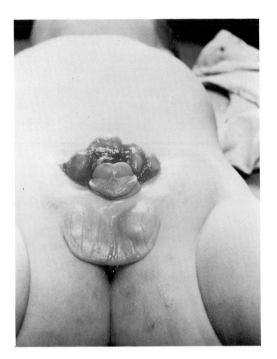

Fig. 15-17. Exstrophy of bladder with complete epispadias. Shows posterior wall of bladder protruding through defect in the anterior abdominal wall below the umbilicus. (Courtesy of Dr. H. Miller.)

urinary infection, surgical reconstruction of the bladder is attempted. Excision of the bladder and transplantation of the ureters into the gut is another method of treatment.

Patent Urachus

In this condition the allantois fails to become obliterated and a fistula persists, connecting the apex of the bladder to the umbilicus. If this should occur in a male child with congenital valvular obstruction of the prostatic urethra, urine starts to drain through the umbilicus soon after birth. In others it may remain undetected throughout life or may appear in the male in old age, when an enlarged prostate obstructs the urethra. Surgical removal of the patent urachus and ligation of the apex of the bladder is the treatment of choice.

Urethra

Congenital anomalies of the urethra will be considered following the discussion of the development of the genital system.

Clinical Problems
Answers on page 445

1. While investigating a 6-year-old boy for multiple congenital defects, it was noted following urography that he did not possess a right kidney. Is this a common congenital anomaly? Is the right ureter likely to be present in this case? Is the left kidney likely to be normal? How can you explain this condition embryologically? What is the prognosis?

2. Following a difficult birth a male child was found to have a greatly enlarged abdomen. On palpation a movable swelling could be felt in each loin. Within 2 days, signs and symptoms of renal dysfunction tem both kidneys were found to be very developed and the child died. At postmor-

much enlarged and on section showed multiple cysts occupying the medulla as well as the cortex. Section of the liver revealed multiple biliary cysts. What is the diagnosis? How can you explain this condition embryologically?

3. A 35-year-old man was seen by his physician because he had hematuria. On questioning, the patient stated that on several occasions he had experienced pain in one or the other of his loins. This pain was in the form of a dull ache which passed off after a few days. On physical examination both kidneys were found to be enlarged and lobulated. An x-ray film taken following an intravenous injection of radiopaque

dye, showed that the kidney pelves on both sides were compressed and the calyces were separated and elongated. Renal function tests revealed a diminution in total renal function. What is the diagnosis? How would you treat this condition? What is the prognosis?

4. A 40-year-old woman was examined by her physician because for 6 months she had been experiencing an aching pain in the umbilical region, which sometimes radiated to both lumbar regions. She also complained of frequency of micturition. There was no history of hematuria or difficulty in micturition. On physical examination, neither kidney could be felt in the costolumbar angle. Fortunately the patient was thin, and on the right side, a firm swelling, which was not mobile, could be felt in the lower lumbar region. An intravenous pyelogram showed that both kidneys were lower in position than normal and much nearer the vertebral column than normal. The downward and medial course of the lower calyces was very obvious. What is the diagnosis? How can you explain this condition on embryological grounds? How would you treat this condition?

5. If a patient is found to have an aberrant renal artery, is this likely to cause any ill effects? If so, why? How can you explain the presence of an aberrant renal artery?

6. A 13-year-old boy was taken to a pediatrician because he had a 3-month history of vague colicky abdominal pain which he sometimes felt in the left renal region or in the anterior abdominal region. Recently, he had had bouts of fever with shivering attacks. On physical examination nothing abnormal was discovered in the right renal region. On the left side of the abdomen a mass was felt which descended on inspiration. An intravenous pyelogram revealed a normal kidney on the right side. On the left side there was poor concentration of the radiopaque material; the renal pelvis and the upper renal calyces were greatly dilated. Close examination showed the presence of two left ureters. Urinalysis revealed bacteriuria and pyuria. What is the diagnosis? How would you treat such a patient? How would you explain this condition from an embryological point of view?

7. A 5-year-old girl underwent a complete urological examination because she had signs and symptoms suggestive of a chronic urinary infection. Following an intravenous pyelogram she was seen to have bilateral megalo-ureters. Can you explain this condition? What is the treatment?

8. Following the birth of a baby boy, a moist, red, protruding area was noted on the lower part of his anterior abdominal wall above the symphysis pubis. On closer examination, jets of urine could be seen discharging through the upper lateral corners of the red protruding area. The skin was seen to be continuous with the margins of this red area. The child had epispadias and bilateral undescended testes. X-ray examination of the lower abdominal area showed separation of the symphysis pubis. What is the diagnosis? How might you explain the embryological cause for this condition? What is the treatment?

9. On physical examination of a 6-year-old boy, a large intra-abdominal mass was found in the midline just above the symphysis pubis. The mass was firm in consistency and relatively fixed. It measured about 4 inches (10 cm) in diameter and was tender on palpation. At operation a large cyst was found which was attached above to the umbilicus and below to the apex of the bladder. What is the diagnosis? How can you explain the presence of this cyst?

REFERENCES

Baxter, T. J. Cysts Arising in the Renal Tubules. *Arch. Dis. Child.* 40:464, 1965.

Begg, R. C. The Urachus: Its Anatomy, Histology and Development. *J. Anat.* 64:170, 1930.

Davidson, W. M., and Ross, G. I. M. Bilateral Absence of Kidneys and Related Congenital Anomalies. *J. Path. Bact.* 68:459, 1954.

Eagle, J. F., and Barrett, G. S. Congenital Deficiency of Abdominal Musculature with Associated Genitourinary Abnormalities: A Syndrome. *Pediatrics* 6:721, 1950.

Fergusson, J. D. Observations on Familial Polycystic Disease of the Kidney. *Proc. Roy. Soc. Med.* 42:806, 1949.

Fraser, E. A. The Development of the Vertebrate Excretory System. *Biol. Rev.* 25:159, 1950.

Frazer, J. E. The Terminal Part of the Wolffian Duct. *J. Anat.* 69:455, 1935.

Glenister, T. W. A Correlation of the Normal and Abnormal Development of the Penile Urethra and of the Infra-Umbilical Abdominal Wall. *Brit. J. Urol.* 30:117, 1958.

Gordon-Taylor, G. On Horseshoes and Horseshoe Kidneys, Concave Downwards. *Brit. J. Urol.* 8:112, 1936.

Gruenwald, P. The Normal Changes in the Position of the Embryonic Kidney. *Anat. Rec.* 85:163, 1943.

Gyllensten, L. Contributions to Embryology of the Urinary Bladder: Development of Definitive Relations Between Openings of the Wolffian Ducts and Ureters. *Acta Anat.* (Basel) 7:305, 1949.

Hamilton, W. J., Boyd, J. D., and Mossman, H. W. *Human Embryology,* 3d ed. Williams & Wilkins, Baltimore, 1962.

Heggo, O., and Natvig, J. B. Microdissection Studies of Structural Changes in Cystic Disease of the Kidneys. *Lancet* 2:616, 1963.

Johnston, J. H. Posterior Urethral Valves: An Operative Technic Using an Electric Auriscope. *J. Pediat. Surg.* 1:583, 1966.

Lambert, P. P. Polycystic Disease of the Kidney. *Arch. Path.* (Chicago) 44:34, 1947.

Lattimer, J. K. Congenital Deficiency of the Abdominal Musculature with Associated Genitourinary Anomalies: A Report of 22 Cases. *J. Urol.* 79:343, 1958.

Lattimer, J. K., and Smith, M. J. V. Exstrophy Closure; A Follow-Up of 70 Cases. *J. Urol.* 95:356, 1966.

Mahoney, P. J., and Ennis, D. Congenital Patent Urachus. *New Eng. J. Med.* 215:193, 1936.

Maloney, P. K., Gleason, D. M., and Lattimer, J. K. Ureteral Physiology and Exstrophy of the Bladder. *J. Urol.* 93:588, 1965.

Marshall, V. F., and Muecke, E. C. Variations in Exstrophy of the Bladder. *J. Urol.* 88:766, 1962.

Metrick, S., Browne, R. H., and Rosenblum, A. Congenital Absence of the Abdominal Musculature and Associated Anomalies. *Pediatrics* 19:1043, 1957.

Nesbit, R. M., McDonald, H. P., and Busby, S. Obstructing Valves in Female Urethra. *J. Urol.* 91:79, 1964.

Norris, R. F., and Herman, L. Pathogenesis of Polycystic Kidneys. *J. Urol.* 46:147, 1941.

Nunn, I. N., and Stephens, F. D. *Congenital Malformations of the Rectum, Anus and Genito-Urinary Tracts.* Livingstone, Edinburgh, 1963.

Osathanondh, V., and Potter, E. L. Pathogenesis of Polycystic Kidneys. *Arch. Path.* (Chicago) 77:459, 1964.

Pathiak, I. G., and Williams, D. I. Multicystic and Cystic Dysplastic Kidneys. *Brit. J. Urol.* 36:318, 1964.

Paul, M., and Kanagasuntheram, R. The Congenital Anomalies of the Lower Urinary Tract. *Brit. J. Urol.* 28:64, 1956.

Potter, E. L. *Pathology of the Fetus and the Infant,* 2d ed. Year Book, Chicago, 1961.

Shikinami, J. Detailed Form of the Wolffian Body in Human Embryos of the First Eight Weeks. *Contrib. Embryol.* 18:49, 1926.

Stephens, F. D. *Congenital Malformations of Rectum, Anus and Genito-Urinary Tract.* Livingstone, Edinburgh, 1963.

Torrey, T. W. The Early Development of the Human Nephros. *Contrib. Embryol.* 35:175, 1954.

Wells, L. J., and Bell, E. T. Functioning of the Fetal Kidney as Reflected by Stillborn Infants with Hydroureter and Hydronephrosis. *Arch. Path.* (Chicago) 42:274, 1946.

Williams, D. I., and Eckstein, H. B. Obstructive Valves in the Posterior Urethra. *J. Urol.* 93:236, 1965.

DEVELOPMENT

Formation of the Gonads

The sex of the embryo is determined genetically at the time of fertilization and depends on the presence or absence of the Y chromosome in the fertilizing sperm. The *primordial sex cells* are first seen in the wall of the yolk sac close to the allantois very early in development. With the formation of the body folds, this part of the yolk sac is taken into the embryo and forms the hindgut. Later these cells migrate via the dorsal mesentery and, by the sixth week, they come to lie beneath the coelomic epithelium on the medial side of the mesonephros (Fig. 16-1). The presence of the primordial sex cells beneath the coelomic epithelium stimulates the epithelial cells to multiply, and cords of epithelial cells now grow down into the underlying mesenchyme. The cords of cells are called *sex cords,* and they come to surround the primordial sex cells, maintaining their connection with the surface epithelium. The proliferation of cells has resulted in the formation of a ridge on the medial side of the mesonephros called the *genital ridge*. At this stage it is not possible to differentiate between the male and female gonad.

Testis

During the seventh week of development, the sex cords become separated from the coelomic epithelium by the proliferation of the mesenchyme (Fig. 16-2). The newly formed mesenchyme now condenses to form a dense fibrous layer, the *tunica albuginea*. During the fourth month, the sex cords become U-shaped and form the *seminiferous tubules*. The free ends of the tubules form the *straight tubules,* which join one another in the mediastinum testis to form the *rete testis*. The primordial sex cells in the seminiferous tubules form the *spermatogonia,* and the sex cord cells form the *cells of Sertoli*. The mesenchyme in the developing gonad forms the connective tissue and fibrous septa. The *interstitial cells* are also formed from mesenchyme. The rete testis becomes canalized, and the tubules extend into the mesonephric tissue, where they join the remnants of the mesonephric tubules; the latter tubules become the *efferent ductules* of the testis. The *duct of the epididymis,* the *vas deferens,* the *seminal vesicle,* and the *ejaculatory duct* are formed from the mesonephric duct (Fig. 16-2). It should be noted that the seminiferous tubules are in fact solid cords until puberty,

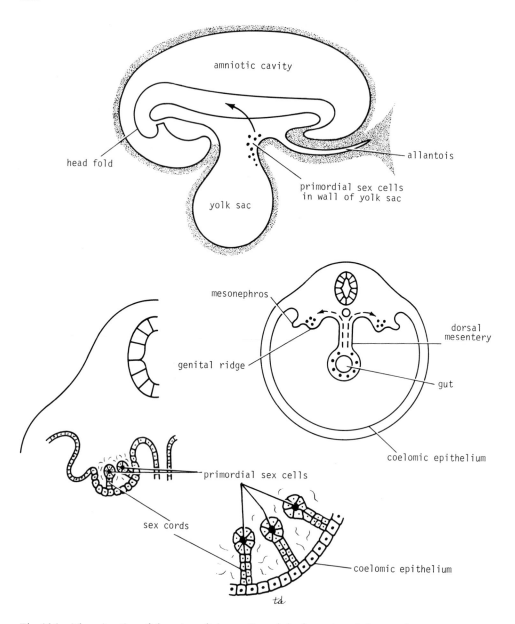

Fig. 16-1.   The migration of the primordial sex cells and the formation of the gonad.

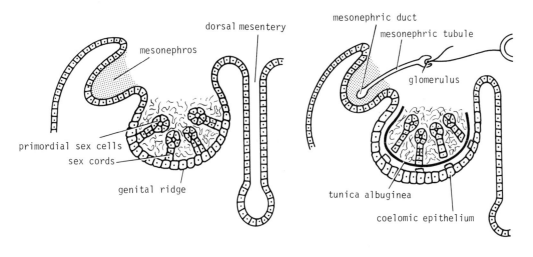

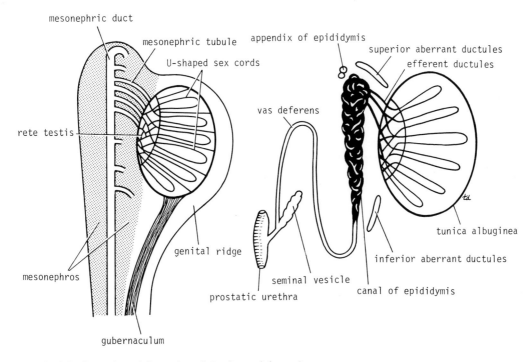

Fig. 16-2.   The formation of the testis and the ducts of the testis.

when, as the result of stimulation by the pituitary gonadotropic hormone, the spermatogonia start to proliferate, the Sertoli cells increase in size, and the tubules acquire a lumen.

Ovary

The female gonad differentiates later than that of the male. The sex cords containing groups of primordial germ cells become broken up into irregular cell clusters by the proliferating mesenchyme (Fig. 16-3). The mesenchyme, however, does not form a thick tunica albuginea, as it does in the male. The primordial germ cells differentiate into *oogonia,* and by the third month they start to undergo a number of mitotic divisions within the cortex of the ovary to form *primary oocytes.* These primary oocytes become surrounded by a single layer of cells derived from the sex cords, called the *granulosa cells.* A *primordial follicle* has now been formed. Many of the primordial follicles degenerate, and some authorities believe that a secondary ingrowth of sex cords takes place from the coelomic epithelium. These sex cord cells again become associated with preexisting primordial germ cells, and additional primordial follicles are formed. The mesenchyme that surrounds the follicles provides the ovarian stroma.

Uterine Tubes, Uterus, and Vagina

Paramesonephric Ducts (Müllerian Ducts)

The paramesonephric ducts appear on the posterior abdominal wall of a 6-week-old embryo. They commence as an invagination of coelomic epithelium into the underlying mesenchyme on the lateral side of the mesonephros (Fig. 16-4). The cranial end of the groove remains as the abdominal *ostium* of the uterine tube and later develops *fimbriae.* The caudal end of the invagination forms a solid bud of cells that grow caudally lateral to the mesonephric duct. On reaching the pelvic region, the paramesonephric duct crosses the mesonephric duct ventrally to reach its medial side. The paramesonephric ducts continue to grow caudally. They now lie close to each other in the midplane, and they fuse to form a solid bud (Fig. 16-4). By the ninth week of development, the caudal tip of the bud reaches the posterior wall of the urogenital sinus. It should be noted that, as the paramesonephric ducts descend through the pelvis anterior to the developing rectum and behind the primitive bladder, they pull toward the midline a transverse fold of coelomic epithelium and underlying mesenchyme on each side, which, when the ducts fuse, forms the *broad ligament.*

Each paramesonephric duct may be divided into three regions: (1) a cranial vertical part, which will form the upper portion of the uterine tube, (2) a middle horizontal part, which will form the lower portion of the uterine tube, and (3) a caudal vertical part, which fuses with its fellow of the opposite side to form a common tube from which will develop the uterus and possibly part of the vagina.

Uterine Tube

The uterine tube on each side is formed from the cranial vertical and middle horizontal parts of the paramesonephric duct (Fig. 16-4). During the fourth and fifth months, marked growth activity is seen to occur in the uterine tube. The tube elongates and becomes coiled. Differentiation of the muscle and mucous membrane takes place, the *fimbriae* develop, and the *infundibulum, ampulla,* and *isthmus* are identifiable.

Uterus

The uterus is derived from the fused caudal vertical parts of the paramesonephric ducts (Fig. 16-4), and the site of their angular junction becomes a convex dome and forms the *fundus.* The fusion between the ducts is at

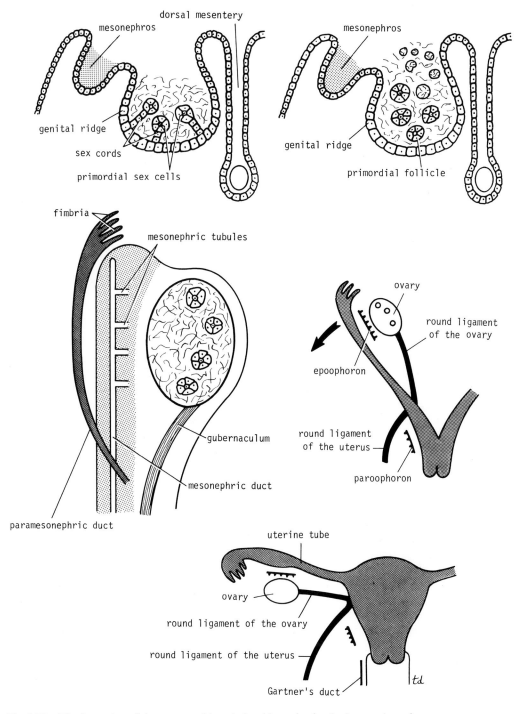

Fig. 16-3. The formation of the ovary and its relationship to the developing uterine tube.

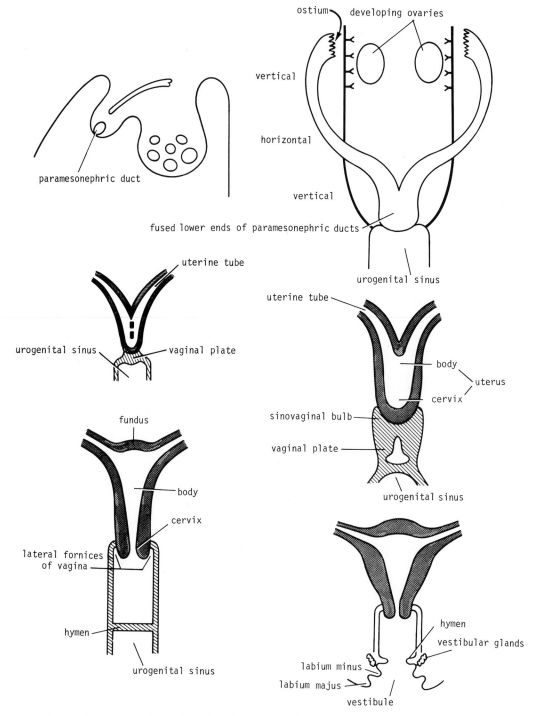

Fig. 16-4. The formation of the uterine tubes, the uterus, and the vagina.

first incomplete, a septum persisting between the lumina. Later the septum disappears so that a single cavity remains. The upper part of the cavity forms the lumen of the *body* and *cervix* of the uterus. The myometrium is formed from the surrounding mesenchyme.

Vagina

Two possible theories exist for the formation of the vagina. The first theory proposes that the upper four-fifths of the vagina are formed from the fused lower ends of the paramesonephric ducts and the lower fifth is of urogenital sinus origin. The second theory, which is the most recent one and the one that is largely accepted, is that the fused lower ends of the paramesonephric ducts form the body and cervix of the uterus only and the vagina is formed from the wall of the urogenital sinus (Fig. 16-4). Once the solid end of the fused paramesonephric ducts reaches the posterior wall of the urogenital sinus, two outgrowths occur from the sinus, called the *sinovaginal bulbs*. The cells of the sinovaginal bulbs rapidly proliferate and form a plate, the *vaginal plate*. By continued cellular proliferation, the vaginal plate extends around the solid end of the fused paramesonephric ducts. At the eleventh week of development, a lumen appears in the caudal end of the vaginal plate. Meanwhile the plate is thickening and elongating. At the fifth month, the plate is completely canalized and the vaginal fornices are formed.

The *hymen* is developed from the distal part of the vaginal plate and the wall of the urogenital sinus (Fig. 16-4).

Fate of the Paramesonephric Ducts in the Male

Degeneration of the ducts occurs during the third month, leaving behind small portions of the upper and lower ends. The cranial end persists as the *appendix of the testis*, while the caudal end forms the *prostatic utricle* (Fig. 16-5).

Summary of the Fate of the Anterior Portion of the Cloaca in Both Sexes

The anterior portion of the entodermal cloaca may be divided into an upper part, the *primitive bladder,* and a lower part, the *urogenital sinus,* by the openings of the caudal ends of the mesonephric ducts.

Primitive Bladder

In the male this structure forms the *bladder* and the *prostatic urethra* as far distally as the openings of the ejaculatory ducts. In the female it forms the *bladder* and the proximal two-thirds of the *urethra*. In both sexes the trigone of the bladder is mesodermal in origin and derived originally from the caudal ends of the mesonephric ducts. In the male the same mesodermal tissue forms the proximal part of the prostatic urethra and in the female the proximal two-thirds of the urethra.

Urogenital Sinus

In the male this forms the *lower part of the prostatic urethra*, the *membranous urethra*, and the greater part of the penile urethra. A series of buds grow into the surrounding mesenchyme from the prostatic urethra and form the *prostate gland*. A pair of solid buds arise from the membranous urethra to form the *bulbo-urethral glands*.

In the female the urogenital sinus forms the *vagina* and the *lower end of the urethra*. A number of entodermal buds grow out from the lower end of the urethra and form the *para-urethral glands*. The lower end of the urogenital sinus opens on the surface as a cleft, the *vestibule*, into which the vagina and urethra open. The *greater vestibular glands*

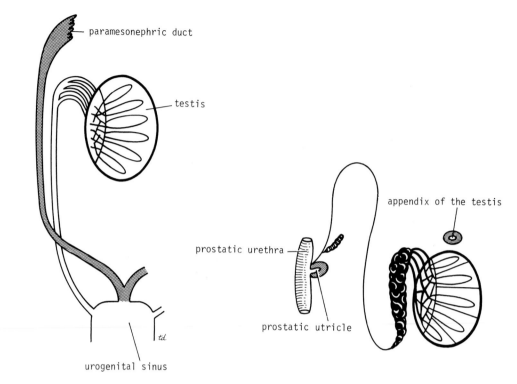

Fig. 16-5. The fate of the paramesonephric ducts in the male.

arise from the vestibule as entodermal outgrowths.

External Genitalia

Early in development, the embryonic mesenchyme arising from the primitive streak grows around the cloacal membrane and causes the overlying ectoderm to be raised up to form three swellings. One swelling occurs between the cloacal membrane and the umbilical cord in the midline and is called the *genital tubercle* (Fig. 16-6). A swelling appears on each side of the membrane, called the *genital fold*. At the seventh week, the genital tubercle elongates to form the *phallus* and develops an expanded end, the *glans*. The anterior part of the cloacal membrane, the *urogenital membrane,* now ruptures so that the urogenital sinus opens onto the surface. The entodermal cells of the urogenital sinus proliferate and grow into the root of the phallus, forming a *urethral plate*. Meanwhile a second pair of lateral swellings appear lateral to the genital folds, called the *genital swellings*. At this stage of development, the genitalia of the two sexes are identical.

Male

The phallus now rapidly elongates and pulls the genital folds anteriorly onto its ventral surface so that they form the lateral edges of a groove, the *urethral groove* (Figs. 16-6 & 16-7). The floor of the groove is formed by the entodermal *urethral plate*. The two genital folds start to fuse together and unite progressively along the shaft of the phallus in the direction of the *glans penis*. In this manner, the penile part of the urethra is formed, but

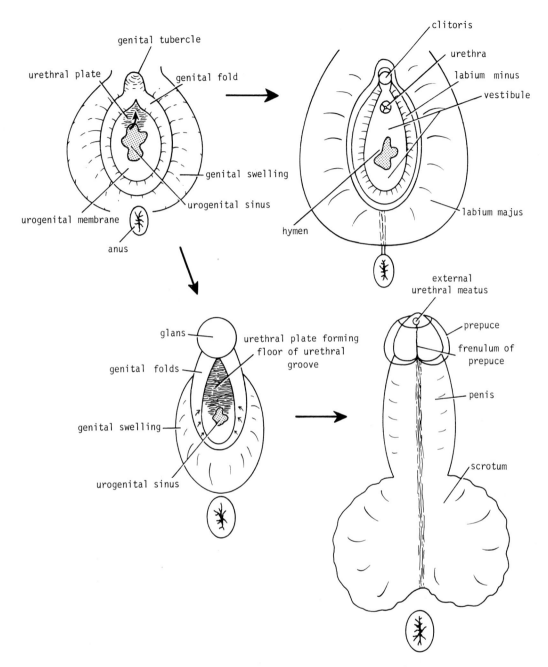

Fig. 16-6. The development of the external genitalia in the female and in the male.

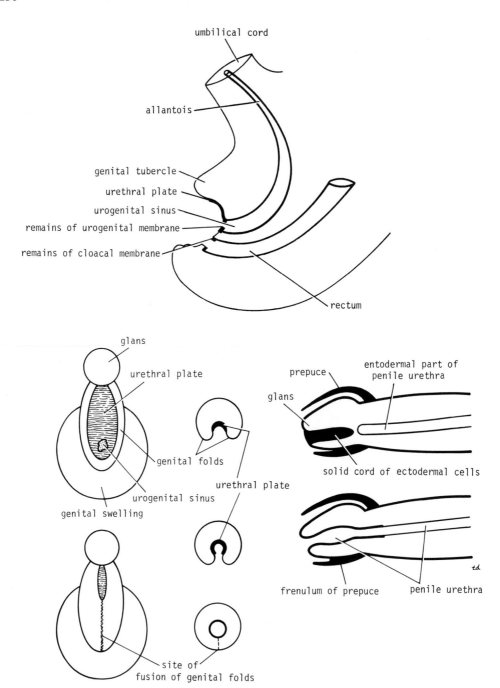

Fig. 16-7. The development of the penile portion of the male urethra.

at this stage it only extends to the root of the glans. During the fourth month, a bud of ectodermal cells from the tip of the glans grows into the substance of the glans and joins the entodermal cells lining the penile urethra. This cord of cells later becomes canalized so that the penile urethra opens at the tip of the glans.

The *prepuce* or *foreskin* is formed from a fold of skin at the base of the glans (Figs. 16-6 & 16-7). This grows over and surrounds the glans as far as the tip. The prepuce now fuses with the skin of the glans. Later, clefts appear in the plane of fusion and the prepuce becomes free once again. The fold of skin remains tethered to the ventral aspect of the root of the glans by the *frenulum*. The erectile tissue, the *corpus spongiosum,* and the *corpora cavernosa* develop within the mesenchymal core of the penis.

Female

The changes in the female are less extensive than those in the male. The phallus becomes bent and forms the *clitoris* (Fig. 16-6). The genital folds do not fuse to form the urethra, as in the male, but develop into the *labia minora*. The genital swellings enlarge to form the *labia majora*. The lower part of the urogenital sinus forms the *vestibule* (Fig. 16-6).

Descent of the Testis

The testis originates within the abdomen and is first seen as a ridge on the dorsal wall of the coelomic cavity, called the *genital ridge* (Fig. 16-2). This is situated on the medial side of the atrophying mesonephros and extends caudally from the diaphragm. Attached to the caudal end of the gonad is a band of mesenchyme that extends to the inguinal region, where it is continuous with the mesenchyme in the area that will form the inguinal canal. Beyond this area, the mesenchyme is continuous with that of the genital swell-ing. This continuous column of mesenchyme extending from the testis to the genital swell-ing is called the *gubernaculum testis* (Figs. 16-2 & 16-8). By the third month of fetal life, the testis has reached a position close to the future deep inguinal ring; the descent of the testis is a result mainly of the differential growth of the trunk rather than its active migration.

Meanwhile the mesenchyme of the inferior part of the anterior abdominal wall is invaded by a diverticulum of coelomic epithelium, the *processus vaginalis* (Fig. 16-8). The processus vaginalis, which is in fact a peritoneal sac, follows the path of the gubernaculum and lies ventral or anterior to it. As the processus passes through the layers of the abdominal wall into the genital swelling, it carries with it a covering derived from each of the layers. In this manner, the *inguinal canal* is formed and the processus acquires the following coats: (1) the *internal spermatic fascia,* derived from the *fascia transversalis;* (2) the *cremasteric fascia,* derived from the *internal oblique muscle* of the abdominal wall; and (3) the *external spermatic fascia,* derived from the *external oblique muscle* of the abdominal wall (Fig. 16-8).

During the seventh month, the testis passes through the inguinal canal following the gubernaculum and lying behind (dorsal to) the processus vaginalis. It takes up its final position in the genital swelling, which has now fused with the swelling of the opposite side to form the *scrotum,* by the end of the eighth month. As this process is taking place, the testicular blood and lymphatic vessels are actively growing to enable the organ to move inferiorly. It is important to remember that these vessels retain their initial origins and terminations high up on the posterior abdominal wall.

On reaching the scrotum, the testis lies posterior to the processus vaginalis and bulges forward into its cavity. Before birth,

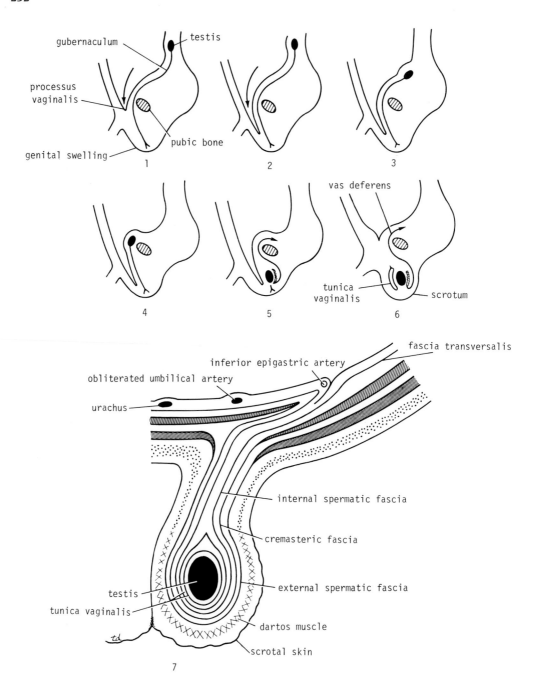

Fig. 16-8. The descent of the testis and the formation of the inguinal canal.

the connection between the expanded lower end of the processus and the peritoneal cavity becomes obliterated, and the now-isolated sac is known as the *tunica vaginalis*. The visceral layer of the tunica vaginalis is closely applied to the anterior and lateral surfaces of the testis and extends posteriorly to cover the sides of the epididymis.

As a result of the testicular descent, the rapidly elongating vas deferens becomes looped over the ureter and passes around the lateral border of the *inferior epigastric artery* before entering the inguinal canal and joining the tail of the epididymis in the scrotum.

The Mechanism of Testicular Descent

It is now generally agreed that the initial change in position of the testis from one high up on the posterior abdominal wall to the inguinal region is brought about by differential growth of the posterior abdominal wall and related structures rather than by active migration. During this period, the gubernaculum does *not* elongate correspondingly and it does *not shorten*.

The final descent of the testis through the inguinal canal to the scrotum is accompanied by shortening and thickening of the gubernaculum. The exact role of the gubernaculum in the descent of the testis is still unknown. Apart from keeping open the path of descent, which is an important function, it does not appear to exert an active role in the mechanism. It certainly *does not pull* the testis down into the scrotum. It is probable that the mechanism of descent, whatever this might be, is under hormonal control. The administration of *gonadotropins* has been shown to induce descent of the testes in a number of cases of *cryptorchidism*.

It is important that at least one testis should descend into the scrotum; otherwise the person will be sterile. The higher temperature existing in the abdominal cavity and in the inguinal canal causes irreversible destructive changes in the seminiferous tubules of the testis.

Descent of the Ovary

As in the male, the caudal end of the developing ovary is connected to the genital swelling by a column of mesenchyme, the *gubernaculum* (Fig. 16-3). As development proceeds, the gubernaculum becomes attached to the developing uterus at its junction with the uterine tube. The part of the gubernaculum that joins the ovary to the uterus becomes the *round ligament of the ovary*. That part which extends from the uterus through the inguinal canal becomes the *round ligament of the uterus*. A *processus vaginalis* is formed in the same manner as in the male, so that an inguinal canal is developed in the female. The processus becomes obliterated by the time of birth.

The ovaries descend to the pelvic brim during the third month. Later they take up their final position on the posterior surfaces of the broad ligament, where they are suspended by the *mesovarium*. The attachment of the round ligament of the ovary to the uterus prevents the extra-abdominal descent of the ovaries into the labia majora.

CONGENITAL ANOMALIES

Testis

Anterior Inversion

This condition is a common anomaly. The epididymis is situated anteriorly, and the testis and the tunica vaginalis posteriorly. No treatment is required, but the condition may cause confusion in the diagnosis of testicular diseases.

Polar Inversion

The testis lies inverted in the scrotum; this is a rare anomaly.

Imperfect Descent of the Testis

This condition may be divided as: (1) incomplete descent and (2) maldescent of the testis.

INCOMPLETE DESCENT. The testis may partially descend along the normal path but fails to reach the floor of the scrotum.

MALDESCENT. The testis descends outside its normal path and does not enter the scrotum.

INCOMPLETE DESCENT OF THE TESTIS. Scorer found that among 3,612 newborn boys, 97.3 percent of full-term infants and 79 percent of premature infants had both testes in the scrotum. Of those testes which were not in the scrotum at birth, some had decended within 1 month, others within 3 months, and a few took up to 9 months of age. Scorer came to the conclusion that if a testis does not reach the floor of the scrotum within 6 weeks of birth in a full-term infant and within 3 months in a premature infant, it remains permanently higher and smaller than normal. Incomplete descent occurs more commonly on the right side.

If a testis is left within the abdomen or in the inguinal canal, the higher temperatures found there will progressively retard its development. At puberty, the testis is softer and smaller than normal, and irreversible destructive changes have occurred in the seminiferous tubules. The production of testosterone by the interstitial cells of the testis occurs normally and, as a result, the accessory organs of reproduction begin to develop and the secondary male sex characteristics make their appearance.

The following varieties of incompletely descended testis may be recognized (Fig. 16-9): (1) *Abdominal:* the testis usually lies just above the deep inguinal ring and is extraperitoneal in position. (2) *Inguinal canal:* the testis lies within the inguinal canal and is extremely difficult to palpate. (3) *Superficial inguinal ring:* the testis has emerged from the inguinal canal and lies superficial to the external oblique muscle of the abdomen. In some cases it is possible to pull such a testis gently down to the floor of the scrotum. The testis, on being released, is immediately drawn up by the cremaster muscle to its original position at the superficial ring. (4) Such a testis is referred to as a *rectractile testis.* The latter variety require no treatment, since normal descent is usual by the time of puberty.

In view of the likelihood of sterility in bilateral cases (*cryptorchidism*) (Fig. 16-10), the increased susceptibility to damage and torsion, and the increased possibility of the development of malignant tumors, incompletely descended testes should be treated surgically and placed in the scrotum (Fig. 16-11). Only very rarely is hormone treatment recommended.

MALDESCENT OF THE TESTIS. Instead of descending by its normal path into the scrotum, the testis may be found at one of the following sites (Fig. 16-12): (1) Abdominal wall:

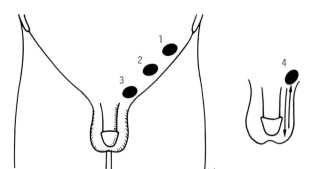

Fig. 16-9. The common sites of incomplete descent of the testis: (1) abdominal, (2) inguinal canal, (3) superficial inguinal ring, and (4) retractile testis.

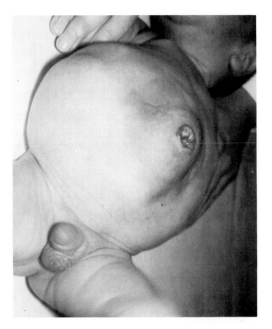

Fig. 16-10. An example of cryptorchidism. Both testes are situated within the abdominal cavity. Note the small size of the empty scrotum. (Courtesy of Dr. G. Avery.)

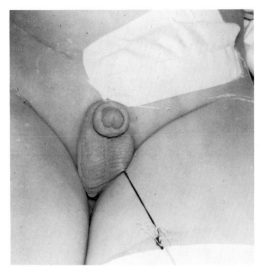

Fig. 16-11. Operative correction of left-sided incomplete descent of the testis. After mobilization of the testis within the inguinal canal, it is tethered to the floor of the scrotum by a black thread passing through the scrotal wall. (Courtesy of Dr. H. Miller.)

the testis lies beneath the superficial fascia and on the external oblique aponeurosis, usually above the superficial inguinal ring. (2) At the root of the penis. (3) In the perineum. (4) In the femoral triangle. Since the testis lies outside the abdomen, it usually develops normally. However, its relatively unprotected position makes it very liable to injury, and for this reason it should be treated surgically and, if possible, placed in the scrotum.

CAUSE OF IMPERFECT DESCENT OF THE TESTIS. Since the normal mechanism for the final descent of the testis is not fully understood, it is difficult to explain imperfect descent of the testis. It is possible that a maldescended testis is caused by the gubernaculum being malformed, or split, or involved in fibrous tissue (Fig. 16-13). Under these circumstances, the testis may be shunted off onto a side pathway during its descent so that it never reaches the scrotum.

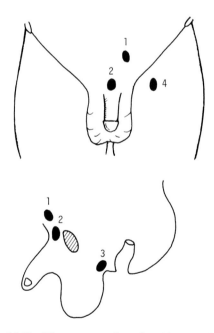

Fig. 16-12. The common sites of maldescent of the testis: (1) abdominal, (2) root of penis, (3) perineum, and (4) femoral triangle.

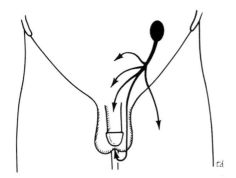

Fig. 16-13. A split gubernaculum. As the testis descends, it may be shunted onto one of the side pathways.

Hydrocele

This is a collection of fluid in the processus vaginalis (Figs. 16-14 & 16-15). Two forms may be considered to be developmental anomalies: (1) congenital hydrocele and (2) encysted hydrocele of the spermatic cord.

CONGENITAL HYDROCELE. In this condition the processus vaginalis remains in communication with the peritoneal cavity by a narrow channel, and peritoneal fluid drains into the processus.

ENCYSTED HYDROCELE OF THE SPERMATIC CORD. In this condition a small segment of the processus remains patent. Later, fluid accumulates in the segment and produces a cystic swelling in the spermatic cord (Fig. 16-12).

In the case of congenital hydrocele, the processus is divided surgically above the tunica vaginalis, and the part between the tunica and the peritoneal cavity is removed. The cyst may also be removed surgically.

Congenital Inguinal Hernia

This is herniation of the abdominal contents into a preformed sac that is a patent processus vaginalis. It differs from congenital hydrocele in that the neck of the processus is wide enough to allow passage of some of the abdominal contents (Figs. 16-14 & 16-16). It is sometimes associated with incomplete descent of the testis.

Normally, that part of the processus vaginalis between the tunica vaginalis and the peritoneal cavity becomes obliterated shortly before birth. This condition is much more common in males than in females. Surgery is the treatment of choice; the hernial contents are returned to the abdomen and the sac is removed.

Male Urethra

Meatal Stenosis

The external urinary meatus is normally the narrowest part of the male urethra, but occasionally the opening is excessively small and may cause back pressure effects on the entire urinary system. In severe cases, dilatation or enlargement of the orifice by incision is necessary.

Posterior Urethral Valves

The valves occur in the prostatic urethra and are situated just below the summit of the urethral crest (verumontanum) (Fig. 16-17). They consist of folds of mucous membrane which are attached to the side walls of the urethra, and between them the urethral lumen forms a narrow slit. Retrograde catheterization of the urethra presents no difficulty, but the valves come together during micturition and cause severe urinary obstruction with devastating back pressure effects on the bladder and both kidneys. The condition is believed to be caused by a failure of the mesonephric ducts to integrate normally with the developing urethral wall. The treatment is surgical removal of the valves.

Urethral Stenosis

This condition is less common than valvular obstruction and is caused by the persistence

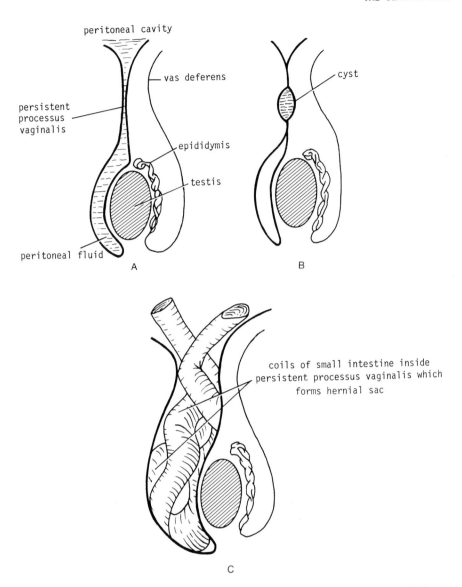

Fig. 16-14. (A) Congenital hydrocele, (B) encysted hydrocele of the spermatic cord, and (C) congenital inguinal hernia.

of a part of the *urogenital membrane* (anterior part of the cloacal membrane). In this condition, there is obstruction to retrograde catheterization as well as urination. Back pressure effects on the urinary system may be serious. The narrowing may be relieved by dilatation or the membrane destroyed by operation.

Hypospadias

This is the commonest congenital anomaly affecting the urethra. The external meatus is situated on the ventral or undersurface of the penis anywhere between the glans and the perineum. Five degrees of severity may occur (type 1 being the commonest): (1) glandu-

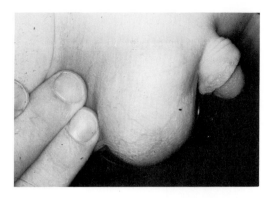

Fig. 16-15. Right-sided congenital hydrocele. (Courtesy of Dr. J. Randolph.)

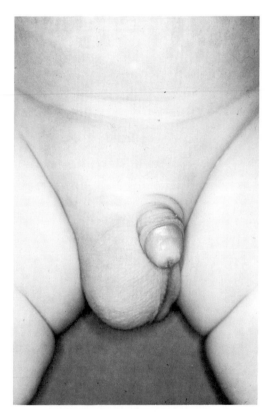

Fig. 16-16. Right-sided congenital indirect inguinal hernia. (Courtesy of Dr. J. Randolph.)

lar, (2) coronal, (3) penile, (4) penoscrotal, and (5) perineal (Figs. 16-18 & 16-19). In all except the first type, the penis is curved in a downward or ventral direction, a condition referred to as *chordee.*

Types 1 and 2 are caused by a failure of the bud of ectodermal cells from the tip of the glans to grow into the substance of the glans and join the entodermal cells lining the penile urethra.

Types 3, 4, and 5 are caused by a failure of the genital folds to unite on the undersurface of the developing penis and so convert the urethral groove into the penile urethra. Also, in the penoscrotal variety, the genital swellings fail to fuse completely, so that the meatal orifice occurs in the midline of the scrotum. Type 1 requires no treatment; for the remainder, plastic surgery is necessary.

Epispadias

This is a relatively rare condition and most commonly found in the male. In the male the external meatus is situated on the dorsal or upper surface of the penis between the glans and the anterior abdominal wall (Figs. 16-20 & 16-21). The most severe type is associated with exstrophy of the bladder (see Chap. 15). In the female the urethra is split dorsally and is associated with a double clitoris. In the mild forms, the child is continent; in the severe forms, the bladder sphincter and the sphincter urethrae may not be adequately developed, and the child will be incontinent. It is thought that epispadias is caused by a slight failure of the embryonic mesenchyme to invade the embryonic disc caudal to the cloacal membrane (see exstrophy of bladder, p. 215). As a result, the inferior part of the anterior abdominal wall in the pubic area possesses no mesenchyme and breaks down along with the cloacal membrane so that the urogenital sinus opens onto the surface on the cranial aspect of the penis. A more extensive failure of the development of the mesenchyme would result in exstrophy of the

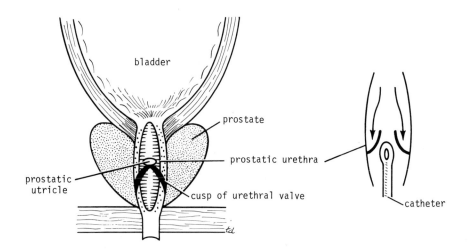

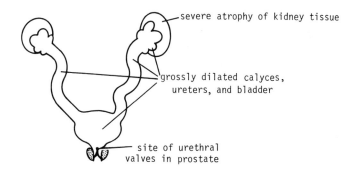

Fig. 16-17. The posterior urethral valves in the prostatic urethra, showing the oblique position of the valves below the verumontanum and the devastating back pressure effects on the bladder, ureters, and kidneys.

Fig. 16-18. The different types of hypospadias: (1) glandular, (2) coronal, (3) penile, (4) penoscrotal, and (5) perineal. Ventral flexion of the penis is also present (chordee).

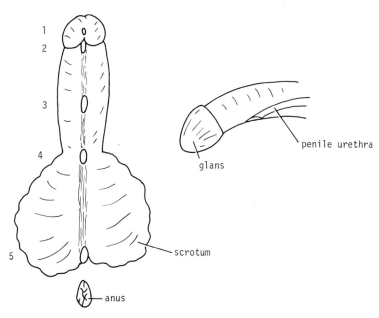

239

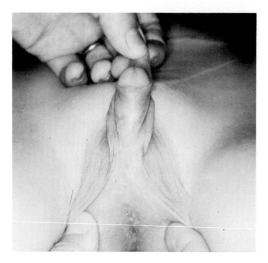

Fig. 16-19. Hypospadias. The urethral orifice is situated on the ventral surface of the root of the penis. (Courtesy of Dr. J. Randolph.)

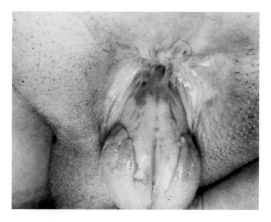

Fig. 16-21. Epispadias. Note that the external urethral meatus is situated between the root of the penis and the anterior abdominal wall. (Courtesy of Dr. H. Miller.)

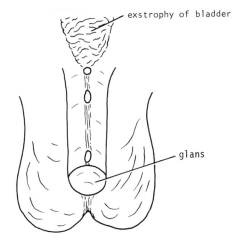

Fig. 16-20. The different types of epispadias.

bladder in addition to epispadias. Plastic surgery is the required treatment.

Ovary

Ovarian Dysgenesis

Complete failure of both ovaries to develop is found in *Turner's syndrome.* The classic features of this syndrome are webbed neck, short stocky build, increased carrying angle of the elbows, lack of secondary sex characteristics, and amenorrhea.

Accessory Ovarian Tissue

This is sometimes found along the course of migration of the gonad.

Imperfect Descent of the Ovary

The ovary may fail to descend into the pelvis or very rarely may be drawn downward with the round ligament of the uterus into the inguinal canal or even into the labium majus.

Uterus

Agenesis of the Uterus

This condition is rare and is caused by a failure of the paramesonephric ducts to develop.

Rudimentary Uterus

This condition consists of a small mass of fibrous tissue without any cavity and is caused by underdevelopment of the fused lower ends of the paramesonephric ducts.

Infantile Uterus

In this condition, in the adult the uterus is much smaller than normal and resembles that present before puberty. Amenorrhea is present, but the vagina and ovaries may be normal.

Failure of Fusion of the Paramesonephric Ducts

In *uterus didelphys,* the uterus is duplicated with two bodies and two cervices. The two external orifices open into the vagina, which may also be double because of the presence of a median septum (Fig. 16-22).

In *uterus bicornis bicollis,* there is a complete septum through the uterus making two uterine cavities and two cervices. This may also be associated with a double vagina (Fig. 16-22).

In *uterus bicornis unicollis,* the ducts have incompletely fused so that there are two separate uterine bodies with one cervix (Fig. 16-22).

In *uterus unicornis,* one paramesonephric duct fails to develop, leaving one uterine tube and half of the body of the uterus. Occasionally a rudimentary horn may be present (Fig. 16-22).

In *uterus septus,* the upper part of the septum persists to a variable extent (Fig. 16-22).

In *uterus arcuatus,* there is a depressed fundus caused by a minor degree of imperfect fusion of the paramesonephric ducts (Fig. 16-22).

Clinically the main problems may be present when pregnancy occurs in a double uterus. Abortion is frequent and the non-pregnant half of the uterus may cause obstruction at labor.

Vagina

Vaginal Agenesis

The paramesonephric ducts fail to develop, causing an absence of the vagina, uterus, and uterine tubes. Plastic surgical construction of a vagina should be attempted.

Double Vagina

This is caused by incomplete canalization of the vaginal plate (Fig. 16-23). The vaginae may be completely separate or more commonly there is present a thin membranous septum, which completely or incompletely divides the vagina into two halves. This condition is frequently associated with severe degrees of uterine malfusion. Surgical division of the septum may be required.

Imperforate Vagina

This is caused by a failure of the cells to degenerate in the center of the vaginal plate (Fig. 16-23) and by a failure of the vaginal canal to open into the urogenital sinus.

Imperforate Hymen

This is caused by a failure of the cells of the lower part of the vaginal plate and the wall of the urogenital sinus to degenerate (Fig. 16-23).

The conditions of imperforate vagina and imperforate hymen lead to retention of the menstrual flow, a clinical condition called *hematocolpos.* Surgical incision of the obstruction, followed by dilatation, relieves the condition.

Cysts of the Mesonephric and Paramesonephric Remnants

Very occasionally cysts may arise in the following remnants (Fig. 16-24).

Mesonephric Origin

In the male the *superior and inferior aberrant ductules of the testis* and the *appendix of the epididymis* may be responsible.

In the female the *tubules* and the *ducts of the epoophoron* and *paraoophoron* may become cystic. *Gartner's duct* may be the origin of a cyst located alongside the vagina.

Paramesonephric Origin

In the male the *appendix of the testis* may become cystic. In the female the parameso-

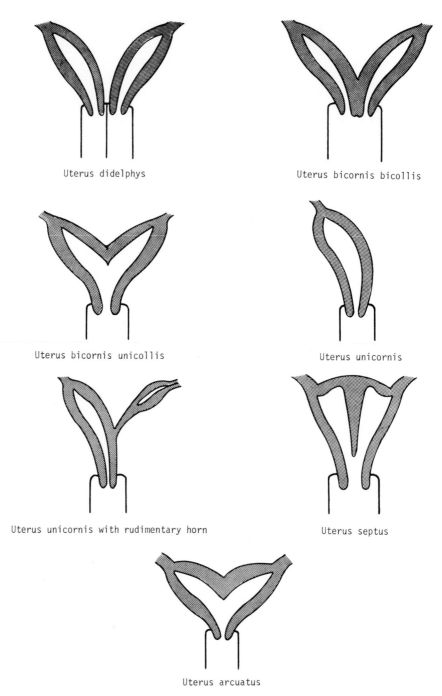

Fig. 16-22. The various types of anomalous uterine development.

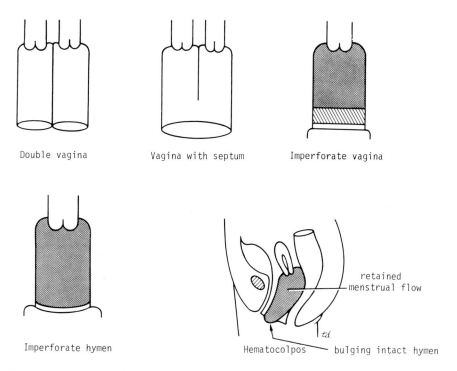

Double vagina   Vagina with septum   Imperforate vagina

Imperforate hymen   Hematocolpos   bulging intact hymen   retained menstrual flow

Fig. 16-23.   The various types of anomalous vaginal development.

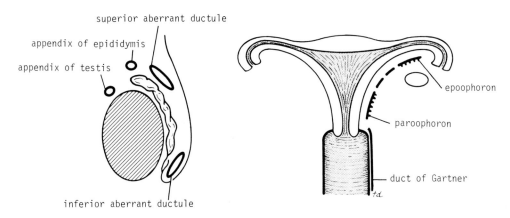

superior aberrant ductule

appendix of epididymis

appendix of testis

inferior aberrant ductule

epoophoron

paroophoron

duct of Gartner

Fig. 16-24.   Remnants of the mesonephric and paramesonephric systems in the male and female. In adult life these may become the sites of cyst formation.

nephric ducts form the uterine tubes and the uterus, and there are no vestigial remnants.

Hermaphroditism

The sex of the embryo is determined genetically at the time of fertilization, and it depends on the presence or absence of the Y chromosome in the fertilizing sperm (see Chap. 1). Certain sex deviations, however, occur; for example, a *true hermaphrodite* is an individual who possesses the gonads and external genitalia of both sexes. Such a condition has never been seen in man, but a few patients have been observed who possess both testicular and ovarian tissue.

Pseudohermaphroditism

This is a condition in which the individual has either a testis (male pseudohermaphrodite) or an ovary (female pseudohermaphrodite) and possesses external genitalia resembling the opposite sex. At birth the sex is often mistaken, and the mistake is only discovered at puberty. The discovery of the darkly staining *sex chromatin body* (one of the two X chromosomes) against the nuclear membrane in female cells has made the recognition of the true sex of an individual a comparatively simple matter.

Adrenogenital Syndrome

The congenital form of this syndrome is the result of an inborn error of metabolism that is determined by an autosomal recessive gene. There is an absence of the enzyme *C-21-hydroxylase,* which is necessary for the production of hydrocortisone. The lack of hydrocortisone results in the pituitary's secreting excess ACTH, thereby causing hypertrophy and hyperplasia of the adrenal cortex, and overproduction of adrenal androgens. In the female pseudohermaphroditism results; the clitoris hypertrophies (Fig.

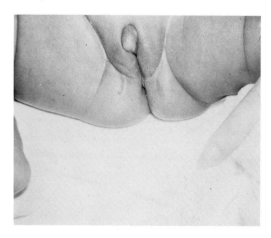

Fig. 16-25. Adrenogenital syndrome in the female showing hypertrophy of the clitoris and enlargement of the labia majora; the latter are not fused in this case. (Courtesy of Dr. G. Avery.)

16-25) and the labia majora fuse to resemble a scrotum. The vaginal orifice may or may not be present, but the upper parts of the vagina, the uterus, and the ovaries are normal. In the male the external genitalia look normal at birth, but between the ages of 1 and 5 years the penis enlarges, pubic hair develops, the child becomes very muscular, and the voice deepens. The testicles remain infantile. During the neonatal period, adrenal failure may develop in both sexes. The excretion of 17-ketosteroids in the urine is raised.

In both sexes continuous cortisone therapy is required for life, and in the female plastic reconstruction of the labia and vagina may be necessary.

Testicular Feminization Syndrome

This is a form of male pseudohermaphroditism in which the external genitalia are those of a normal female, but the gonads are testes and are frequently found in the inguinal canal. The condition is rare and inherited, and it is determined by a recessive gene. The child is brought up as a girl until puberty, when amenorrhea is discovered.

Clinical Problems
Answers on page 447

1. An 18-year-old male was having a physical examination prior to entering the army when the physician noted the presence of an abnormal intrascrotal mass in front of the left testis. On the right side, the vas deferens, epididymis, and testis were normal. On the left side, the vas deferens and testis felt normal, but the epididymis could not be palpated behind the testis. Using your knowledge of anatomy and embryology, can you explain the structure present in front of the left testis? Is this a common congenital anomaly?

2. A mother brought her 3-month-old son to a pediatrician because she had noticed that the right testis was not in the scrotum. This fact had been called to her attention while bathing her baby, when she noted that the right side of the scrotum looked collapsed and empty. Physical examination confirmed the mother's observations. A small, firm ovoid swelling was, however, palpated about halfway along the right inguinal canal. What is your diagnosis? What is the cause of this condition? How would you treat this patient?

3. An 8-year-old boy was examined by a pediatrician and found to have a small, firm ovoid swelling in his perineum between the anus and the scrotum. On examination of the scrotum the left testis was found to be normal in size and position; however, there was no evidence of a testis in the right side of the scrotum. What is the diagnosis? How would you explain this condition? Is surgical treatment required?

4. A 2-year-old boy was taken to a pediatrician because his mother had noticed a swelling of the right side of the scrotum. The swelling was noted to be larger at the end of the day and smaller the following morning. On examination of the child the right side of the scrotum was noted to be swollen, and the swelling enlarged slightly when the child cried. The swelling was situated anterior to the right testis and was oval in shape, fluctuant, and transilluminated. Both testes were normal and in their correct position within the scrotum. No inguinal hernia was present. What is the diagnosis? How would you explain the cause of this condition? How would you treat this patient?

5. In a 20-year-old man a swelling developed above the medial end of the right inguinal ligament. It was associated with a dull, aching pain, but it did not expand on coughing. On palpation, the swelling appeared to fluctuate, and on grasping the right testis through the scrotal wall and gently pulling it inferiorly, the swelling moved medially along the inguinal canal. What was the swelling? How can you explain the swelling, using your knowledge of embryology? Why did the swelling move with the testis? How would you treat this patient?

6. A 4-week-old boy was admitted to the hospital with a swelling in the right groin that extended down into the upper part of the scrotum. The mother reported that during the previous week the child had become fretful, had had an attack of screaming, which lasted for an hour, and showed loss of appetite. On examination it was found that gentle palpation of the swelling caused it to become reduced in

size, and the procedure was accompanied by a gurgling noise. When the child cried, the swelling enlarged. In embryological terms, explain what is wrong with this child. Do you think there is a possible association between the swelling and the screaming attack of the previous week? How would you treat this child?

7. A 6-year-old boy was taken to a pediatrician because he continually wet his bed at night (nocturnal enuresis). The mother said that she had noticed that during the daytime he had difficulty in starting to micturate and that he had a weak stream of urine. At the end of micturition he tended to have a dribbling incontinence. On examination the child was seen to be poorly developed and undernourished. The bladder could be felt as a rounded mass above the pubis, which could be easily emptied by passing a catheter. An intravenous pyelogram showed poor concentration of the radiopaque material in the calyces. The calyces and ureters on both sides showed marked dilatation. The injection of a solution of a radiopaque material into the bladder and an x-ray film made while the child was attempting to micturate showed a dilated proximal part of the urethra and an obstruction halfway down the prostatic urethra. Urethroscopy revealed the cause of the obstruction in the prostatic urethra. What is your diagnosis? Using your knowledge of embryology, how would you explain this obstruction? How would you treat this patient?

8. While bathing her 6-month-old boy a mother noticed that his penis tended to curve downward. On examination by a pediatrician, it was noted that not only did the penis have a definite downward curvature (chordee), but the external urethral meatus opened halfway along the under-surface of the penis. What is your diagnosis? How would you explain the formation of this deformity? How would

you treat this patient? At what age would you start the treatment?

9. A mother took her 15-year-old daughter to a physician because she had failed to start to menstruate. On examination the child was noted to be short and stocky with a webbed neck. She had an abnormally large carrying angle of the elbows (cubitus valgus), a broad chest with lack of breast development, and an absence of pubic and axillary hair. No further abnormalities were found on physical examination. What is your diagnosis? What investigations would you undertake to confirm your diagnosis? How would you treat this patient?

10. A 16-year-old girl visited a gynecologist because she was experiencing increasing degrees of pain with each menstruation. On questioning she stated that even with her first period at the age of 12 years she had had severe discomfort. The pain was cramp-like and gradually increased in severity for 4 days and then subsided. Recently she had noticed that the pain was getting much worse, and nothing seemed to relieve it. Her menstrual flow was sometimes excessive (menorrhagia) and irregular. On bimanual vaginal examination a lateral mass could be felt through the right lateral fornix of the vagina. It was rubbery in consistency, mobile, and attached to the uterus. On admission to the hospital a hysterosalpingogram was made. A small quantity of a radiopaque material was injected into the uterine cavity through the cervix. The x-ray film showed a small uterine cavity and a normal left uterine tube; there was no evidence of the presence of a right uterine tube. What is the possible diagnosis? How would you treat this girl? How can you explain the condition embryologically?

11. A 12-year-old girl was taken to a pediatrician because she experienced cyclic monthly pain, but there was no actual menstrual flow. On physical examination

of the vulva, the hymen was seen as a bulging septum. No vaginal orifice could be detected. What is your diagnosis? How would you explain this condition embryologically? How would you treat this patient?

12. A 40-year-old man visited his physician because he had noticed a swelling in the right side of his scrotum. On physical examination a small fluctuant swelling about the size of a pea could be identified just above the upper pole of the right testis. It was freely movable and not attached to the skin. What embryological remnant situated above the testis is likely to be the cause of this swelling? How would you treat this patient?

13. An 11-year-old boy was examined by a physician prior to his returning to school after a summer vacation. On examination of the genitalia it was noted that pubic hair was already present. The penis was small and had the appearance of a hypospadic penis. The scrotum was represented by two rugose folds which were incompletely fused in the midline. The testes could not be felt within the scrotal folds. Below the penis and urethral orifice and between the scrotal folds was a definite depression or dimple. A buccal smear revealed the presence of female sex chromatin. What is the diagnosis? How can you explain the clinical findings in this interesting case?

14. A 17-year-old girl was taken to a gynecologist because her mother was concerned that her daughter had not started to menstruate. On physical examination the girl was seen to be a most attractive female of normal height with normal body development. She had good breast development and normal distribution of pubic hair. A pelvic examination revealed that the vagina was shorter than normal and there was no uterus. Buccal smear examination showed an absence of the sex chromatin. What further examinations or tests would you undertake in this case? What is the diagnosis? How would you treat this patient?

REFERENCES

Antell, L. Hydrocolpos in Infancy and Childhood. *Pediatrics* 10:306, 1952.

Arey, L. B. *Developmental Anatomy,* 7th ed. Saunders, Philadelphia, 1966.

Backhouse, K. M., and Butler, H. The Development of the Coverings of the Testis Cord. *J. Anat.* 92:645, 1958.

Bounoure, L. *The Origin of Reproductive Cells and the Problem of Germinal Lineage.* Gauthier-Villars, Paris, 1939.

Brunet, J., DeMowbray, R. R., and Bishop, P. M. F. Management of the Undescended Testis. *Brit. Med. J.* 1:1367, 1958.

Bulmer, D. The Development of the Human Vagina. *J. Anat.* 91:490, 1957.

Chiquoine, A. D. Identification, Origin and Migration of the Primordial Germ Cells. *Anat. Rec.* 110:135, 1954.

Farrow, G. A., and Thompson, S. Five Years' Survey of Inguinal Hernia in Childhood. *Canad. J. Surg.* 6:63, 1963.

Ford, C. E., Jones, K. W., Polani, P. E., De Almeida, J. C., and Briggs, J. H. A Sex-Chromosome Anomaly in a Case of Gonadal Dysgenesis (Turner's Syndrome). *Lancet* 1:711, 1959.

Gillman, J. The Development of the Gonads in Man with a Consideration of the Role of Fetal Endocrines and Histogenesis of Ovarian Tumors. *Contrib. Embryol.* 32:81, 1948.

Glenister, T. W. Determination of Sex in Early Human Embryos. *Nature* (London) 177:1135, 1956.

Glenister, T. W. A Correlation of the Normal and Abnormal Development of the Penile Urethra and of the Infra-Umbilical Abdominal Wall. *Brit. J. Urol.* 30:117, 1958.

Greene, R., Mathews, D., Hugesden, P. E., and Howard, A. A Case of True Hermaphroditism. *Brit. J. Surg.* 40:263, 1954.

Griboff, S. I., and Lawrence, R. The Chromosomal Etiology of Congenital Gonadal Defects. *Amer. J. Med.* 30:544, 1961.

Gruenwald, P. The Development of the Sex Cords

in the Gonads of Man and Mammals. *Amer. J. Anat.* 70:359, 1942.

Hamilton, W. J., Boyd, J. D., and Mossman, H. W. *Human Embryology,* 3d ed. Williams & Wilkins, Baltimore, 1962.

Hamlett, G. W. Primordial Germ Cells in a 4.5 mm Human Embryo. *Anat. Rec.* 61:273, 1935.

Hayles, A. B., and Nolan, R. B. Masculinization of Female Fetus, Possibly Related to Administration of Progesterone During Pregnancy: Report of Two Cases. *Mayo Clin. Proc.* 33:200, 1958.

Hunter, R. H. Observations on the Development of the Human Female Genital Tract. *Contrib. Embryol.* 22:91, 1930.

Jeffcoate, T. N. A., Fliegner, J. R. H., Russell, S. H., Davis, J. C., and Wade, A. P. Diagnosis of the Adrenogenital Syndrome Before Birth. *Lancet* 2:553, 1965.

Johnston, J. H. Posterior Urethral Valves; An Operative Technic Using an Electric Auriscope. *J. Pediat. Surg.* 1:583, 1966.

Jones, H. W., and Scott, W. W. *Hermaphroditism, Genital Anomalies and Related Endocrine Disorders.* Williams & Wilkins, Baltimore, 1958.

Jones, W. S. Obstetric Significance of Female Genital Anomalies. *Obstet. Gynec.* 10:113, 1957.

Jost, A. Embryonic Sexual Differentiation. In *Hermaphroditism, Genital Anomalies and Related Endocrine Disorders,* edited by H. W. Jones and W. W. Scott. Williams & Wilkins, Baltimore, 1958.

Jost, A. The Role of Fetal Hormones in Prenatal Development. *Harvey Lect.* 55:201, 1961.

Koff, A. K. Development of the Vagina in the Human Fetus. *Contrib. Embryol.* 24:61, 1933.

Lowsley, O. S. The Development of the Human Prostate Gland with Reference to the Development of Other Structures at the Neck of the Urinary Bladder. *Amer. J. Anat.* 13:299, 1912.

Mancini, R. E., Narbaitz, R., and Lavieri, J. C. Origin and Development of the Germinative Epithelium and Sertoli Cells in the Human Testis: Cytological, Cytochemical and Quantitative Study. *Anat. Rec.* 136:477, 1960.

Marshall, V. F., and Muecke, E. C. Variations in Exstrophy of the Bladder. *J. Urol.* 88:766, 1962.

McKelvey, J. L., and Baxter, J. S. Abnormal Development of the Vagina and Genito-Urinary Tract. *Amer. J. Obstet. Gynec.* 29:267, 1935.

Miller, O. J. Developmental Sex Abnormalities. In *Recent Advances in Human Genetics,* edited by L. S. Penrose. Churchill, London, 1961.

Mintz, B. Embryological Phases of Mammalian Gametogenesis. *J. Cell. Comp. Physiol.* 56:31, 1960.

Mitchell, G. A. G. The Condition of the Peritoneal Vaginal Process at Birth. *J. Anat.* 73:658, 1939.

Monie, S. W., and Sigurdson, L. A. A Proposed Classification for Uterine and Vaginal Anomalies. *Amer. J. Obstet. Gynec.* 59:696, 1950.

Morris, J. M. Syndrome of Testicular Feminization in Male Pseudo-Hermaphrodites. *Amer. J. Obstet. Gynec.* 65:1192, 1953.

Muecke, E. C. The Role of the Cloacal Membrane in Exstrophy: The First Successful Experimental Study. *J. Urol.* 92:659, 1964.

Nesbit, R. M., McDonald, H. P., and Busby, S. Obstructing Valves in Female Urethra. *J. Urol.* 91:79, 1964.

Patten, B. M., and Barry, A. Genesis of Exstrophy of the Bladder and Epispadias. *Amer. J. Anat.* 90:35, 1952.

Scorer, C. G. Incidence of Incomplete Descent of the Testicle at Birth. *Arch. Dis. Child.* 31:198, 1956.

Scorer, C. G. The Descent of the Testis. *Arch. Dis. Child.* 39:605, 1964.

Segal, S. J., and Nelson, W. O. Developmental Aspects of Human Hermaphroditism: The Significance of Sex Chromatin Patterns. *Metabolism* 17:676, 1957.

Spaulding, M. H. The Development of the External Genitalia in the Human Embryo. *Contrib. Embryol.* 13:67, 1921.

Villumsen, A. L., and Zachau-Christiansen, B. Spontaneous Alterations in Position of the Testes. *Arch. Dis. Child.* 41:198, 1966.

Wells, L. J. Descent of the Testis: Anatomical and Hormonal Considerations. *Surgery* 14:436, 1943.

Wilkins, L. Masculinization of Female Fetus due to Use of Orally Given Progestins. *J.A.M.A.* 172:1028, 1960.

Wilkins, L. *The Diagnosis and Treatment of Endocrine Disorders in Childhood and Adolescence,* 3d ed. Thomas, Springfield, Ill., 1965.

Williams, D. I., and Eckstein, H. B. Obstructive Valves in the Posterior Urethra. *J. Urol.* 93:236, 1965.

Wilson, K. W. Origin and Development of the Rete Ovarii and the Rete Testis in the Human Embryo. *Contrib. Embryol.* 17:69, 1926.

Witchi, E. Migrations of Germ Cells of Human Embryos from the Yolk Sac to the Primitive Gonadal Folds. *Contrib. Embryol.* 32:67, 1948.

Wyburn, G. M. The Development of the Infra-Umbilical Portion of the Abdominal Wall, with Remarks on the Aetiology of Ectopia Vesicae. *J. Anat.* 71:201, 1937.

Wyndham, N. R. A Morphological Study of Testicular Descent. *J. Anat.* 77:179, 1943.

DEVELOPMENT

The Blood

At about the fourth week of embryonic life, the first blood cells and blood vessels develop in the extra-embryonic mesoderm in the wall of the yolk sac and allantoic diverticulum. Clusters of mesodermal cells called *blood islands* give rise to groups of central cells that become free and form the *primitive blood cells* (Figs. 17-1 & 17-2). The peripheral cells of each blood island proliferate and become flattened to form endothelial lined tubes or vessels. The primitive blood cells are suspended in *blood plasma,* which is apparently produced by the cells of the blood island. As the blood islands increase in number, they fuse to form a network of small blood vessels called the *area vasculosa,* which eventually covers the whole yolk sac. Meanwhile additional blood vessels are being formed in the extra-embryonic mesoderm of the chorion and the body stalk. It is thus seen that in the earliest stages blood formation takes place outside the embryo.

During the second month of development, blood formation commences in the embryonic mesenchyme within the embryo. This occurs chiefly in the liver and later also in the spleen, thymus, and lymph nodes, when these develop. At the same time, blood vessels are forming throughout the body of the embryo from embryonic mesenchyme, the heart has already started to beat, and the blood begins to circulate. A primitive intra-embryonic and extra-embryonic vascular system has now been established (see p. 81).

At the fourth month of development, the red bone marrow starts to take over the function of blood-cell formation, and by the fifth month the red marrow is the main source of blood cells. Although in this description the formation of blood cells has been divided into three distinct periods, it is important to realize that considerable overlap in the activities of these sources of cells takes place (Fig. 17-3).

After birth the red marrow is the only place where erythrocytes and granular leukocytes are formed, although the liver of premature and full-term infants may contain active intralobular blood islands at birth and occasionally up to the fifteenth day of life. If an infant suffers from great blood loss or severe anemia, the liver and the spleen may again assume blood-forming activity.

From birth until about the age of four, all the bones in the body contain red hematopoietic marrow. In the shafts of long bones, this activity diminishes at about 7 years of

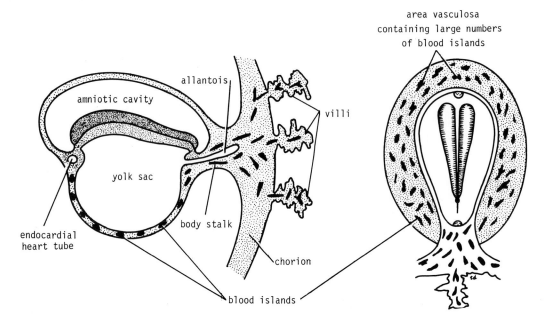

Fig. 17-1. Longitudinal section of embryo showing the appearance of blood islands in the splanchnic mesoderm of the wall of the yolk sac; similar islands are appearing in the body stalk. Both will ultimately join and form with the capillaries in the chorionic villi the extra-embryonic circulation.

Fig. 17-2. Embryonic disc as seen from above. The amnion has been cut away and removed.

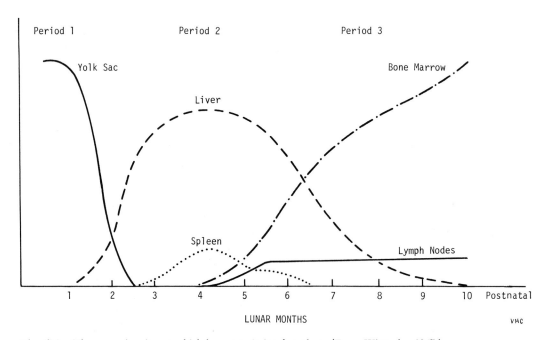

Fig. 17-3. The successive sites at which hematopoiesis takes place. (From Wintrobe, 1967.)

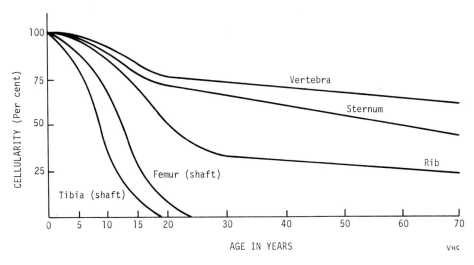

Fig. 17-4. The amount of red marrow in different bones at different ages. (From Wintrobe, 1967.)

age. At puberty, yellow marrow starts to replace red marrow at the distal ends of long bones. This replacement gradually extends proximally until the age of twenty, when all the marrow in long bones is yellow with the exception of the upper end of the humerus and femur. In the adult, red marrow is confined to the bones of the skull, thorax, vertebrae, clavicles, scapulae, and pelvis, and also the upper ends of the humerus and femur (Fig. 17-4). In the adult, when there is severe blood loss or severe anemia, the yellow marrow rapidly becomes converted into red marrow. The various sites in the formation of blood cells in the embryo, fetus, and child are shown in Figure 17-3.

Formation of Blood Cells

The stem cell, from which all blood cells are thought to differentiate, is called the *hemocytoblast.* This is a large ameboid cell with finely granular basophilic cytoplasm.

Formation of Erythrocytes

These arise in the blood islands of the yolk sac, embryonic mesenchyme, liver, lymphoid tissue, and bone marrow as the result of mitotic division of the hemocytoblasts. In the blood islands, the first series of cells to be formed are the *primitive erythroblasts,* which are themselves capable of multiplying by mitosis (Fig. 17-5). As the primitive erythroblasts mature, *hemoglobin* appears in their cytoplasm and the cells are now called *primitive erythrocytes* (Fig. 17-6). Up until the middle of the second month, the primitive erythrocytes are all nucleated.

At about the sixth week of development, the hemocytoblasts in the blood islands of the yolk sac, and later in the liver, and later still in the spleen and bone marrow give rise to a new series of cells called *definitive erythroblasts,* which are smaller than the primitive erythroblasts. The definitive erythroblast series now dominates the red cells in the blood, and the primitive erythroblasts and erythrocytes cease to be produced. As the definitive erythroblasts mature, they acquire hemoglobin and eventually become *definitive erythrocytes,* which are smaller and more circular than the primitive erythrocytes. By the fifth month of development, the red bone

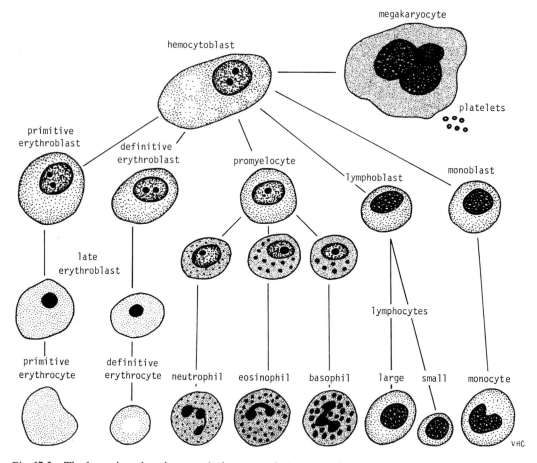

Fig. 17-5. The formation of erythrocytes, leukocytes, and platelets in the embryo and fetus.

marrow becomes the major source of erythrocytes; most definitive erythrocytes are nonnucleated.

The erythrocyte count at the end of the second month has been estimated to number about 1 million per cubic millimeter of blood. This count increases rapidly as development proceeds, and at birth the erythrocyte count may be as high as 5 to 6 million per cubic millimeter. At the same time, as the count increases, the size and hemoglobin content of the corpuscles decrease. Great variation in cell size characterizes fetal blood. Half the cells measure about 8 μ in diameter, the remainder measure from 7 to 17 μ.

It should be noted that in the newborn *reticulocytes* are present in the blood in higher numbers (2 to 6 percent) than are found in the adult (less than 2 percent).

Fetal Hemoglobin

Fetal hemoglobin (Hb-F) differs in physicochemical properties from adult hemoglobin (Hb-A). The basis for the difference lies in the globin portion of the molecule rather than the heme portion. Hb-F contains isoleucine, which is not present in Hb-A and differs in other respects in amino acid composition. Hb-F is more stable to alkali than Hb-A, and this fact is used as a means of estimat-

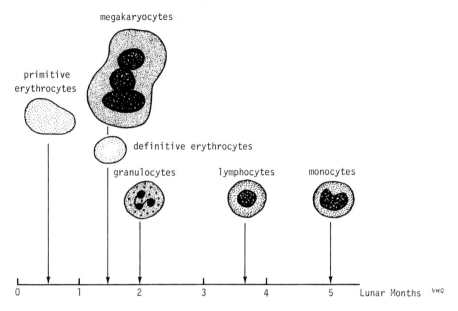

Fig. 17-6.   The successive appearance of the different forms of blood cells.

ing the amounts of Hb-F present in a blood sample. The physiological importance of Hb-F, as compared with Hb-A, seems to be its greater affinity for oxygen. However, it is not certain whether this difference is a result of the molecule itself or of the ionic environment, erythrocyte permeability, and blood pH.

At birth, Hb-F comprises 63 to 91 percent of blood hemoglobin, but in the majority of children very little can be detected by the end of the first year of life.

Formation of Leukocytes

The *granulocytes* are first formed from the hemocytoblast in the mesenchyme of the liver during the second month of development (Fig. 17-6). *Promyelocytes* are the first cells to appear, and these become neutrophilic, eosinophilic, or basophilic (Fig. 17-5). Later, the promyelocytes divide and give origin to the three forms of granular leukocytes. As development proceeds, the formation of the granular leukocytes is taken over entirely by the red bone marrow.

The *lymphocytes* arise from hemocytoblasts or directly from mesenchymal cells in the connective tissue around lymph vessels. The *lymphoblast* is the stem cell and can form either *large* or *small lymphocytes* (Fig. 17-5). Lymphocytes are formed in the lymph nodes, spleen, and for a limited period in the liver and bone marrow. They appear in the fetal blood during the third month (Fig. 17-6). Recently evidence has been adduced to show that the thymus is an important source for the production of lymphocytes (see below).

The *monocytes* arise from the hemocytoblasts during the fifth month. The first cell of the series is the *monoblast,* which gives rise to the monocyte with its characteristic kidney-shaped nucleus (Figs. 17-5 & 17-6).

Formation of Megakaryocytes and Platelets

Megakaryocytes are formed very early in development from hemocytoblasts and are found in association with blood vessels in different parts of the embryo (Fig. 17-6). By the fourth month, the red bone marrow becomes the source and site of these cells. Platelets arise by fragmentation of the cytoplasm of the megakaryocytes (Fig. 17-5).

The Lymphatic System

Lymphatic Vessels

These originate as small spaces in the mesenchyme; the lining cells become flattened so that each space acquires an endothelial lining.

With continued growth, adjacent spaces fuse so that a network of lymphatic capillaries is formed. During the course of development, a number of *lymph sacs* appear as the result of dilatation and fusion of several mesenchymal spaces (Fig. 17-7). A pair of lymph sacs is found in the neck, the *jugular lymph sacs;* a pair in the pelvic region, the *iliac lymph sacs;* a single sac is found on the posterior abdominal wall near the midline, the *retroperi-*

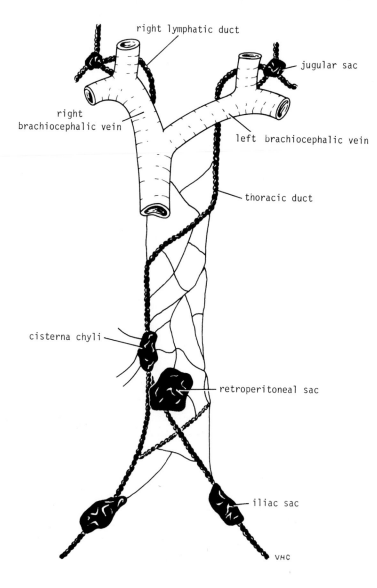

Fig. 17-7. The position of the lymph sacs and the formation of the thoracic duct.

right lymphatic duct

jugular sac

right brachiocephalic vein

left brachiocephalic vein

thoracic duct

cisterna chyli

retroperitoneal sac

iliac sac

VHC

toneal lymph sac; a further single sac is found in the region of the developing diaphragm, the *cisterna chyli*.

As the result of continued elongation, growth, and branching of the lymphatic capillaries, lymphatic vessels are found in most tissues of the body. They tend to be distributed along the main veins but they are never found in the following tissues: the central nervous system, the meninges, the eyeball and cornea, the internal ear, cartilage, epidermis, and the spleen. By the second month of development, the lymphatic vessels have acquired valves.

Meanwhile each lymph sac has become associated with the lymphatic vessels draining specific areas. The jugular lymph sacs send out lymphatic capillary plexuses which spread to the tissues of the head and neck and arms. The iliac lymph sacs send out lymphatic vessels to the lower part of the trunk and legs. The retroperitoneal lymph sac sends out vessels to the gut via the dorsal mesentery, and the cisterna chyli sends out vessels which join with others on the posterior abdominal wall.

The caudal end of each jugular lymph sac becomes joined to the cisterna chyli by channels which eventually form paired primitive *thoracic ducts*. These are united by many transverse branches, and ultimately the upper or cephalic part of the *thoracic duct* is formed from the left primitive thoracic duct. The jugular sacs become connected with the brachiocephalic veins on each side (Fig. 17-7). Later, all the lymph sacs are replaced by lymphatic vessels. It is thus seen that a valved system of vessels is formed, which closely follows the course of the venous system and assists in returning tissue fluid to the bloodstream.

Lymph Nodes

These arise as the result of proliferation of mesenchymal cells in relation to lymphatic capillary plexuses. Some of the mesenchymal cells differentiate into lymphoblasts, which in turn will give rise to lymphocytes. Other mesenchymal cells form connective tissue cells so that a fibrous capsule is developed, and trabeculae and a reticular net are laid down. During the early stages of development, hemocytoblasts and erythroblasts are present within the nodes. Later, erythrocyte formation is confined to the red bone marrow. The organization of the lymphoid tissue into *cortical nodules* and *medullary cords* is not complete until after birth.

Spleen

This organ develops as a circumscribed thickening of mesenchyme in the dorsal mesentery, which enlarges and projects from its left surface (Fig. 17-8). In the earliest stages, the spleen consists of a number of mesenchymal masses that later fuse, so by the third month it has acquired its characteristic shape. The notches along its anterior border are permanent and indicate that the mesenchymal masses never completely fuse.

The part of the dorsal mesentery that extends between the hilum of the spleen and the greater curvature of the stomach is called the *gastrosplenic omentum* or *ligament,* and the part that extends between the spleen and the left kidney on the posterior abdominal wall is called the *lienorenal ligament* (Fig. 17-8).

The mesenchymal cells in the developing spleen differentiate and form the capsule, the trabeculae, and the reticular framework. Lymphoblasts appear early and start to produce lymphocytes. During the fourth and fifth months of intra-uterine life, erythroblasts, myeloblasts, and megakaryocytes are present in the spleen, so that erythrocytes and granular leukocytes and platelets are produced in the spleen for a period of time. By the eighth month, the formation of erythrocytes and granular leukocytes ceases. The splenic tissue is supplied by a branch of the foregut artery (celiac artery), the *splenic artery*.

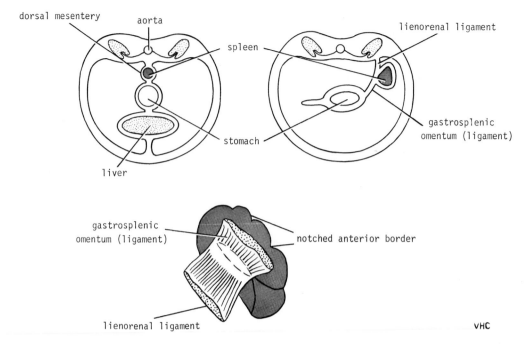

Fig. 17-8. The formation of the spleen in the dorsal mesentery. The persistent notches on the anterior border are also shown.

Thymus

The thymus arises as an entodermal diverticulum from each third pharyngeal pouch (see Chap. 10). Each diverticulum grows inferiorly in the neck to reach the anterior aspect of the aorta. It is at first hollow, but later, due to cellular proliferation, it becomes a solid bar. The two thymic bars fuse in the superior mediastinum and sever their connection with the third pharyngeal pouches. The entodermal cells multiply to form solid clusters, the *corpuscles of Hassall.* By the end of the third month, the thymus is invaded by surrounding mesenchymal cells, and these differentiate and form a reticular framework. At the same time, increasing numbers of lymphocytes appear within the reticulum. Meanwhile a capsule and trabeculae are being formed from the mesenchyme, and the organ becomes subdivided into *lobules.* The higher concentration of lymphocytes in the periphery of each lobule makes it possible to recognize a denser *cortex* and a looser *medulla.* The thymus at birth is relatively a very large organ and extends from the region of the thyroid cartilage in the neck through the superior mediastinum anterior to the great vessels to reach the anterior surface of the pericardium (Fig. 17-9). The thymus continues steadily to enlarge but at a slower rate than the rest of the body. At puberty it has reached its maximum size, but usually it is restricted to the superior mediastinum. Thereafter, the thymus begins to regress and is gradually replaced by fibro-fatty connective tissue. However, even in adults thymic tissue can be demonstrated histologically.

There is considerable experimental evidence to show that small lymphocytes of the peripheral lymphoid tissues originate in the thymus during intra-uterine life. While the thymus is developing, the spleen, lymph nodes, and other areas of lymphoid tissue are

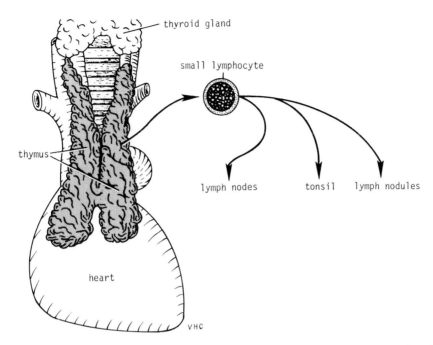

Fig. 17-9. The large size of the thymus is shown in relation to the other structures in the neck and superior mediastinum. Also shown is the distribution of the small lymphocytes from the thymus to other lymphoid organs.

forming, but initially they consist only of a reticular framework, and small lymphocytes are absent. It is believed that small lymphocytes leave the thymus and populate the peripheral lymphoid tissue. It is possible also that the thymus influences the development of peripheral lymphoid tissue by a humeral mechanism.

Tonsils

The *palatine tonsils* develop as solid buds of entodermal cells from the second pharyngeal pouch. The buds extend into the underlying mesenchyme, and the central cells of each bud break down so that *tonsillar crypts* are formed. Meanwhile the mesenchymal cells form a reticular framework around the crypts, and by the third month lymphocytes appear in the reticulum and become arranged as nodules. The capsule of the tonsil is formed from a condensation of mesenchyme.

The *nasopharyngeal tonsil* develops in the roof and posterior wall of the nasopharynx by the accumulation of lymphocytes in the connective tissue of the mucous membrane. The mesenchymal cells lay down a reticular framework, and the lymphocytes become organized into nodules.

Solitary Lymph Nodules

In the mucous membrane of the respiratory and digestive systems, these nodules develop in an identical manner to that seen in the formation of the nasopharyngeal tonsil.

CONGENITAL ANOMALIES

Erythrocytes

Congenital Hypoplastic Anemia

This is rare and is caused by chronic red marrow hypoplasia involving erythropoietic tissue; the leukocytes and platelets are un-affected. Spontaneous cure may take place or life may be sustained with repeated blood transfusions.

Congenital Malformation of Erythrocytes

HEREDITARY SPHEROCYTOSIS. This condition is transmitted as a mendelian dominant trait. The gene defect results in production of small spherical cells, the life span of which is short. The treatment is blood tranfusion when necessary.

Congenital Coagulation Defects

HEMOPHILIA. This disease is caused by a sex-linked recessive gene. In all cases, the disease is carried on the X chromosome and is thus handed down from unaffected carrier females to affected sons. The genetic fault in hemophilia is probably the result of a fault in a single enzyme that plays a vital part in the synthesis of antihemophilic globulin. Habit-ual hemorrhage, from various parts of the body, either spontaneous or following slight trauma, is the main symptom of the disease. All the lesions are caused by the relative failure of blood coagulation, resulting from antihemophilic globulin deficiency.

In a severe hemophiliac individual, the first 6 to 9 months of life are usually without symptoms. Then, following a slight injury or occurring spontaneously, a deep tissue hemorrhage may occur. Later, when the child walks, hemorrhage into a joint may take place. The mortality from continued hemorrhage is very high during the first year. The treatment is directed toward protection of the child from wounds or abrasions and avoidance of even the most trivial operations. Transfusions of concentrated antihemophilic globulin may be given.

A number of very rare congenital coagula-tion defects also occur, such as congenital afibrinogenemia and congenital prothrombin deficiency; the student is referred to a text-book of hematology for a description of these conditions.

Erythroblastosis Fetalis (Hemolytic Disease of the Newborn)

This disease occurs in the fetus or in the first few days of life. Under certain conditions of mating, antibodies are elaborated by the mother that pass across the placental barrier and produce excessive destruction of the erythrocytes. The bone marrow, liver, and spleen, and even the lymph nodes, thymus, and kidneys, engage in active erythropoiesis, and large numbers of nucleated red cells appear in the peripheral blood (erythro-blasts). The hemolysis of the fetal blood is a result of isoimmunization of the mother by a corpuscular factor in the fetus which leads to the production of maternal agglutinins potentially active on the fetal blood. The condition occurs most commonly when the mother is Rh-negative and the father and fetus are Rh-positive. It would appear that in this condition small numbers of fetal red cells containing the antigen manage to cross the placental barrier. The following varieties of the condition occur:

FETAL HEMOLYTIC DISEASE. Death occurs early in utero and a *macerated fetus* is de-livered. This rarely occurs in the first preg-nancy unless the mother has been sensitized by a previous blood transfusion. In *hydrops fetalis* the infant is stillborn or dies within a few hours of birth. The liver and spleen are grossly enlarged, and the fetus and placenta are edematous.

ICTERUS GRAVIS NEONATORUM. This is a form of hemolytic disease of the newborn in which there is severe, often fatal, jaundice caused by excessive destruction of the erythro-cytes. The treatment is exchange transfusion with Rh-negative blood of group O or of its own group. Direct compatibility tests, using the mother's serum, should always be carried out.

Hereditary Disorders Associated with Abnormal Hemoglobin

SICKLE CELL ANEMIA. This is a hereditary and familial form of chronic hemolytic anemia, occurring almost exclusively in Negroes. It is distinguished morphologically by the presence of sickle-shaped erythrocytes (Figs. 17-10 & 17-11), as well as signs of excessive blood destruction and active blood formation. There is considerable evidence to support the theory that when the gene for sickling is heterozygous, only the sickle cell trait is found, whereas the homozygous state produces sickle cell anemia.

The sickle shape of the erythrocytes is caused by the presence of abnormal hemoglobin "S," which, by reason of insolubility in the reduced state at the lower ranges of oxygen tension found in the body, causes the corpuscles to assume this characteristic shape. With sickle cell trait, only a small proportion of the corpuscular hemoglobin is of the "S" type, and it is not sufficient to change the

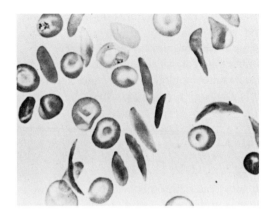

Fig. 17-10. Sickle cell anemia. A blood film showing the presence of sickle-shaped erythrocytes. (Courtesy of Dr. L. Lessin.)

shape of the erythrocytes at low oxygen tensions.

THALASSEMIA. This is a form of hemolytic anemia found typically in people living in the region of the Mediterranean and is caused by a dominant mendelian inherited abnormality of hemoglobin resulting from abnormalities of globin production. Such persons continue to produce fetal hemoglobin (Hb-F). The

Fig. 17-11. Sickle cell anemia. A scanning electron micrograph of a blood film showing examples of sickle-shaped erythrocytes. (Courtesy of Dr. P. Klug.)

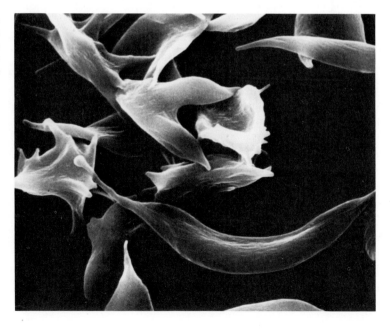

disease may be of a major form that is serious and often fatal. The minor form is often symptomless and discovered by chance.

Other hereditary disorders associated with abnormal hemoglobins occur, and a textbook of hematology should be consulted.

Platelets

Congenital Thrombocytopenia

In most cases, thrombocytopenic purpura is present in the mother and probably is a result of transplacental passage of the factor responsible for the thrombocytopenia in the mother, e.g., antiplatelet agglutinins for the baby's platelets in a manner similar to Rh iso-immunization. In some cases the red marrow shows an absence or reduced number of megakaryocytes. Most cases recover spontaneously.

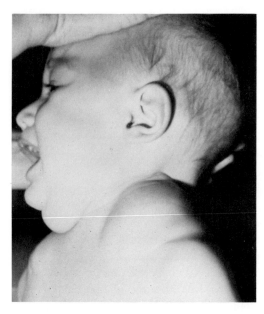

Fig. 17-12. Cystic hygroma in the left side of the neck. (Courtesy of Dr. R. Chase.)

Lymphatic System

Lymphatic Vessels

CYSTIC HYGROMA. If, in the formation of lymphatic vessels, the mesodermal spaces fail to unite and join with the central system, a cystic hygroma results (Fig. 17-12). The cystic hygroma gradually enlarges because the lymph collecting in the cystic spaces cannot drain away due to atresia of the collecting vessels, which commonly occur in the neck and also in the axilla, mediastinum, and tongue (see Fig. 10-10). The treatment is operative removal (Fig. 17-13).

IDIOPATHIC HEREDITARY LYMPHEDEMA (MILROY'S DISEASE). This is a firm edema of one or more extremities often noticed at birth. The leg is involved much more commonly than the arm (Fig. 17-14). This condition is both congenital and familial. The peripheral lymph vessels may be aplastic or hypoplastic, and some may show varicosity. There is no satisfactory treatment.

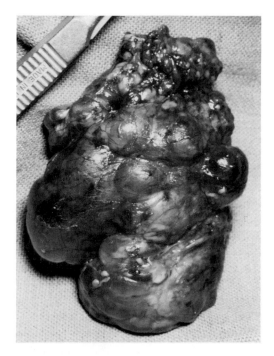

Fig. 17-13. Specimen of cystic hygroma removed from patient seen in Fig. 17-12. (Courtesy of Dr. R. Chase.)

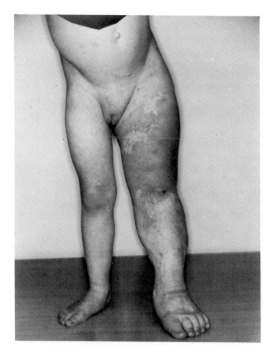

Fig. 17-14. Idiopathic hereditary lymphedema. Shows gross enlargement of the left leg. (Courtesy of Dr. L. Thompson.)

Lymphatic Tissue

SUPERNUMERARY SPLEENS. In 10 percent of persons, one or more supernumerary spleens may be present, either in the gastrosplenic ligament or the lienorenal ligament. Their clinical importance lies in the fact that they may hypertrophy after removal of the major spleen and be responsible for a recurrence of symptoms of the disease for which splenectomy was initially performed.

CONGENITAL ABSENCE OF THE SPLEEN. This is a rare condition and often associated with severe malformations of other organ systems.

THYMUS. The thymus may fail to descend into the thorax and remain in the neck, where it can rarely produce obstructive symptoms. Lobules of thymus may be seen in the thyroid gland. It is believed that several forms of impairment of formation of the thymus are associated with immunological deficiency states, for example, *agammaglobulinemia with lymphopenia.*

Clinical Problems

Answers on page 450

1. A 4-year-old boy was taken to a pediatrician because his mother had noticed a large bruise developing on the lateral surface of his right thigh. On questioning, the mother said that the child had not fallen and she just could not understand why such a large bruise had formed. On further questioning the mother said that a similar large bruise had developed without apparent cause on the back of the left calf about 3 months previously. On examination, a large bruise was found on the lateral surface of the middle third of the right thigh. The area was swollen and obviously very tender to touch. The child had no clinical evidence of anemia. Further questioning of the mother revealed that she had a 10-year-old son who had a similar history of bruising easily and a strong tendency to bleed excessively from minor cuts or scratches. Her husband was perfectly normal. What is your diagnosis? Is this condition likely to be present in all the sons of this mother? Are the daughters likely to have this condition? Can the disease be transmitted by the sons? Would you advise this child to participate in sports when he goes to school? Is this disease likely to get better or worse with age?

2. An expectant mother had a sample of her

blood tested for A, B, O, and Rh groups. The woman was found to be Rh-negative. It was decided to test the woman for the presence of Rh antibodies. Why? If Rh antibodies are found in a mother's serum, the Rh genotype of the husband should be ascertained. Why? Is it important to know whether or not an Rh-negative mother has been transfused in the past with Rh-positive blood?

3. A 25-year-old Negro visited his physician because of weakness, breathlessness, vomiting, and severe pains in the epigastrium. On examination the patient was found to be anemic and exhibited yellowish discoloration of his sclera. His liver could be palpated beneath the costal margin. On further questioning, the patient said that sometimes the abdominal pain was agonizing and often occurred at different sites. The pain tended to subside within 3 or 4 days. Sometimes the pain was accompanied by fever. He also stated that he had had a large skin ulcer over the medial malleolus of his left leg 3 years previously and that it had taken 6 months to heal. Examination of the blood film revealed a normocytic anemia. The hemoglobin concentration was 5 gm per 100 ml. There was a reticulocytosis present. What is your diagnosis? How would you confirm the diagnosis?

4. A 7-year-old boy was examined by a pedia-

trician because of a large swelling in the left armpit. The mother had noticed the swelling while bathing her son 2 years previously. Since that time the swelling had progressively increased in size. On examination, a soft, painless, poorly defined mass about 3 in. (4.5 cm) in diameter was noted to be present in the left axilla. The swelling was fluctuant on palpation and could be transilluminated. The swelling extended up into the axilla towards the apex. Nothing abnormal could be palpated in the root of the neck on the left side. What is your diagnosis? How would you explain this congenital anomaly? How would you treat this patient?

5. A 25-year-old woman was seen by her physician because she had a swollen right leg. On questioning, she stated that for as long as she could remember her right leg had always been larger and heavier than her left leg. On examination, the right leg was found to be considerably larger in diameter as compared with the left leg. The enlargement included the right foot and involved the whole leg but did not extend proximal to the inguinal ligament. The skin felt thickened and firm and did not pit on pressure. The left leg was normal. What is your diagnosis? How would you explain this congenital anomaly? How would you treat this patient?

REFERENCES

Ackerman, G. A. The Lymphocyte: Its Morphology and Embryological Origin. In *The Lymphocyte in Immunology and Haemopoiesis,* edited by J. M. Yoffey. Arnold, London, 1967. P. 11.

Allen, D. W., Wyman, J., Jr., and Smith, C. A. The Oxygen Equilibrium of Fetal and Adult Human Hemoglobin. *J. Biol. Chem.* 203:81, 1953.

Beaven, G. H., Ellis, M. J., and White, J. C. Studies on Human Foetal Haemoglobin. *Brit. J. Haemat.* 6:1, 201, 1960.

Bloom, W., and Bartelmez, G. W. Hematopoiesis in Young Human Embryos. *Amer. J. Anat.* 67:21, 1940.

Chernoff, A. I., and Singer, K. Studies on Abnormal Hemoglobins. IV. Persistence of Fetal Hemoglobin in the Erythrocytes of Normal Children. *Pediatrics* 9:469, 1952.

Gilmour, J. R. Normal Haemopoiesis in Intra-Uterine and Neonatal Life. *J. Path. Bact.* 52:25, 1941.

Huntington, G. S. The Development of the Mammalian Jugular Lymph Sac of the Tributary Primitive Ulnar Lymphatic and of the Thoracic Duct from the Viewpoint of Recent Investigations of Vertebrate Lymphatic Ontogeny, Together with a Consideration of the Genetic Relations of Lymphatic and Haemal Vascular Channels in the Embryos of Amniotes. *Amer. J. Anat.* 16:259, 1914.

Kampmeier, O. F. *Evolution and Comparative Morphology of the Lymphatic System.* Thomas, Springfield, Ill., 1969.

Kissane, J. M., and Smith, M. G. *Pathology of Infancy and Childhood.* Mosby, St. Louis, 1967.

Rusznyak, I., Foldi, M., and Szabo, G. *Lymphatics and Lymph Circulation,* 2d ed. Pergamon, New York, 1967.

Sabin, F. R. A Critical Study of the Evidence Presented in Several Recent Articles on the Development of the Lymphatic System. *Anat. Rec.* 5:417, 1911.

Sabin, F. R. The Origin and Development of the Lymphatic System. *Johns Hopkins Hosp. Reports* 17:347, 1916.

Thompson, E. L. Time and Rate of Loss of Nuclei by the Red Blood Cells of Human Embryo. *Anat. Rec.* 111:317, 1951.

Walker, J., and Turnbull, E. P. N. Haemoglobin and Red Cells in the Human Foetus. *Lancet* 2:312, 1953.

Whitby, L. E. H., and Britton, C. J. C. *Disorders of the Blood,* 10th ed. Grune & Stratton, New York, 1969.

Wintrobe, M. M. *Clinical Hematology,* 7th ed. Lea & Febiger, Philadelphia, 1974.

Wiseman, B. K. The Origin of the White Blood Cells. *J.A.M.A.* 103:1523, 1934.

Yoffey, J. M., and Courtice, F. C. *Lymphatics, Lymph and the Lymphomyeloid Complex.* Academic, New York, 1970.

Zilliacus, H. Human Embryo Haemoglobin. *Nature* (London) 188:1102, 1960.

DEVELOPMENT

Hypophysis

The hypophysis, or *pituitary gland,* develops from two sources: (1) a small ectodermal diverticulum, *Rathke's pouch,* which grows superiorly from the roof of the stomodeum immediately anterior to the buccopharyngeal membrane, and (2) a small ectodermal diverticulum, the *infundibulum,* which grows inferiorly from the floor of the diencephalon.

During the second month of development, Rathke's pouch comes into contact with the anterior surface of the infundibulum, and its connection with the oral epithelium elongates, narrows, and finally disappears (Fig. 18-1). Rathke's pouch is now a vesicle that flattens itself around the anterior and lateral surfaces of the infundibulum. The cells of the anterior wall of the vesicle proliferate and form the *pars anterior* of the hypophysis, and from its upper part there is a cellular extension that grows superiorly and around the stalk of the infundibulum, forming the *pars tuberalis.* The cells of the posterior wall of the vesicle never develop extensively; they form the *pars intermedia;* some of the cells later migrate anteriorly into the pars anterior. The cavity of the vesicle is reduced to a narrow cleft that may completely disappear.

Meanwhile the infundibulum has differentiated into the *stalk* and *pars nervosa* of the hypophysis (Fig. 18-1). The neuroglial cells of the pars nervosa differentiate into *pituicytes.* Nerve cells in the hypothalamic nuclei give rise to many nerve fibers that grow inferiorly into the pars nervosa by way of the stalk, and neurosecretory activity begins in late fetal life.

During the third and fourth months, the cells of the pars anterior differentiate into *chromophobe cells, acidophil cells,* and *basophil cells.* At the same time, the cells become arranged in columns around the blood sinusoids. Meanwhile the organ becomes vascularized, and a portal system of blood vessels is established.

Pineal Gland

The pineal gland develops as a small ectodermal diverticulum in the posterior part of the roof of the diencephalon during the seventh week of development (Fig. 18-2). As the result of cellular proliferation in its walls, the diverticulum eventually becomes a solid bud. The neuroglia differentiates into *pineal cells,* and nerve fibers invade the pineal from the epithalamus. The pineal gland is rich in *serotonin* and in *melatonin,* but the precise

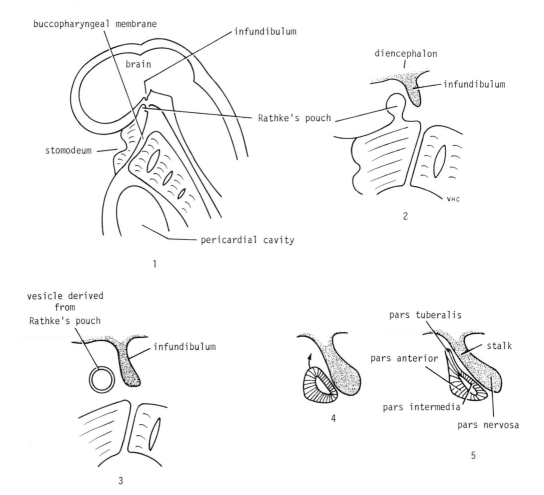

Fig. 18-1. The different stages in the development of the pituitary gland.

role of these substances has not been clearly defined. It is possible that the pineal gland exerts an inhibitory effect on sexual maturation; and it may also influence the activity of the suprarenal cortex.

Thyroid Gland

The thyroid gland begins during the third week as an entodermal thickening in the midline of the floor of the pharynx between the tuberculum impar and the copula (Fig. 18-3). Later this thickening becomes a diverticulum that grows inferiorly into the underlying mesenchyme and is called the *thyroglossal duct*. As development continues, the duct elongates and its distal end becomes bilobed. Soon the duct becomes a solid cord of cells, and as a result of epithelial proliferation the bilobed terminal swellings expand to form the thyroid gland.

The thyroid gland now migrates inferiorly in the neck and passes either anterior to, or through, the developing body of the hyoid bone, or posterior to it. By the seventh week, it reaches its final position in relation to the larynx and trachea. Meanwhile the solid cord connecting the thyroid gland to the tongue

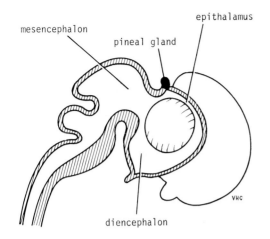

Fig. 18-2. The development of the pineal gland from the posterior part of the diencephalon.

small median isthmus and two large lateral lobes (Fig. 18-3).

In the earliest stages, the thyroid gland consists of a solid mass of cells. Later, as a result of invasion by surrounding vascular mesenchymal tissue, the mass becomes broken up into plates and cords and finally into small clusters of cells. By the third month, colloid starts to accumulate in the center of each cluster so that *follicles* are formed. The fibrous capsule and connective tissue develop from the surrounding mesenchyme.

The *ultimobranchial bodies* (see Chap. 10) are believed to be incorporated into the thyroid gland, where they form the *parafollicular cells,* which produce *calcitonin.*

Parathyroid Glands

The initial development of the four parathyroid glands is described in Chapter 10.

fragments and disappears. The site of origin of the thyroglossal duct on the tongue remains as a pit called the *foramen cecum.* The thyroid gland may now be divided into a

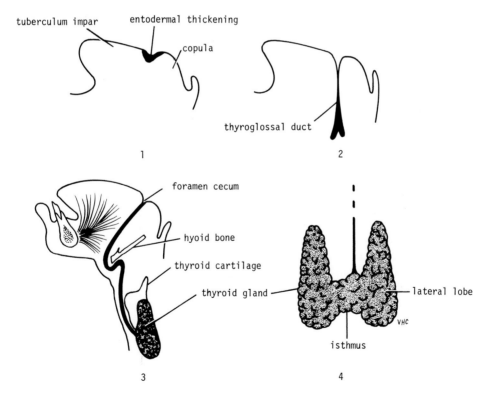

Fig. 18-3. The different stages in the development of the thyroid gland.

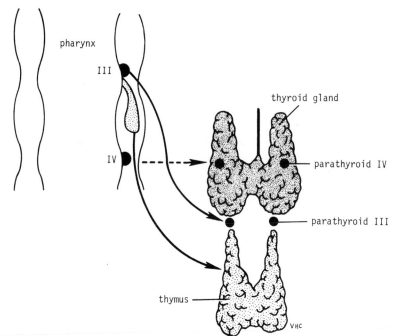

Fig. 18-4. The four parathyroid glands taking up their final positions in the neck.

The pair of *inferior parathyroid glands,* known as *parathyroids III,* develop as a result of proliferation of entodermal cells in the third pharyngeal pouch on each side. As the thymic diverticulum on each side grows inferiorly in the neck, it pulls the inferior parathyroid with it so that it finally comes to rest on the posterior surface of the lateral lobe of the thyroid gland near its lower pole and becomes completely separate from the thymus (Fig. 18-4).

The pair of *superior parathyroid glands, parathyroids IV,* develop as a proliferation of entodermal cells in the fourth pharyngeal pouch on each side. These loosen their connection with the pharyngeal wall and take up their final position on the posterior aspect of the lateral lobe of the thyroid gland on each side, at about the level of the isthmus (Fig. 18-4).

In the earliest stages, each gland consists of a solid mass of clear cells, the *chief cells.* In late childhood acidophilic cells, the *oxyphil cells,* appear. The connective tissue and vascular supply are derived from the surrounding mesenchyme. It is believed that *parathormone* is secreted early in fetal life by the chief cells to regulate calcium metabolism. The oxyphil cells are thought to be nonfunctioning chief cells.

Suprarenal Glands

The suprarenal glands develop from two sources: (1) a mesodermal part, which forms the *cortex* of the gland, and (2) an ectodermal part, which forms the *medulla.*

The cortex develops during the sixth week from the coelomic mesothelium covering the posterior abdominal wall between the root of the dorsal mesentery and the mesonephros. The mesothelial cells proliferate and grow down into the underlying mesenchyme, where they differentiate into large acidophilic cells that form the *fetal cortex* (Fig. 18-5). Later, a further mesothelial proliferation occurs and smaller cells are formed that cover the outer surface of the fetal cortex. As development proceeds, the outer smaller cells become arranged into the *zona glomerulosa*

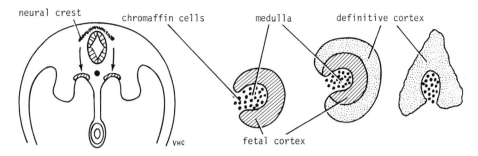

Fig. 18-5. The different stages in the development of the suprarenal gland.

and the *zona fasciculata* of the *definitive cortex*. The surrounding mesenchyme forms the capsule and connective tissue of the cortex. After birth the fetal cortex retrogresses and its involution is largely completed in the first few weeks of life.

Meanwhile the neural crest cells that form the sympathochromaffin cells of the medulla migrate ventrally and invade the cortex on its medial aspect (Fig. 18-5). By the tenth week of development, catecholamines are present in the cells of the medulla, and later epinephrine and norepinephrine can be identified. As further invasion of the cortex continues, the chromaffin cells of the medulla come to occupy a central position and are arranged in cords and clusters. Preganglionic myelinated sympathetic nerve fibers grow into the medulla and, by means of the chemical transmitter acetylcholine, they influence the activity of the medullary cells. The medulla remains relatively undeveloped at birth and attains maturity during the first 3 years of postnatal life.

At birth the suprarenal glands are relatively very large because of the presence of the fetal cortex; later, when this part of the cortex involutes, the glands become reduced in size. Hyperemia precedes the normal involution of the fetal cortex in the newborn child, and the large area formed by the delicate cortex within the glands renders them very liable to damage and severe hemorrhage at this time.

The function of the fetal cortex is not completely known. Several investigators have shown that *hydrocortisone, corticosterone,* and other steroids can be synthesized in this part of the cortex. It has been recently shown that the fetal cortex produces large amounts of *estrogen* and thus assists the placenta in the formation of this hormone.

Accessory Medullary Tissue

Pieces of chromaffin tissue occur on the posterior abdominal wall outside the suprarenal medulla; they are known as the *aortic bodies* and lie along the anterior surface of the aorta. Small pieces of tissue may also be found in relation to the sympathetic trunk. Although well defined in the fetus and in the newborn, they largely disappear during childhood.

Islets of Langerhans of the Pancreas

The development of the pancreas is described in Chapter 11. The pancreatic islets arise as small buds of entodermal cells from the developing ducts (Fig. 18-6). Later these cells lose their connection with the duct system and form isolated groups of cells which start to secrete *insulin* at about the fifth month. Throughout life, the concentration of pancreatic islets is greatest in the tail of the pancreas, intermediate in the body, and least in the head. Three types of islet cells have been described: *alpha, beta,* and *delta cells.* The alpha cells produce *glucagon,* which is an active hyperglycemic agent. The granular

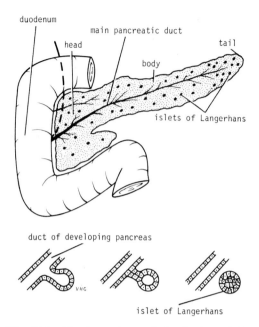

Fig. 18-6. The formation and distribution of the islet cells in the pancreas.

beta cells are the site of formation and storage of insulin. The function of the delta cells is unknown.

Interstitial Cells of the Testis

The development of the testis is described in Chapter 16. The interstitial cells are derived from the mesenchymal cells lying between the developing seminiferous tubules. Between the third and the fifth months, the interstitial cells show marked activity, developing into large polyhedral cells, the cytoplasm of which contains lipid droplets. It is believed that the production of male hormones by the fetal testis is important in the development of male internal and external genitalia. These hormones are secreted locally and cause *induction* of the mesonephric duct system with the formation of the efferent ductules of the testis, the epididymis, the vas deferens, and the seminal vesicles; they cause *regression* of the paramesonephric duct system (the uter-

ine tubes and uterus). After birth the interstitial cells regress and remain in this state until stimulated by the gonadotropic hormones of the pituitary at puberty to secrete *testosterone* and *androstenedione*. It is also known that these cells produce small amounts of estrogens.

Ovary

The development of the ovary is described in Chapter 16. It is believed that the theca interna cells and the granulosa cells, which are derived from mesenchyme, are the main sources of *estrogens* produced by the ovary. The corpus luteum produces both *progesterone* and *estrogen*.

CONGENITAL ANOMALIES

Hypophysis

Absence of the Hypophysis

Congenital absence of the hypophysis in the presence of a normally developed brain is rare and incompatible with life. Infants born with no pars anterior have maldeveloped adrenals, thyroid, and testes, demonstrating the dependence of these organs on the pars anterior in fetal life.

Congenital absence of the cell responsible for the secretion of a specific pituitary hormone is now recognized; for example, hereditary growth hormone deficiency is inherited as an autosomal recessive trait.

Pharyngeal Hypophysis

As Rathke's pouch becomes detached from the roof of the pharynx, a fairly common remnant is left attached to the pharyngeal wall, called the *pharyngeal hypophysis*. Pars anterior tissue has also been found in the body of the sphenoid bone. A *craniopharyngioma* is a form of cystic epidermoid tumor that is believed to arise from remnants of Rathke's pouch.

Thyroid Gland

Agenesis of the Thyroid

Failure of development of the thyroid gland may occur and is the commonest cause of *cretinism*.

Incomplete Descent of the Thyroid

The descent of the thyroid may be arrested at any point between the base of the tongue and the trachea (Fig. 18-7). *Lingual thyroid* is the commonest form of incomplete descent (Fig. 18-8). The mass of tissue is found just beneath the foramen cecum and may be sufficiently large to obstruct swallowing in the infant.

Ectopic Thyroid Tissue

This occasionally is found in the thorax in relation to the trachea or bronchi or even the esophagus. One must assume that this thyroid tissue arose from entodermal cells

Fig. 18-7. A thyroglossal cyst in the midline in the neck and a thyroglossal fistula.

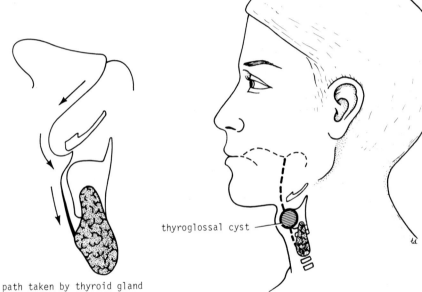

path taken by thyroid gland
as it descends in the neck

thyroglossal cyst

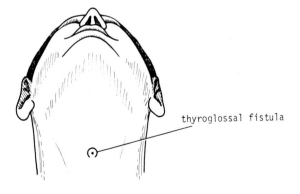

thyroglossal fistula

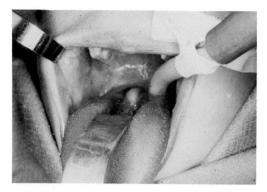

Fig. 18-8. Lingual thyroid. (Courtesy of Dr. J. Randolph.)

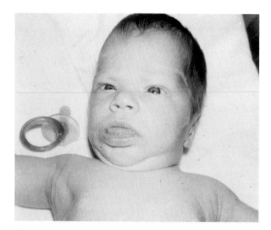

Fig. 18-9. Cretinism. Note the large protruding tongue. (Courtesy of Dr. G. Avery.)

displaced during the formation of the laryngotracheal tube or from entodermal cells of the developing esophagus.

Cretinism

This condition results from inadequate production of thyroid hormone during intrauterine life (Fig. 18-9). A few cases have occurred following the ingestion of goitrogens such as *thiouracil* by the mother during pregnancy. The majority are caused by lack of development of thyroid tissue. *Familial goitrous cretinism* is a condition which appears to result from a congenital impairment

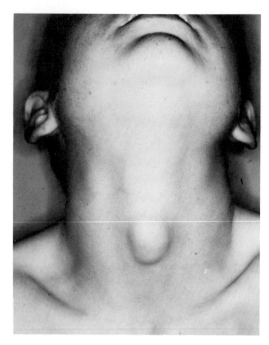

Fig. 18-10. Thyroglossal cyst. (Courtesy of Dr. L. Thompson.)

of the ability of the thyroid gland to synthesize thyroxin.

Neonatal Thyrotoxicosis

This is thought to result from the transplacental passage of *long-acting thyroid stimulator* from the maternal circulation, the mother having thyrotoxicosis.

Thyroglossal Duct

Conditions related to a persistence of the thyroglossal duct usually appear in childhood, in adolescence, or in young adults.

Thyroglossal Cyst

These may occur at any point along the thyroglossal tract (Figs. 18-7 & 18-10). They occur most commonly in the region below the hyoid bone. Such a cyst occupies the midline and develops as a result of persistence of a small amount of epithelium that continues to secrete mucus. As the cyst en-

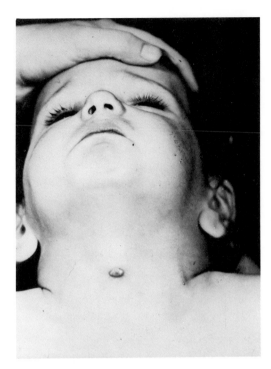

Fig. 18-11. Thyroglossal fistula. (Courtesy of Dr. J. Randolph.)

larges, it is prone to become infected, and for this reason it should be removed surgically. Since remnants of the duct often traverse the body of the hyoid bone, this may have to be excised also to prevent recurrence.

Thyroglossal Sinus (Fistula)

Occasionally a thyroglossal cyst ruptures spontaneously, producing a sinus. Usually this is a result of an infection of a cyst (Fig. 18-11). All remnants of the thyroglossal duct should be removed surgically.

Parathyroid Glands

Absence and Hypoplasia of the Parathyroid Glands

This has been demonstrated in individuals with idiopathic hypoparathyroidism.

Ectopia

The close relationship between the parathyroids III and the developing thymus explains the frequent finding of parathyroid tissue in the superior mediastinum (Fig. 18-4). If the parathyroid glands remain attached to the thymus, they may be pulled inferiorly into the lower part of the neck or thoracic cavity. Moreover, this also explains the variable position of the inferior parathyroid glands in relation to the lower poles of the lateral lobes of the thyroid gland.

Suprarenal Glands

Agenesis

Agenesis, or hypoplasia of the suprarenal cortex, frequently occurs in anencephaly associated with pituitary deficiency.

Ectopic Suprarenal Glands

Very occasionally suprarenal tissue is found beneath the capsule of the kidney.

Accessory Cortical Tissue

This has been found closely associated with the main gland and also in many situations on the posterior abdominal wall and pelvis behind the peritoneum. Such accessory cortical tissue is not usually associated with medullary tissue.

Adrenogenital Syndrome

This is described in Chapter 16.

Islets of Langerhans

Neonatal Pseudodiabetes Mellitus

In newborn infants, a rare transient diabetes-like condition occurs with hyperglycemia and glycosuria. The child recovers spontaneously in 2 to 3 weeks as his beta cells begin to function.

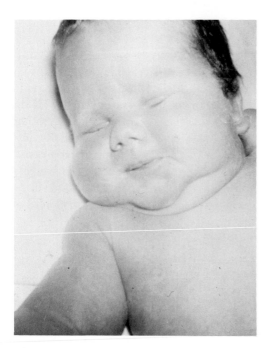

Fig. 18-12. Obese baby born to a diabetic mother. (Courtesy of Dr. G. Avery.)

Diffuse Islet Hyperplasia

Hypertrophy and hyperplasia of pancreatic islets occur in babies born to diabetic mothers. The total amount of islet tissue may be as much as three times that found in a normal child. This condition is brought on by the maternal hyperglycemia causing fetal hyperglycemia. The high level of blood sugar stimulates the fetal pancreatic islet cells. The increased insulin production in the presence of a plentiful supply of glucose results in fetal obesity (Fig. 18-12).

Testis and Ovary

The congenital anomalies of the testis and ovary are described in Chapter 16.

Clinical Problems

Answers on page 451

1. A 5-year-old girl died; she had the symptoms and signs of an intracranial tumor. During the last 2 months of her life she had bitemporal hemianopia and diabetes insipidus, indicating that pressure was being exerted on the optic chiasma and the pituitary gland. At postmortem a large cystic tumor was found in the floor of the sella turcica, involving the body of the sphenoid bone. The diagnosis was a craniopharyngioma. Do you know of any embryological remnants that may be present in the body of the sphenoid bone and could give rise to such a tumor?

2. An 8-year-old boy was examined by a physician because he said he could feel a lump in his tongue. On physical examination, a rounded mass about ½ in. (1.25 cm) in diameter could be felt in the tongue beneath the foramen cecum. Examination of the neck resulted in a failure to feel the thyroid gland. What is the differential diagnosis? How would you treat this patient?

3. A 6-month-old girl was seen by a pediatrician because the mother was concerned that the child was constipated. She had also noticed that the baby slept a great deal and hardly ever cried. "She never seems to be hungry," the mother said. On physical examination it was noted that the child had a lethargic expression, flat nose, and a large protruding tongue. The skin was dry and yellow in color and the hairline was low

on the forehead. The hair on the head was dry and thin. The abdomen was distended, and a small umbilical hernia was present. Fatty pads were present in the neck above both the clavicles. The extremities were short and the muscles hypotonic. The hands were broad and the fingers short. Using your knowledge of embryology, make the diagnosis. How would you treat this patient?

4. An 18-year-old woman went to her physician because she had noticed a swelling in the midline of her neck. She said she had first noticed this swelling 3 years previously and it had gradually increased in size. On physical examination a small swelling was found in the midline of the neck measuring about ½ in. (1.25 cm) in diameter. It was situated just below the body of the hyoid bone, was fluctuant, and moved upward on swallowing. Nothing else abnormal was discovered. What is your diagnosis? How would you treat this patient?

5. A 30-year-old woman had been treated for 5 years for recurrent renal calculi in both kidneys. Recently a diagnosis of adenoma of the parathyroid gland had been made. The presence of this tumor was responsible for the high blood calcium level in this case, which in turn was the cause of the multiple renal calculi. Before the operation for removal of the adenoma the surgeon expressed concern that he might experience difficulty in finding the tumor. Why do you think the surgeon might have difficulty? Where are the parathyroid glands formed?

REFERENCES

Aceto, T., MacGillivray, M. H., Caprano, V. J., Munschauer, R. W., and Raiti, S. Congenital Virilizing Adrenal Hyperplasia Without Acceleration of Growth or Bone Maturation. *J.A.M.A.* 198:1341, 1966.

Adams, D. D., Lord, J. M., and Stevely, H. A. A. Congenital Thyrotoxicosis. *Lancet* 2:497, 1964.

Ainger, L. E., and Kelly, V. C. Familial Athyrotic Cretinism: A Report of 3 Cases. *J. Clin. Endocr.* 15:469, 1955.

Akerren, Y. Prolonged Jaundice in the Newborn Associated with Congenital Myxoedema. *Acta Paediat.* (Uppsala) 43:411, 1954.

Ariens Kappers, J. Development of the Human Paraphysis. *J. Comp. Neurol.* 102:425, 1955.

Baird, J. D., and Farquhar, J. W. Insulin-Secreting Capacity in Newborn Infants of Normal and Diabetic Women. *Lancet* 1:71, 1962.

Benner, M. C. Studies on the Involution of the Fetal Cortex of the Adrenal Glands. *Amer. J. Path.* 16:787, 1940.

Birke, G., Diczfalusy, E. Plantin, L. O., Robbe, H., and Westman, H. Familial Congenital Hyperplasia of the Adrenal Cortex. *Acta Endocr.* (Kobenhavn) 29:55, 1958.

Blizzard, R. M., and Alberts, M. Hypopituitarism, Hypoadrenalism and Hypogonadism in the Newborn Infant. *J. Pediat.* 48:782, 1956.

Blizzard, R. M., Chandler, R. W., Landing, B. H., Pettit, M. D., and West, G. D. Maternal Autoimmunization to Thyroid as a Probable Cause of Athyrotic Cretinism. *New Eng. J. Med.* 263: 327, 1960.

Blotner, H. The Inheritance of Diabetes Insipidus. *Amer. J. Med. Sci.* 204:261, 1942.

Boyd, J. D. Development of the Thyroid and Parathyroid Glands and the Thymus. *Ann. Roy. Coll. Surg. Eng.* 7:455, 1950.

Brewer, D. Congenital Absence of the Pituitary Gland and Its Consequences. *J. Path. Bact.* 73: 59, 1967.

Bruce, J., and Strong, J. A. Maternal Hyperparathyroidism and Parathyroid Deficiency in the Child. *Quart. J. Med.* 24:307, 1955.

Carr, E. A., Beierwaltes, W. H., Raman, G., Dodson, V. N., Tanton, J., Betts J. S. and Stambaugh, R. A. The Effect of Maternal Thyroid Function on Fetal Thyroid Function and Development. *J. Clin. Endocr.* 19:1, 1959.

Chapman, E. M., Comer, G. N., Robinson, D., and Evans, R. D. The Collection of Radioactive Iodine by the Human Foetal Thyroid. *J. Clin. Endocr.* 8:717, 1948.

Corcoran, W. J., and Strauss, A. A. Suprarenal Hemorrhage in the Newborn. *J.A.M.A.* 82:626, 1924.

Dunn, J. M. Anterior Pituitary and Adrenal Absence in a Live-Born Normocephalic Infant. *Amer. J. Obstet. Gynec.* 96:893, 1966.

Eberlein, N. R. *Fetal Adrenal Function in Congenital Hyperplasia: Excerpta Med.* (Amsterdam) International Congress Series, No. 132, 1967. P. 687.

Ellis, R. W. B., and Mitchell, R. G. *Disease in Infancy and Childhood,* 7th ed. Livingstone, Edinburgh, 1973.

Falin, L. I. The Development of the Human Hypophysis and Differentiation of Cells of Its Anterior Lobe During Embryonic Life. *Acta Anat.* 44:188, 1961.

Gilmour, J. R. The Embryology of the Parathyroid Glands, the Thymus and Certain Associated Rudiments. *J. Path. Bact.* 45:507, 1937.

Goetsch, E. Lingual Goiter. *Ann. Surg.* 127:291, 1948.

Greig, W. R., Henderson, A. S., Boyle, J. A., McGirr, E. M., and Hutchison, J. H. Thyroid Dysgenesis in Two Pairs of Monozygotic Twins and in a Mother and Child. *J. Clin. Endocr.* 26: 1309, 1966.

Hamilton, W. J., and Mossman, H. W. *Human Embryology,* 4th ed. Williams & Wilkins, Baltimore, 1972.

Hubble, D. *Paediatric Endocrinology.* Blackwell, Oxford, 1969.

Hunter, R. B., MacGregor, A. R., Shepherd, D. M., and West, G. B. Noradrenaline in Human Foetal Adrenals and Organs of Zuckerkandl. *J. Pharm. Pharmacol.* 6:407, 1953.

Jeffcoate, T. N. A., Fliegner, J. R. H., Russell, S. H., Davis, J. C., and Wade, A. P. Diagnosis of the Adrenogenital Syndrome Before Birth. *Lancet* 2:553, 1965.

Jost, A. Problems of Fetal Endocrinology: The Gonadal and Hypophyseal Hormones. *Recent Progr. Hormone Res.* 8:379, 1953.

Kingsbury, B. F. The Question of a Lateral Thyroid in Mammals with Special Reference to Man. *Amer. J. Anat.* 65:333, 1939.

Marshall, S. F., and Beeker, W. F. Thyroglossal Cysts and Sinuses. *Ann. Surg.* 129:642, 1949.

McClintock, J. C., and Mahaffey, D. E. Thyroglossal Tract Lesions. In *Transactions of the American Goiter Association.* Thomas, Springfield, Ill., 1950.

McKenzie, J. M. Neonatal Grave's Disease. *J. Clin. Endocr.* 24:660, 1964.

Montgomery, M. L. Lingual Thyroid: A Comprehensive Review. *Western J. Surg.* 44:54, 1936.

Mosier, H. D., Blizzard, R. M., and Wilkins, L. Congenital Defects in the Biosynthesis of Thyroid Hormone: Report of Two Cases. *Pediatrics* 21:248, 1958.

Norris, E. H. The Parathyroid Glands and the Lateral Thyroid in Man: Their Morphogenesis, Histogenesis, Topographic Anatomy and Prenatal Growth. *Contrib. Embryol.* 26:247, 1937.

Norris, E. H. Anatomical Evidence of Pre-Natal Function of the Human Parathyroid Glands. *Anat. Rec.* 96:129, 1946.

Ross, M. H. Electron Microscopy of the Human Foetal Adrenal Cortex. In *The Human Adrenal Cortex,* edited by A. R. Currie. Livingstone, Edinburgh, 1962. P. 558.

Scammon, R. E. The Prenatal Growth and Natal Involution of the Human Suprarenal Gland. *Proc. Soc. Exp. Biol. Med.* 23:809, 1926.

Sgalitzer, K. E. Contribution to the Study of the Morphogenesis of the Thyroid Gland. *J. Anat.* 75:389, 1941.

Shanklin, W. M. Differentiation of Pituicytes in the Human Fetus. *J. Anat.* 74:459, 1940.

Sutherland, J. M., Esselborn, V. M., Burket, R. L., Shillman, T. B., and Benson, J. T. Familial Non-Goiterous Cretinism Apparently Due to Maternal Anti-Thyroid Antibody. *New Eng. J. Med.* 263:336, 1960.

Taitz, L. S., Zarate-Salvador, C., and Schwarz, E. Congenital Absence of the Parathyroid and Thymus Glands in an Infant (3–4 Pharyngeal Pouch Syndrome). *Pediatrics* 38:412, 1966.

Tilney, F. Development and Constituents of the Human Hypophysis. *Bull. Neurol. Inst. N. Y.* 5:387, 1936.

Tweedie, A. R., and Keith, A. Ectopia of the Pituitary with Other Congenital Anomalies of the Nose, Palate and Upper Lip. *Proc. Roy. Soc. Med.* 4:47, 1911.

Van Dyke, J. H. Behavior of the Ultimobranchial Tissue in the Postnatal Thyroid Gland. *Amer. J. Path.* 76:201, 1945.

Weller, G. L. Development of the Thyroid, Parathyroid and Thymus Glands in Man. *Contrib. Embryol.* 24:93, 1933.

For purposes of description, the nervous system may be divided into two main parts: (1) the central nervous system, consisting of the spinal cord and brain and (2) the peripheral nervous system (see Chap. 20), consisting of the cranial and spinal nerves and ganglia.

DEVELOPMENT

During the third week of development, the ectoderm on the dorsal surface of the embryo between the primitive knot and the buccopharyngeal membrane becomes thickened to form the *neural plate* (Fig. 19-1). The plate, which is pear-shaped and wider cranially, develops a longitudinal *neural groove*. The groove now deepens so that it is bounded on either side by *neural folds*. With further development, the neural folds fuse, converting the neural groove into a *neural tube*. Fusion starts about the midpoint along the groove and extends cranially and caudally so that in the earliest stage the cavity of the tube remains in communication with the amniotic cavity through the *anterior* and *posterior neuropores*. The anterior neuropore closes first, and two days later the posterior neuropore closes. Meanwhile the neural tube has sunk beneath the surface ectoderm.

During the invagination of the neural plate to form the neural groove, the cells forming the lateral margin of the plate do not become incorporated in the neural tube but form a strip of ectodermal cells that lie between the neural tube and the covering ectoderm. This strip of ectoderm is called the *neural crest* (Fig. 19-1), and subsequently this group of cells will migrate ventrolaterally on each side around the neural tube. Ultimately the neural crest cells will differentiate into the cells of the *posterior root ganglia*, the *sensory ganglia of the cranial nerves, autonomic ganglia, Schwann cells, the cells of the suprarenal medulla*, and the *melanocytes*. It is also believed that these cells give rise to mesenchymal cells in the head and neck.

Meanwhile the cephalic end of the neural tube dilates to form *three primary brain vesicles*, the *forebrain vesicle*, the *midbrain vesicle*, and the *hindbrain vesicle* (Fig. 19-2). The remainder of the tube elongates and remains smaller in diameter and will form the *spinal cord*.

Spinal Cord

The wall of the neural tube consists of a thick layer of pseudostratified epithelium, the *neuroepithelium* (Fig. 19-2). At their luminal

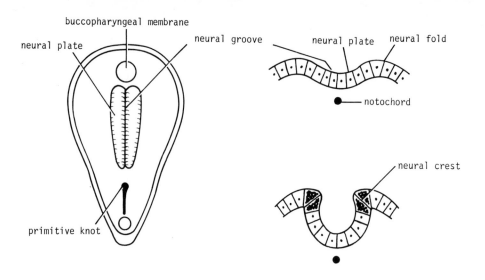

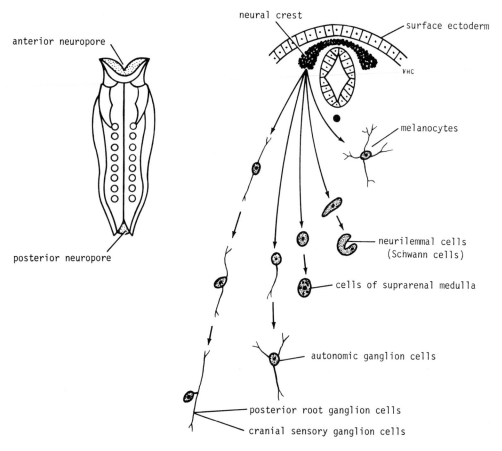

Fig. 19-1. The formation of the neural plate, neural groove, and neural tube. The cells of the neural crest differentiate into the cells of the posterior root ganglia, the sensory ganglia of cranial nerves, autonomic ganglia, neurilemmal cells (Schwann cells), the cells of the suprarenal medulla, and melanocytes.

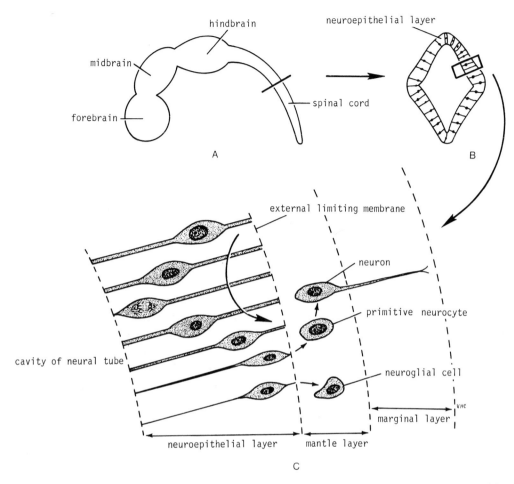

Fig. 19-2. (A) Expansion of the cephalic end of the neural tube to form the forebrain, midbrain, and hindbrain vesicles. (B) and (C) Cross section of the developing neural tube in the region of the spinal cord. The cells of the neuroepithelial layer have been widely separated for clarity.

ends, the cells are connected to each other by terminal bars. The outer surfaces of the cells are bound by an external limiting membrane. While proliferation of the neuroepithelium is taking place, the nuclei of the cells undergo a cyclic change in position. During the interphase, when DNA synthesis occurs, the nucleus lies in the outer part of the cell away from the lumen of the neural tube. During the premitotic phase, the nucleus progressively approaches the luminal end of the cell. Mitosis now takes place. Once cell division

has occurred, each daughter nucleus moves toward the outer part of the cell. The repeated division of the neuroepithelial cells results in an increase in length and diameter of the tube, which remains lined by a pseudostratified epithelium. Eventually cells are formed that are incapable of further division. These cells, the *primitive neurocytes,* migrate peripherally to form a zone which surrounds the neuroepithelial layer, and this zone is known as the *mantle layer* (Fig. 19-2). The mantle layer will later form the *gray matter*

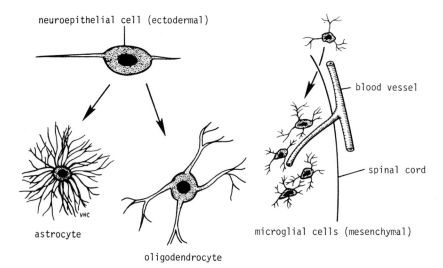

neuroepithelial cell (ectodermal)

blood vessel

spinal cord

astrocyte

oligodendrocyte

microglial cells (mesenchymal)

Fig. 19-3. Origin of the neuroglial cells.

of the spinal cord. The primitive neurocytes now give rise to nerve fibers which grow peripherally and form a layer external to the mantle layer called the *marginal layer*. The nerve fibers in the marginal layer become myelinated and have a white appearance. For this reason, the marginal layer is known as the *white matter* of the spinal cord.

While the primitive neurocytes are being formed, the neuroepithelial cells also give rise to two types of *neuroglial cells,* the *astrocytes* and the *oligodendrocytes* (Figs. 19-2 & 19-3). These new cells migrate from the neuroepithelial layer and take up their final positions as supporting cells in the white and gray matter of the spinal cord. Later a third type of neuroglial cell, the *microglial cells,* which are thought to be members of the reticuloendothelial system and are derived from the surrounding mesenchyme, migrate into the developing spinal cord along with blood vessels (Fig. 19-3) and also take up positions in the white and gray matter.

Finally the neuroepithelial cells differentiate into a single layer of ciliated columnar cells which line the neural tube and are known as *ependymal cells.*

As a result of the development that is taking place in the wall of the neural tube, the cavity of the tube becomes narrowed to form a dorsoventral cleft with thick lateral walls and a thin floor and roof (Fig. 19-4). The latter are referred to as the *floor* and *roof plates,* respectively, and they consist only of neuroglial cells, the narrow marginal layer providing a pathway for commissural fibers.

With the continuous addition of new primitive neurocytes to the mantle layer of the lateral wall of the neural tube, a large ventral and later a smaller dorsal thickening become apparent. The ventral or anterior thickenings are known as the *basal plates,* and the neurocytes will become the *motor anterior horn* cells (Fig. 19-4). The dorsal or posterior thickenings are known as the *alar plates,* and the neurocytes will become the sensory cells of the *posterior horns.* The two thickenings are separated on each side by a longitudinal groove, the *sulcus limitans,* and this serves to mark the junction between the anterior motor (basal plate) and posterior sensory (alar plate) areas of the mantle layer (Fig. 19-4).

As a result of continued growth of the basal plates, they extend forward on each side of the midline, forming a deep longitudinal groove on the anterior surface of the spinal cord, called the *anterior median fissure* (Fig. 19-4). The alar plates also increase in size and extend medially, compressing the posterior

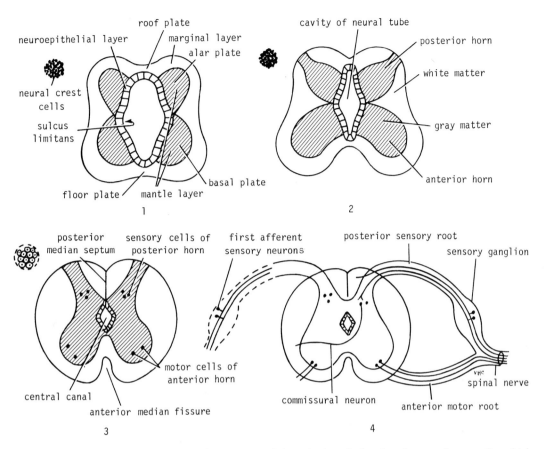

Fig. 19-4. The different stages in the development of the spinal cord, showing the neural crest cells, which will form the first afferent neurons in the sensory pathway.

part of the lumen of the neural tube. Ultimately the walls of the posterior portion of the neural tube come into apposition and fuse to form the *posterior median septum*. The remaining ventral part of the lumen of the neural tube is now known as the *central canal* of the spinal cord (Fig. 19-4). The most caudal portion of the central canal is slightly dilated and is known as the *terminal ventricle*.

Further Development of the Motor Neurons in the Anterior Horn

The primitive neurocytes of the anterior horn develop first, and only when most of these have migrated into the anterior horn does the

development of primitive neurocytes for the posterior horn commence. In the early stages, the primitive neurocyte has no processes, but later, as development proceeds, a number of short processes arise at one end of the cell, known as *dendrites,* and a long process develops at the opposite pole of the cell and is known as the *axon* (Fig. 19-5). The entire cell with all its processes is referred to as a *neuron*. Since the neuron has many processes arising from different points on the cell surface, it is commonly called a *multipolar neuron.*

With further development, the multipolar neurons in the anterior horn become very large, and it is possible to divide them into

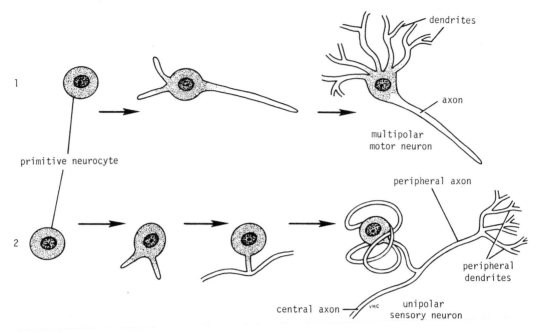

Fig. 19-5. The successive stages in the development of (1) a multipolar motor neuron found in the anterior horn, and (2) a unipolar sensory neuron found in a sensory ganglion.

(1) a medial group, the axons of which leave the anterior surface of the spinal cord and are distributed as motor fibers to the musculature of the body, and (2) a lateral group, the axons of which also leave the anterior surface of the spinal cord as autonomic preganglionic fibers. The fibers leaving the anterior surface of the spinal cord are collectively known as the *anterior root of the spinal nerve* (Fig. 19-4). Between the first thoracic and second or third lumbar segments of the mature spinal cord, the lateral group of anterior horn cells have developed into a distinctive column of gray matter, which is now referred to as the *lateral horn* (Fig. 19-6).

Further Development of the First Afferent Neurons in the Sensory Pathway

The first neurons in this pathway have their cell bodies situated outside the spinal cord and are derived from the neural crest (Fig. 19-4.) The neural crest cells migrate to a posterolateral position on either side of the developing spinal cord and become segmented into cell clusters. Some of the cells in each cluster now differentiate into primitive neurocytes (Fig. 19-5). Each primitive neurocyte develops two processes, a peripheral process and a central process. The peripheral processes grow out laterally to become typical axons of sensory nerve fibers. The central processes, also axons, grow into the posterior part of the developing spinal cord and either end in the posterior horn or ascend through the marginal layer (white matter) to one of the higher brain centers. These central processes are referred to collectively as the *posterior root of the spinal nerve* (Fig. 19-4). The peripheral processes join the anterior nerve root to form the trunk of the *mixed spinal nerve.*

The primitive neurocyte is now known as a *unipolar neuron,* and collectively these cells form the posterior root ganglia (see

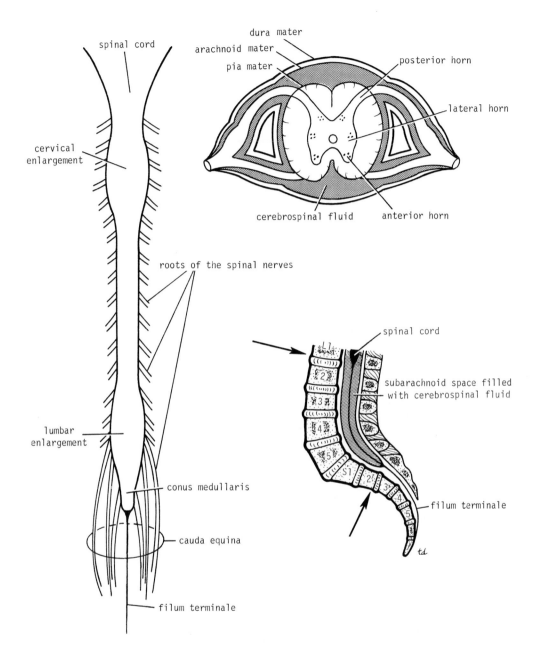

Fig. 19-6. The spinal cord and its meninges. In the adult, the lower end of the spinal cord lies at the level of the lower border of the body of the first lumbar vertebra (*arrow*) and the subarachnoid space ends at the lower border of the body of the second sacral vertebra (*arrow*).

Chap. 20). Not all the neural crest cells in the ganglia differentiate into neurocytes. Some cells develop into *capsule cells,* which surround each of the nerve cells in a ganglion (Fig. 20-5).

Further Development of the Sensory Neurons in the Posterior Horn

The primitive neurocytes, which have entered the alar plates, now develop processes that enter the marginal layer (white matter) of the cord on the same side and either ascend or descend to a higher or lower level and are known as *association neurons.* Other cells send processes to the opposite side of the cord through the floor plate, where they ascend or descend for variable distances and are known as *commissural neurons* (Fig. 19-4).

Myelination in the Spinal Cord

In the spinal cord the nerve fibers are heavily myelinated or slightly myelinated. The myelin sheath is formed and maintained by the *oligodendrocytes* of the neuroglia. The cervical portion of the cord is the first part to develop myelin, and from here the process extends caudally. The fibers of the anterior nerve roots are myelinated before those of the posterior nerve roots. The process of myelination begins within the cord at about the fourth month, and the sensory fibers are affected first. The descending motor fibers are the last to myelinate, which process does not begin until term; it continues during the first 2 years of postnatal life.

The Development of the Meninges and the Relation of the Spinal Cord to the Vertebral Column

In the spinal region, the neural tube is surrounded by loose mesenchymal tissue derived from the sclerotomes. This differentiates into the three *meninges* of the spinal cord, the *pia mater,* the *arachnoid mater,* and the *dura mater.*

The inner vascular membrane, the pia mater, is adherent to the underlying nervous tissue and sends fibrous septa into the spinal cord (Fig. 19-6). The middle delicate nonvascular membrane, the arachnoid mater, envelops the spinal cord and extends laterally to form sheaths around the roots of the spinal nerves. At the caudal end of the fully developed spinal cord, the arachnoid extends beyond the lower limit of the cord to the level of the second sacral vertebra. A cavity develops between the pia and arachnoid and is called the *subarachnoid space,* which becomes filled with *cerebrospinal fluid* (Fig. 19-6). The outer tough fibrous membrane, the dura mater, also envelops the spinal cord and extends from the foramen magnum of the skull superiorly, where it is continuous with the dura covering the brain, to the level of the second sacral vertebra inferiorly. Each nerve root also receives an investment of dura, which is continuous with the epineurium of the spinal nerve. The fibrous trabeculae in the subarachnoid space and the *ligamentum denticulatum* develop from areas of condensation of mesenchyme.

During the first two months of intra-uterine life, the spinal cord is the same length as the vertebral column. Thereafter the developing vertebral column grows more rapidly than the spinal cord, so that at term the coccygeal end of the cord lies at the level of the third lumbar vertebra. *In the adult, the lower end of the spinal cord lies at the level of the lower border of the body of the first lumbar vertebra.* As a result of this disproportion in the rate of growth of the vertebral column and spinal cord, the anterior and posterior roots of the spinal nerves below the first lumbar segment of the spinal cord descend within the vertebral canal until they reach their appropriate exits through the intervertebral foramina. Moreover the pia mater, which attached the coccygeal end of the spinal cord to the coccyx, now extends down as a slender fibrous strand from the lower end of the cord to the coccyx and is called the *filum terminale* (Fig. 19-6). The obliquely coursing anterior and posterior roots of the spinal nerves and the filum terminale, which now occupy the lower end of the vertebral canal, are collectively called the *cauda equina* (Fig. 19-6).

It is important to realize that the cauda equina is enclosed within the subarachnoid space down as far as the level of the second sacral vertebra. It is in this region, below the lower end of the spinal cord, that samples of cerebrospinal fluid may be obtained by *lumbar puncture*.

In the earliest stages, the developing spinal cord is a thick-walled tube that gradually tapers at its caudal end. In the fourth month, as the result of the development of the limb buds and the additional sensory and motor neurons at these levels, the cord becomes swollen in the cervical and lumbar regions to form the *cervical* and *lumbar enlargements* (Fig. 19-6).

The Brain*

Once the neural tube has closed, the *three primary brain vesicles*—the *forebrain vesicle,* the *midbrain vesicle,* and the *hindbrain vesicle*—complete their development (Fig. 19-7). The forebrain vesicle will form the forebrain (*prosencephalon*), the midbrain vesicle will form the midbrain (*mesencephalon*), and the hindbrain vesicle will form the hindbrain (*rhombencephalon*).

By the fifth week the forebrain and hindbrain vesicles divide into two secondary vesicles (Fig. 19-7). The forebrain vesicle forms (1) the *telencephalon,* with its primitive cerebral hemispheres, and (2) the *diencephalon,* which develops optic vesicles. The hindbrain vesicle forms (1) the *meten-*

* Only those aspects of brain development which are considered to be important for a student of medicine are considered here. If further details are required, consult the references for this chapter.

cephalon, the future pons and cerebellum, and (2) the *myelencephalon,* or medulla oblongata.

The basic pattern of the ventricular system is now established. The cavity in each cerebral hemisphere is known as the *lateral ventricle.* The cavity of the diencephalon is known as the *IIIrd ventricle.* With continued growth, the cavity of the midbrain vesicle becomes small and forms the *aqueduct of Sylvius.* The cavity of the entire hindbrain vesicle forms the *IVth ventricle.* The IVth ventricle is continuous with the central canal of the spinal cord. The lateral ventricles communicate with the IIIrd ventricle through the *interventricular foramina of Monro.* The ventricular system and the central canal of the spinal cord are lined with ependyma and are filled with *cerebrospinal fluid.* In the earliest stages, the cerebrospinal fluid within the ventricular system is not continuous with that of the subarachnoid space.

Early in development, the embryonic disc is flat and the neural tube is straight. Later with the development of the head fold and tail fold, the neural tube becomes gently curved. As the head fold increases, the hindbrain vesicle becomes bent acutely forward on the neural tube, forming the *cervical flexure.* Largely as the result of unequal growth in different areas of the brain vesicles, another *ventral flexure* appears in the mesencephalon, and a *dorsal flexure* (pontine) follows in the hindbrain. Finally another *dorsal flexure* appears in the forebrain.

Medulla Oblongata (Myelencephalon)

The walls of the vesicle show initially the typical organization seen in the neural tube with ventral or anterior thickenings, the *basal plates,* and dorsal or posterior thickenings, the *alar plates,* the two being separated by the *sulcus limitans* (Fig. 19-8). As development proceeds, the lateral walls are moved laterally (like an opening clamshell) at higher levels by the expanding IVth ventricle. As a

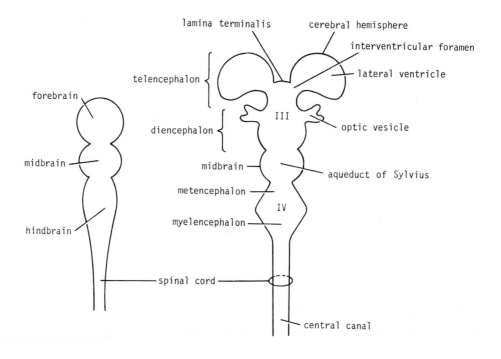

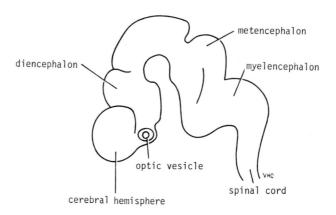

Fig. 19-7. The division of the forebrain vesicle into the telencephalon and the diencephalon, and the hindbrain vesicle into the metencephalon and myelencephalon. Also shown is the way in which the cerebral hemisphere on each side develops as a diverticulum from the telencephalon.

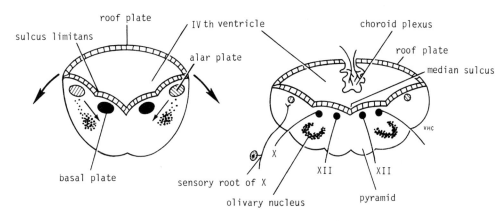

Fig. 19-8. The development of the medulla oblongata (myelencephalon).

result, the alar plates come to lie lateral to the basal plates. The neurons of the basal plate form the motor nuclei of the cranial nerves IX, X, XI, and XII and are situated in the floor of the IVth ventricle medial to the sulcus limitans. The neurons of the alar plate form the sensory nuclei of cranial nerves V, VIII, IX, and X and the *gracile* and *cuneate nuclei*. Other cells of the alar plate migrate ventrolaterally and form the *olivary nuclei*.

The roof plate becomes stretched into a thin layer of ependymal tissue. The vascular mesenchyme lying in contact with the outer surface of the roof plate forms the pia mater, and the two layers together form the *tela choroidea*. Vascular tufts of tela choroidea project into the cavity of the IVth ventricle to form the *choroid plexus* (Fig. 19-8). Between the fourth and fifth months, local resorptions of the roof plate occur, forming paired lateral foramina, *foramina of Luschka,* and a median foramen, the *foramen of Magendie.* These apertures are extremely important and allow the cerebrospinal fluid produced within the ventricles of the brain to escape into the subarachnoid space (Fig. 19-11).

The floor plate remains narrow and forms the region of the *median sulcus.*

In the marginal layer on the ventral aspect of the medulla, descending axons from cells in the motor cortex produce prominent swellings called the *pyramids*.

Pons (Ventral Part of Metencephalon)

The pons arises from the ventral or anterior part of the metencephalon (Fig. 19-9), but it also receives a cellular contribution from the alar part of the myelencephalon.

The neurons of the basal plates form the motor nuclei of cranial nerves V, VI, and VII. The neurons of the ventromedial part of each alar plate form the main sensory nucleus of cranial nerve V, a sensory nucleus of cranial nerve VII, and the vestibular and cochlear nuclei of cranial nerve VIII; they also form the *pontine* nuclei. The axons of the pontine nuclei grow transversely to enter the developing cerebellum of the opposite side, thus forming the *transverse pontine fibers* and the *middle cerebellar peduncle.*

Cerebellum (Dorsal Part of Metencephalon)

The cerebellum is formed from the dorsal part of the alar plates of the metencephalon. On each side, the alar plates bend medially to form the *rhombic lips* (Fig. 19-10). As they enlarge, the lips project caudally over the roof plate of the IVth ventricle and unite with each other in the midline to form the cere-

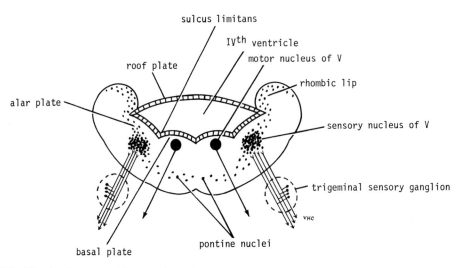

Fig. 19-9. The development of the pons from the ventral part of the metencephalon.

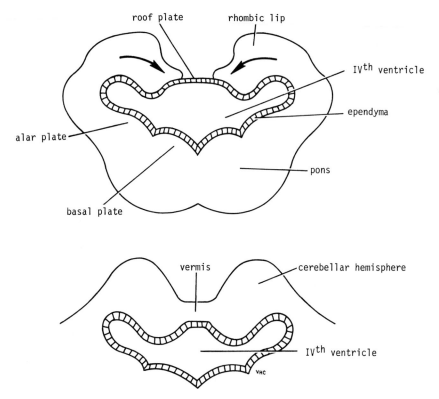

Fig. 19-10. The development of the cerebellum. Also shown is the fusion of the rhombic lips in the midline to form the dumbbell-shaped cerebellum.

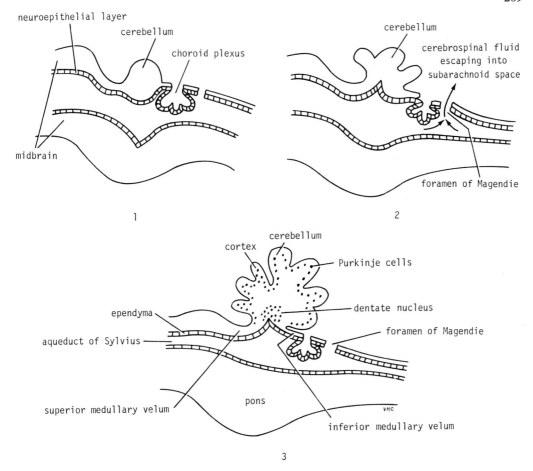

Fig. 19-11. Sagittal sections of the developing cerebellum.

bellum (Figs. 19-11 & 19-12). At the twelfth week, a small midline portion, the *vermis,* and two lateral portions, the *cerebellar hemispheres,* may be recognized. At about the end of the fourth month, fissures develop on the surface of the cerebellum and the characteristic folia of the adult cerebellum gradually develop.

The primitive neurocytes derived from the neuroepithelium migrate toward the surface of the cerebellum and eventually give rise to the neurons forming the *cortex* of the cerebellum. Other primitive neurocytes remain close to the ventricular surface and differentiate into the *dentate* and other deep cerebellar nuclei. With further development, the axons of neurons forming these nuclei grow out into the mesencephalon (midbrain) to reach the forebrain and these fibers will form the greater part of the *superior cerebellar peduncle.* Later, the growth of the axons of the *pontocerebellar fibers* and the *corticopontine fibers* will connect the cerebral cortex with the cerebellum, and so the *middle cerebellar peduncle*s will be formed. The *inferior cerebellar peduncle* will be largely formed by the growth of sensory axons from the spinal cord, the vestibular nuclei, and the olivary nuclei.

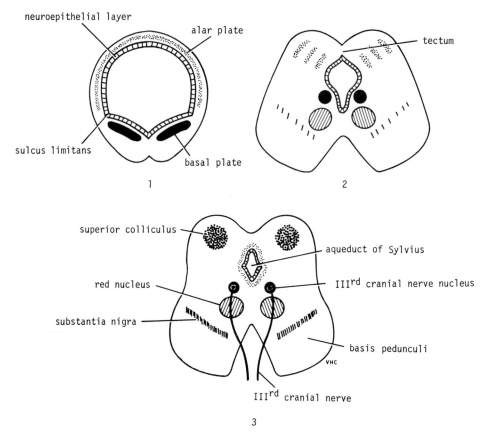

Fig. 19-12.   The successive stages in the development of the midbrain.

Superior and Inferior Medullary Vela

These are formed from the roof plate of the IVth ventricle (Fig. 19-11).

Midbrain (Mesencephalon)

The midbrain develops from the midbrain vesicle, the cavity of which becomes much reduced to form the *cerebral aqueduct of Sylvius* (Fig. 19-12). The sulcus limitans separates the alar plate from the basal plate on each side, as seen in the developing spinal cord. The primitive neurocytes in the basal plates will differentiate into the neurons forming the nuclei of the *IIIrd* and *IVth cranial nerves* and possibly the *red nuclei,* the substantia nigra, and the *reticular formation.* The marginal layer of each basal plate enlarges considerably and forms the *basis pedunculi.* These are formed by nerve fibers descending from the cerebral cortex to the lower centers in the pons and spinal cord, i.e., the *corticopontine, corticobulbar,* and *corticospinal tracts.*

The two alar plates and the original roof plate form the *tectum.* The primitive neurocytes in the alar plates differentiate into the sensory neurons of the *superior* and *inferior colliculi* (Fig. 19-12). In the earliest stages, the dorsal surface of the midbrain shows two longitudinal elevations separated by a median depression. Later a transverse depression appears so that the four swellings representing the four colliculi can be recognized on the dorsal surface of the midbrain. The superior colliculi are associated with visual reflexes and the inferior colliculi are associated with auditory reflexes.

With further development, the fibers of the IVth cranial nerve emerge on the dorsal surface and the fibers of the IIIrd cranial nerve emerge on the ventral surface of the midbrain.

Forebrain (Prosencephalon)

The forebrain develops from the forebrain vesicle. The roof and floor plates remain thin, while the lateral walls become thick, as in the developing spinal cord. At an early stage a lateral diverticulum appears on each side of the forebrain, called the *optic vesicle.* That part of the forebrain that lies cephalic to the optic vesicle is for practical purposes the *telencephalon,* and the remainder of the forebrain is the diencephalon (Fig. 19-13). The optic vesicle and stalk will ultimately form the retina and optic nerve.

The telencephalon now develops a lateral diverticulum on each side of the *cerebral hemisphere,* and its cavity is known as the *lateral ventricle.* The anterior part of the IIIrd ventricle is therefore formed by the medial part of the telencephalon and ends at the *lamina terminalis,* which represents the cephalic end of the neural tube. The opening into each lateral ventricle is the future *interventricular foramen of Monro.*

Fate of the Diencephalon

The cavity of the diencephalon forms the greater part of the IIIrd ventricle (Fig. 19-13). Its roof shows a small diverticulum immediately anterior to the midbrain; this is the beginning of the development of the *pineal gland* (see Chap. 18). The remainder of the roof is devoid of primitive neurocytes and forms the ependyma, which becomes invaded by vascular mesenchyme to form the *choroid plexus* of the IIIrd ventricle (Fig. 19-14). In the lateral wall of the IIIrd ventricle the *thalamus* arises as a thickening of the alar plate on each side. Posterior to the thalamus, the *medial* and *lateral geniculate bodies* develop as solid buds. With the continued growth of the two thalami, the ventricular cavity becomes narrowed, and in some individuals the two thalami may meet and fuse in the midline to form the *interthalamic adhesion* of gray matter which crosses the IIIrd ventricle (Fig. 19-15).

Fig. 19-13. The division of the forebrain vesicle into the telencephalon and the diencephalon.

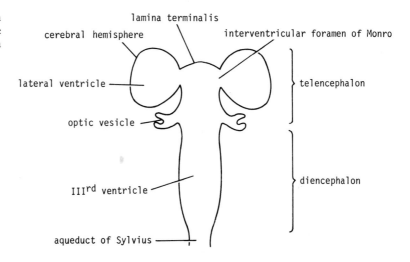

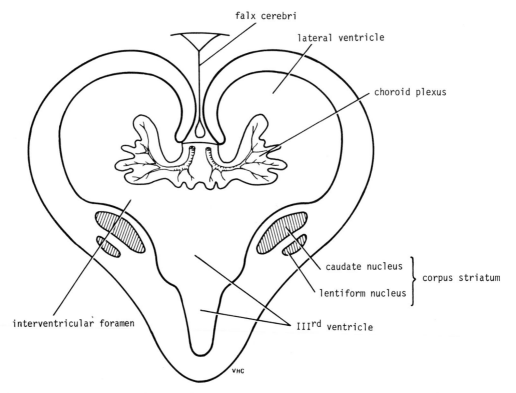

Fig. 19-14. Coronal section of the cerebral hemispheres showing the developing choroid plexuses in the IIIrd and lateral ventricles.

The lower part of the alar plate on each side will differentiate into a large number of *hypothalamic nuclei.* One of these becomes conspicuous on the ventral surface of the hypothalamus and forms a rounded swelling on each side of the midline called the *mammillary body* (Fig. 19-16).

The *infundibulum* develops as a diverticulum from the floor of the diencephalon and will give origin to the *stalk* and *pars nervosa of the hypophysis* (Fig. 19-16). The development of the hypophysis is considered in detail in Chapter 18.

Fate of the Telencephalon

The telencephalon forms the anterior end of the IIIrd ventricle, which is closed by the lamina terminalis, while the diverticulum on either side forms the cerebral hemisphere.

Cerebral Hemispheres

Each hemisphere arises at the beginning of the fifth week of development. As it expands superiorly, its walls thicken and the interventricular foramen becomes reduced in size (Figs. 19-13—19-15). The mesenchyme between each cerebral hemisphere condenses to form the *falx cerebri.* As development proceeds, the cerebral hemispheres grow and expand rapidly, first anteriorly to form the *frontal lobes,* then laterally and superiorly to form the *parietal lobes,* and finally posteriorly and inferiorly to produce the *occipital* and *temporal lobes.* As the result of this great ex-

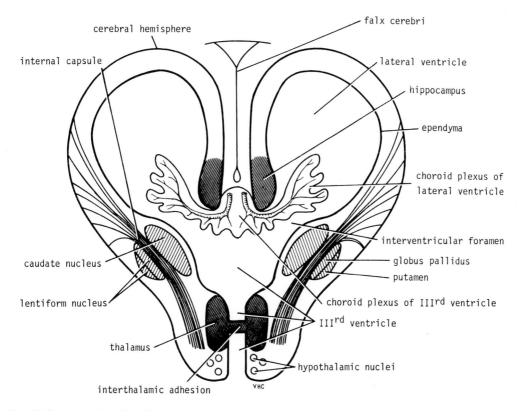

Fig. 19-15. Coronal section of the cerebral hemispheres showing the choroid plexuses in the IIIrd and lateral ventricles. Also shown are the caudate and lentiform nuclei and the thalami. The ascending and descending nerve tracts can be seen passing between the masses of gray matter to form the internal capsule.

pansion, the hemispheres cover the midbrain and hindbrain (Fig. 19-17).

The medial wall of the cerebral hemisphere remains thin and is formed by ependymal cells. This area becomes invaginated by vascular mesoderm, which forms the *choroid plexus of the lateral ventricle* (Fig. 19-15). The occipital lobe of the cerebral hemisphere is separated from the cerebellum by mesenchyme, which condenses to form the *tentorium cerebelli.*

Meanwhile the neuroepithelium lining the floor of the vesicle proliferates, producing large numbers of primitive neurocytes. These collectively form a projection that encroaches on the cavity of the lateral ventricle and is known as the *corpus striatum* (Fig. 19-14).

Later this differentiates into two parts: the dorsomedial portion, the *caudate nucleus,* and a ventrolateral part, the *lentiform nucleus;* the latter becomes subdivided into a lateral part, the *putamen,* and a medial part, the *globus pallidus* (Fig. 19-15). As each hemisphere expands, its medial surface approaches the lateral surface of the diencephalon so that the caudate nucleus and thalamus come in close contact.

Superior to the region of the choroid plexus, a further thickening occurs in the wall of the vesicle, which protrudes as a longitudinal elevation into the lateral ventricle. This is called the *hippocampus* (Fig. 19-15).

While these various masses of gray matter

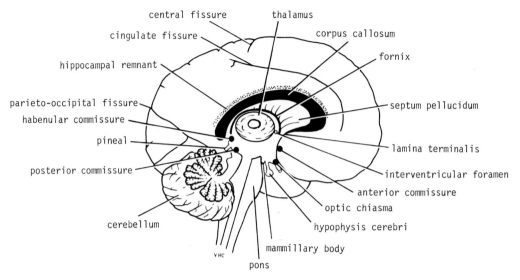

Fig. 19-16. Sagittal section of fully developed brain.

are developing within each cerebral hemisphere, maturing neurons in different parts of the nervous system are sending axons either to or from the differentiating cortex. These axons form the large ascending and descending tracts, which, as they develop, are forced to pass between the thalamus and caudate nucleus medially and the lentiform nucleus laterally. The compact bundle of ascending and descending tracts is known as the *internal capsule* (Fig. 19-15). The *external capsule* consists of a few cortical projection fibers, which pass lateral to the lentiform nucleus.

Cerebral Cortex

As each cerebral hemisphere rapidly expands, a great many *convolutions* or *gyri* separated by *fissures* or *sulci* become evident on its surface. The cortex covering the lentiform nucleus remains as a fixed area called the *insula* (Fig. 19-17). Later this region becomes buried in the *lateral fissure* as the result of overgrowth of adjacent temporal, parietal, and frontal lobes.

The neuroepithelial cells lining the cavity of the cerebral hemisphere produce large numbers of primitive neurocytes and *neuroglial cells* that migrate out into the marginal layer. The remaining neuroepithelial cells will ultimately form the *ependyma,* which lines the lateral ventricle. In the twelfth week, the cortex becomes very cellular because of the migration of large numbers of primitive neurocytes. At term, the neurocytes have become differentiated and have assumed a stratified appearance as the result of the presence of incoming and outgoing fibers. Different areas of the cortex soon show specific cell types; thus the motor cortex contains a large number of *pyramidal cells,* while the sensory areas are mainly characterized by *granular cells.*

Commissures

The *lamina terminalis,* which is the cephalic end of the neural tube, forms a bridge between the two cerebral hemispheres and enables nerve fibers to pass from one cerebral hemisphere to the other (Fig. 19-13).

The first commissure to develop within the lamina terminalis is the *anterior commissure.*

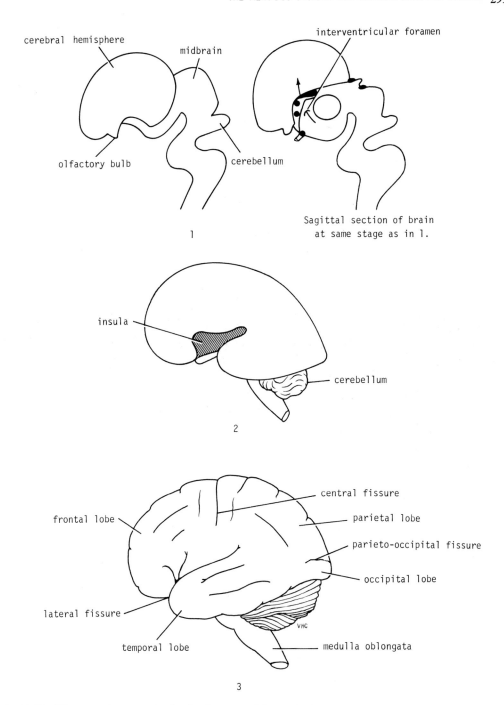

Fig. 19-17. The successive stages in the development of the cerebral cortex.

This connects the olfactory bulb and temporal lobe of the cortex of one side with the same structures of the opposite hemisphere (Fig. 19-16).

The second commissure to develop is the *fornix* (Fig. 19-16), which connects the cortex of the hippocampus in each hemisphere.

The third commissure to develop, the *corpus callosum,* becomes the largest and most important (Fig. 19-16). Its first fibers connect the frontal lobes of both sides and later the parietal lobes. As the corpus callosum increases in size because of increased numbers of fibers, it arches back over the roof of the developing IIIrd ventricle. The remains of the lamina terminalis, which lies between the corpus callosum and the fornix, become stretched out to form a thin septum, the *septum pellucidum.* The *optic chiasma* (Fig. 19-16) is formed in the inferior part of the lamina terminalis and contains fibers from the medial halves of the retinae, which cross the midline to join the optic tract of the opposite side and so pass to the *lateral geniculate body* and the *superior colliculus.*

Myelination in the Brain and the Onset of Function

Myelination in the brain begins at about the sixth month of fetal life but is restricted to the fibers of the basal ganglia. Later the sensory fibers passing up from the spinal cord myelinate, but the progress is slow so that at birth the brain is still largely unmyelinated. In the newborn there is very little cerebral function; motor reactions such as respiration, sucking, and swallowing are essentially reflex. After birth the corticobulbar, corticospinal fibers, and the tectospinal and corticopontocerebellar fibers begin to myelinate. This process of myelination is not haphazard but systematic, occurring in different nerve fibers at specific times. The corticospinal fibers, for example, start to myelinate at about 6 months after birth, and the process is largely com-

plete by the end of the second year. It is believed that some nerve fibers in the brain and spinal cord do not complete myelination until puberty.

CONGENITAL ANOMALIES OF THE CENTRAL NERVOUS SYSTEM

Practically any part of the nervous system may show defects of development, and these produce a wide variety of clinical signs and symptoms. Only the most severe defects will be discussed here. Anencephalia, hydrocephalus, and spina bifida each occur about six times per thousand births and are therefore the more common congenital anomalies.

Spinal Cord

Spina Bifida

The spines and arches of one or more adjacent vertebrae fail to develop. The condition occurs most commonly in the lower thoracic, lumbar, and sacral regions. Beneath this defect the meninges and spinal cord may or may not be involved to varying degrees. The condition is a result of failure of the embryonic mesenchyme, which grows in between the neural tube and the surface ectoderm, to form the vertebral arches in the affected region. Some authorities believe that local overgrowth of the neural plate in the early stages of development might be a factor in the production of spina bifida. The types of spina bifida are as follows:

SPINA BIFIDA OCCULTA. The spines and arches of one or more vertebrae, usually in the lumbar region, are absent, and the vertebral canal remains open posteriorly (Fig. 19-18). The spinal cord and nerve roots are usually normal. The defect is covered by the postvertebral muscles and cannot be seen from the surface. A small tuft of hair or a fatty tumor may be present over the defect.

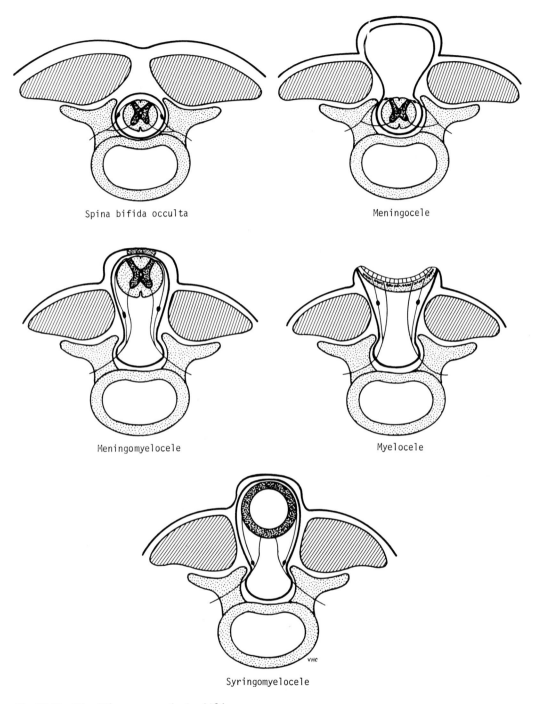

Spina bifida occulta

Meningocele

Meningomyelocele

Myelocele

Syringomyelocele

Fig. 19-18.   The different types of spina bifida.

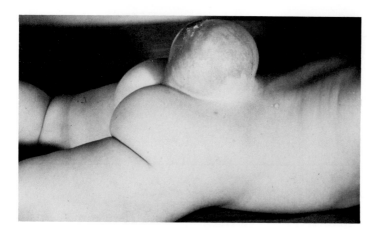

Fig. 19-19. Meningocele in the lumbar-sacral region. (Courtesy of Dr. L. Thompson.)

Most cases are symptomless and are diagnosed by chance when the vertebral column is x-rayed.

MENINGOCELE. The meninges project through the defect in the vertebral arches, forming a cystic swelling beneath the skin and containing cerebrospinal fluid which communicates with the subarachnoid space (Figs. 19-18 & 19-19). The spinal cord and nerves are usually normal.

MENINGOMYELOCELE. The normal spinal cord, or cauda equina, lies within the meningeal sac, which projects through the vertebral arch defect (Figs. 19-18 & 19-20). The spinal cord or nerve roots are adherent to the inner wall of the sac.

MYELOCELE. The neural tube fails to close in the region of the defect (Fig. 19-18). An oval raw area is found on the surface; this represents the neural groove that is not united. The central canal discharges clear cerebrospinal fluid onto the surface.

SYRINGOMYELOCELE. This is rare. A meningomyelocele is present, and in addition the central canal of the spinal cord at the level of the bony defect is grossly dilated (Fig. 19-18).

Spina bifida occulta is the commonest defect. The next most common defect is myelocele, and many afflicted infants are born dead. If the child is born alive, death from infection of the spinal cord occurs within a few days.

Most cases of spina bifida occulta require no treatment. A meningocele should be removed surgically within a few days of birth. Cases of meningomyelocele should also be

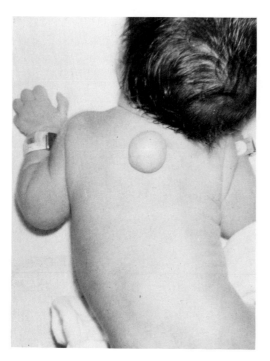

Fig. 19-20. Meningomyelocele in the upper thoracic region. (Courtesy of Dr. G. Avery.)

treated surgically. The sac is opened and the spinal cord or nerves are freed and carefully replaced in the vertebral canal. The meninges are sutured over the cord and the postvertebral muscles are approximated.

Brain

Hydrocephalus

This is an abnormal increase in the volume of cerebrospinal fluid within the skull. The condition may be associated with spina bifida and meningocele. Hydrocephalus alone may be caused by stenosis of the aqueduct of Sylvius or, more commonly, by the normal single channel being represented by many inadequate minute tubules. Another cause, which is progressive, is the overgrowth of neuroglia around the aqueduct. Inadequate development or failure of development of the interventricular foramen, or the foramina of Magendie and Luschka, may also be responsible.

In cases of hydrocephalus with spina bifida, the *Arnold-Chiari* malformation may occur.

During development, the cephalic end of the spinal cord is fixed by virtue of the brain's residing in the skull, and in the presence of spina bifida the caudal end of the cord may also be fixed. The longitudinal growth of the vertebral column is more rapid and greater than that of the spinal cord, and this results in traction pulling the medulla and part of the cerebellum through the foramen magnum. This displacement of the hindbrain downward obstructs the flow of cerebrospinal fluid through the foramina in the roof of the IVth ventricle.

Hydrocephalus may occur before birth, and if it is advanced, it could obstruct labor. It is usually noticed during the first few months of life because of the enlarging head, which may attain a huge size and measure more than 30 inches in diameter (Figs. 19-21 & 19-22). The brow overhangs the roof of the orbits, the cranial sutures are widely separated, and the anterior fontanelle is much enlarged. The veins of the scalp are distended and the eyes look downward. Cranial nerve paralyses are common. The cerebral ventri-

Fig. 19-21. Hydrocephalus. Note the large size of the head, the prominent brow, the downward-looking eyes, and the distended veins of the scalp. (Courtesy of Dr. G. Avery.)

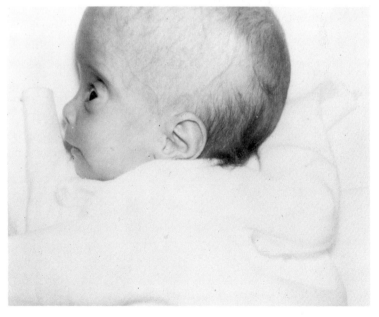

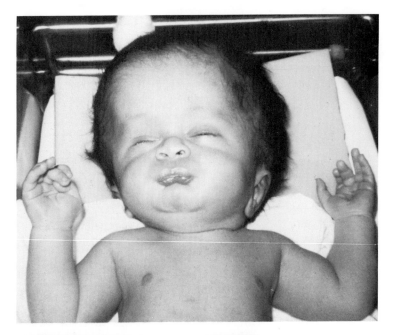

Fig. 19-22. Hydrocephalus. Note the large size of the head. (Courtesy of Dr. G. Avery.)

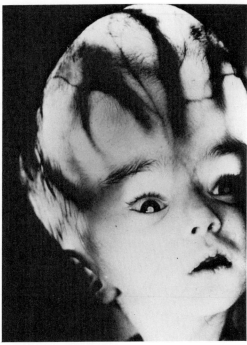

Fig. 19-23. Hydranencephaly. The absence of the cerebral hemispheres allows the light to pass easily through the head when the latter is transilluminated. (Courtesy of Dr. M. Platt.)

cles can become markedly dilated. This ventricular expansion occurs largely at the expense of the white matter, and the neurons of the cortex are mostly spared. This results in the preservation of cerebral function, but the destruction of the tracts, especially the corticobulbar and corticospinal tracts, produces a progressive loss of motor function.

The surgical treatment of congenital hydrocephalus has been disappointing. However, the recent introduction of a drainage system using a nonreturn valve, which allows the cerebrospinal fluid to flow directly from the cerebral ventricles into the internal jugular vein in the neck, should give improved results.

Hydranencephaly

There is a complete or almost complete absence of the cerebral hemispheres; the lateral and IIIrd ventricles are absent, but the basal ganglia are normal. The cause of the failure of the cerebral hemispheres to develop is unknown. In most cases the skull is excessively large (Fig. 19-23), but in some it may be very small. Cases have been reported where the children "live" for as long as 5 years.

Anencephalia

In this condition the greater part of the brain and the vault of the skull are absent (Fig. 19-24). The anomaly is caused by the complete or almost complete failure of the cephalic part of the neural tube to develop, and as a consequence its cavity remains open at the cephalic end. In place of the normal neural tissue are thin-walled vascular channels resembling the choroid plexus and masses of neural tissue. Although the eyes are present, the optic nerves are absent. The condition commonly involves the spinal cord, which remains open in the cervical region. There are frequently multiple anomalies of other organs. Since the fetus cannot swallow, *hydramnios* often occurs. The condition is usually diagnosed before birth, when x-ray study shows absence of the vault of the skull. Most anencephalic infants are stillborn or die shortly after birth.

Arhinencephalia

In this condition the olfactory bulbs, tracts, and corpus striatum fail to develop. The corpus callosum is absent and a single unpaired ventricle is present. Other areas of the brain are poorly developed or absent.

Microcephaly

In this condition the skull and the cerebral hemispheres are small, and the gyri and sulci have a simple pattern (Fig. 19-25). The cerebellum and brain stem are normal. This condition may be familial and is usually associated with mental deficiency.

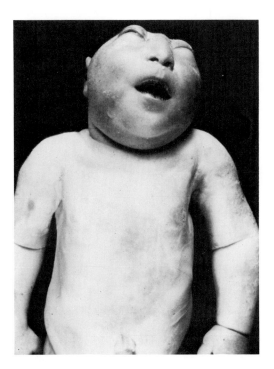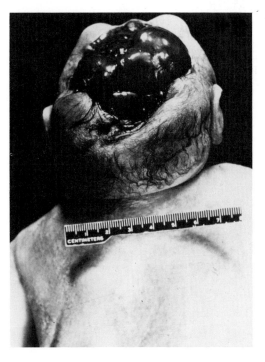

Fig. 19-24. An example of anencephalia. Note that the greater part of the brain and the vault of the skull are absent. In the posterior view, the remainder of the brain is exposed. (Courtesy of Dr. M. Platt.)

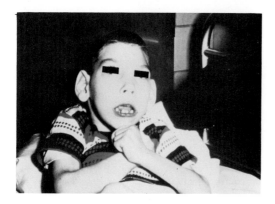

Fig. 19-25. Microcephaly. (Courtesy of Dr. M. Platt.)

Megalencephaly

This is rarer than microcephaly. The brain may be generally enlarged or show enlargement of one portion at the expense of another. The condition is associated with mental deficiency.

Porencephaly

A wide circumscribed defect is present in the wall of the cerebral hemisphere. The condition is associated with severe mental deficiency and cerebral palsy.

Cyclopia

This is rare, and it involves the entire forebrain (Fig. 19-26). The forebrain consists of a single ventricle surrounded by cerebral cortex. The corpus callosum, septum pellucidum, and fornix are absent. Other anomalies include defects in the formation of the eyes. Commonly a single median globe with paired or fused corneas, pupils, and lenses is present. In this condition the ventricular cavity is formed from the original forebrain vesicle, and only portions of the hemispheric vesicles develop.

Cortical Agenesis

Different degrees of cortical agenesis occur, which result in various forms of congenital

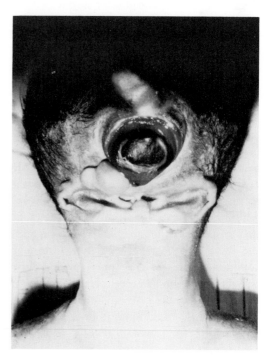

Fig. 19-26. An example of cyclopia. The anomalies include a single median eye with fused corneas and pupils. (Courtesy of Dr. M. Platt.)

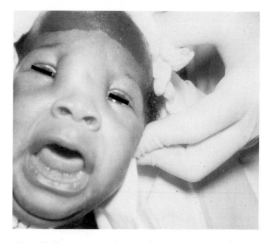

Fig. 19-27. Cranioschisis. The meninges and parts of the frontal lobes of the brain are protruding forward in the midline between the frontal and nasal bones (meningoencephalocele). (Courtesy of Dr. G. Avery.)

idiocy. If the motor cortex is involved, a *spastic monoplegia* or *diplegia* occurs.

Agenesis of the Corpus Callosum

This may be complete or partial. The lesion may exist without neurological signs or symptoms.

Cerebellar Agenesis

One or both hemispheres are absent, and the pons is poorly developed. Few if any neurological signs or symptoms are present.

Cranioschisis

This condition is characterized by a defect in the membranous bones of the skull through which meninges or meninges and neural tissue may protrude (Fig. 19-27). It usually occurs in the midline in the occipital region or between the frontal and nasal bones. The condition is probably the result of anomalous formation and separation of the neural tube from the surface ectoderm of the embryo. In cephalic *meningocele,* where there is herniation of the meninges and no neural tissue is included in the protuberance, the chances of a successful surgical excision are good. In *meningoencephalocele,* where a portion of the brain is included, the prospects of successful surgery are greatly reduced and hydrocephalus commonly results.

Clinical Problems
Answers on page 452

---

1. A 15-year-old boy fell off his bicycle and hurt his back. Following a physical examination by a physician, an x-ray film of the vertebral column was made. Examination of the film revealed the complete absence of the spine and laminae of the fifth lumbar vertebra. A thorough neurological examination showed no abnormal signs. What is the diagnosis? How would you explain the presence of the bony defect?

2. Following a normal delivery of a male child, a large swelling was noted over the lower part of his lumbar vertebral column. On closer examination, the summit of the swelling had an oval raw area from which a clear fluid was discharging. The legs showed hyperextension at the knees, and the feet were held in the position of talipes calcaneus. What is the diagnosis? How would you explain the congenital defect on the back?

3. A 3-month-old boy was taken to the clinic because his mother had noticed that his head seemed to be larger than normal. "He looks top-heavy," she said. On physical examination the enlarged head was seen to be globular in shape and the forehead bulged forward. The anterior fontanelle was greatly enlarged and extended posteriorly to the enlarged posterior fontanelle. The large head contrasted markedly with the small face. Some congested veins could be seen running down the front and sides of the scalp, and the child's eyes tended to look downward. Neurological examination revealed some evidence of optic atrophy on both sides and increased tone in the muscles of the lower limbs. What is the diagnosis? How can you explain this congenital anomaly? What is the prognosis if the patient is left untreated?

4. A 6-month-old girl was seen by a plastic surgeon because of the presence of a swelling at the root of the nose. The mother said that she had noticed the swelling at birth and that since then it had gradually increased in size. On examination a fluctuant swelling was found at the root of

the nose in the midline, situated between the frontal and nasal bones. It was pulsatile, and the pulse coincided with the heart rate and with that felt over the anterior fontanelle. What is the diagnosis?

REFERENCES

Abbie, A. A. The Origin of the Corpus Callosum and the Fate of the Structures Related to It. *J. Comp. Neurol.* 70:9, 1939.

Adams, R. D., Schatzki, R., and Scoville, W. B. The Arnold-Chiari Malformation. *New Eng. J. Med.* 225:135, 1941.

Angevine, J. B. The Time of Neuron Origin in the Hippocampal Region: An Autoradiographic Study in the Mouse. *Exp. Neurol.* (Suppl.) 2:1, 1965.

Angevine, J. B., and Sidman, R. L. Autoradiographic Study of Cell Migration During Histogenesis of Cerebral Cortex in the Mouse. *Nature* (London) 192:766, 1961.

Aronson, N. Hydrocephalus. In *Pediatric Surgery,* edited by C. D. Benson et al. Year Book, Chicago, 1962.

Barcroft, J., and Barron, D. H. Observations on the Functional Development of the Foetal Brain. *J. Comp. Neurol.* 77:431, 1942.

Bartelmez, G. W., and Dekaban, A. S. The Early Development of the Human Brain. *Contrib. Embryol.* 37:13, 1962.

Bering, E. A. Pathophysiology of Hydrocephalus. In *Workshop in Hydrocephalus,* edited by K. Shulman. Children's Hospital, Philadelphia, 1965.

Boris, M., Blumberg, R., Feldman, D. B., and Sellers, J. E. Increased Incidence of Myelomeningocele. *J.A.M.A.* 184:768, 1963.

Conel, J. L. *Postnatal Development of the Human Cerebral Cortex: The Cortex of the Newborn,* vol. 1. Harvard University Press, Cambridge, 1939.

Conel, J. L. The Origin of the Neural Crest, *J. Comp. Neurol.* 76:191, 1942.

Connolly, C. J. Development of the Cerebral Sulci. *Amer. J. Phys. Anthrop.* 26:113, 1940.

Crone, L., and Sylvester, P. E. Hydranencephaly. *Arch. Dis. Child.* 33:235, 1958.

Dekaban, A. S., and Bartelmez, G. W. Complete Dysraphism in 14 Somite Human Embryo: A Contribution to Normal and Abnormal Morphogenesis. *Amer. J. Anat.* 115:27, 1964.

De Robertis, E., Gerschenfeld, H. M., and Weld, F. Cellular Mechanism of Myelination in the Central Nervous System. *J. Biophys. Biochem. Cytol.* 4:651, 1958.

Detwiler, S. R., and Kehoe, K. Further Observations on the Origin of the Sheath Cells of Schwann. *J. Exp. Zool.* 81:415, 1939.

Eckstein, H. B. Management of Hydrocephalus. In *Proceedings of a Symposium on Spina Bifida.* National Foundation for Research into Poliomyelitis and Other Crippling Diseases, London, 1965.

Eckstein, H. B., and MacNab, G. H. Myelomeningocele and Hydrocephalus. *Lancet* 1:842, 1966.

Elliott, H. C. Studies on the Motor Cells of the Spinal Cord. II. Distribution in the Normal Human Fetal Cord. *Amer. J. Anat.* 72:29, 1943.

Forrest, D. M., Hole, R., and Wynne, J. M. Treatment of Infantile Hydrocephalus Using the Holter Valve. *Develop. Med. Child. Neurol.* (Suppl. 11) 27, 1966.

Fujita, S. Analysis of Neuron Differentiation in the Central Nervous System by Tritiated Thymidine Autoradiography. *J. Comp. Neurol.* 112:311, 1964.

Gilbert, M. S. The Early Development of the Human Diencephalon. *J. Comp. Neurol.* 62:81, 1935.

Harrison, R. G. The Croonian Lecture: On the Origin and Development of the Nervous System Studied by the Methods of Experimental Embryology. *Proc. Roy. Soc.* [Biol.] 118:155, 1935.

Harvey, S., and Burr, H. Development of the Meninges. *Arch. Neurol. Psychiat.* 15:545, 1926.

Hess, A. The Ground Substance of the Developing Central Nervous System. *J. Comp. Neurol.* 102:65, 1955.

Hewitt, W. The Development of the Human Internal Capsule and Lentiform Nucleus. *J. Anat.* 95:191, 1961.

Hicks, S. P. Migrating Cells in the Developing Nervous System Studied by Their Radiosensitivity and Tritiated Thymidine Uptake. *Brookhaven Sympos. Biol.* 14:246, 1961.

Hines, M. Studies in the Growth and Differentiation of the Telencephalon in Man: The Fissura Hippocampi. *J. Comp. Neurol.* 34:73, 1922.

Horstadius, S. *The Neural Crest*. Oxford University Press, London, 1950.

Hoytema, G. J., and Van Den Berg, R. Embryological Studies of the Posterior Fossa in Connection with Arnold-Chiari Malformation. *Develop. Med. Child. Neurol.* (Suppl. 11) 61, 1966.

Ingraham, F. D., and Scott, H. W. Spina Bifida and Cranium Bifidum. *New Eng. J. Med.* 229: 108, 1943.

Kershman, J. Genesis of Microglia in the Human Brain. *Arch. Neurol. Psychiat.* 41:24, 1939.

Labrum, T., and Wood, C. Congenital Malformations of the Central Nervous System. *Obstet. Gynec.* 18:430, 1961.

Langworthy, O. R. Development of Behavior Patterns and Myelinization of the Nervous System in the Human Fetus and Infant. *Contrib. Embryol.* 24:1, 1933.

Larsell, O. Development of Cerebellum in Man in Relation to Its Comparative Anatomy. *J. Comp. Neurol.* 87:85, 1947.

Laurence, K. M., and Tew, B. J. Follow-Up of 65 Survivors from the 425 Cases of Spina Bifida Born in South Wales Between 1956 and 1962. *Develop. Med. Child. Neurol.* (Suppl. 13) 1, 1967.

Martin, A., and Langman, J. The Development of the Spinal Cord Examined by Autoradiography, Pt. 1. *J. Embryol. Exp. Morph.* 14:25, 1965.

Morton, W. R. M. Arhinencephaly and Multiple Developmental Anomalies Occurring in a Human Full-Term Foetus. *Anat. Rec.* 98:45, 1947.

Rawles, M. E. Origin of Pigment Cells from Neural Crest in the Mouse Embryo. *Physiol. Zool.* 20:248, 1947.

Romanes, G. L. The Development of the Spinal Cord. In *Spinal Cord (Ciba Foundation Symposium)*, edited by G. E. W. Wolstenholme et al. Churchill, London, 1953.

Russell, D. S. *Observations on the Pathology of Hydrocephalus.* (*Medical Research Council Special Report No. 265*). Medical Research Council, London, 1949.

Sensenig, E. C. The Early Development of the Meninges of the Spinal Cord in Human Embryos. *Contrib. Embryol.* 34:147, 1951.

Shaner, R. F. Development of Nuclei and Tracts of Mid-Brain. *J. Comp. Neurol.* 55:493, 1932.

Sharp, J. A. The Junctional Region of the Cerebral Hemisphere and the Third Ventricle in Mammalian Embryos. *J. Anat.* 93:159, 1959.

Sidman, R. L., Miale, T., and Feber, N. Cell Proliferation and Migration in the Primitive Ependymal Zone. *J. Exp. Nerv.* 1:322, 1959.

Wilson, J. T. On the Nature and Mode of Origin of the Foramen of Magendie. *J. Anat.* 71:423, 1937.

The peripheral nervous system consists of the cranial nerves, the spinal nerves, and the ganglia.

DEVELOPMENT

Cranial Nerves

Olfactory Nerve

Primitive neurocytes derived from olfactory epithelial cells, which line the upper part of the developing nasal cavity, differentiate into nerve cells. These give origin to axons, the *olfactory fibers,* which grow through the cartilaginous roof of the nasal cavity and reach the apical region of the temporal lobe of each cerebral hemisphere. At the same time, an olfactory diverticulum grows out of the temporal lobe on each side and becomes expanded at its end to form the *olfactory bulb* (Fig. 20-1). The stalk of the olfactory bulb forms the *olfactory tract,* and the extension of the ventricular cavity into it becomes obliterated. The olfactory fibers synapse on the cells of the olfactory bulb; these cells in turn give origin to the secondary olfactory fibers. These axons grow through the olfactory tract and end in the pyriform cortex.

Optic Nerve

The ganglion cells of the retina give rise to axons that pass to the brain along the *optic stalk.* Once the inner and outer walls of the optic stalk fuse, the *optic nerve* is formed (see Chap. 21). On reaching the *optic chiasma,* those nerve fibers, which originated from the medial halves of the retinae, cross the midline to join the optic tract of the opposite side (Fig. 20-2). The nerve fibers ultimately reach the *lateral geniculate bodies,* the *superior colliculi,* and the *pretectum.*

Oculomotor or Third Cranial Nerve

This motor nerve has a large somatic efferent component and a smaller visceral efferent component (parasympathetic). The neurons differentiate from the primitive neurocytes in the basal plates of the developing midbrain at the level of the superior colliculi. The axons emerge on the ventral aspect of the midbrain between the cerebral pedicles (Fig. 19-12); the somatic fibers supply all the extrinsic muscles of the eye (except the *superior oblique* and the *lateral rectus muscles*), and the parasympathetic fibers supply the *constrictor pupillae muscle* of the iris and the *ciliary muscle.*

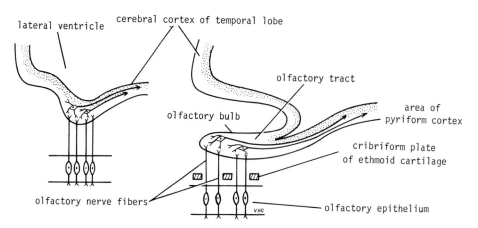

Fig. 20-1. The development of the olfactory nerves.

Trochlea or Fourth Cranial Nerve

This motor nerve has a somatic efferent component only. The neurons differentiate from the primitive neurocytes in the basal plates of the developing midbrain at the level of the inferior colliculi. The axons emerge on the dorsal aspect of the midbrain after decussating completely in the tectum, and eventually they supply the *superior oblique muscle* of the eye.

Trigeminal or Fifth Cranial Nerve

This large nerve has a motor efferent component and two sensory afferent components. The motor neurons differentiate from the primitive neurocytes in the basal plates of the developing pons and form the *motor nucleus*. The axons emerge on the ventral surface of the pons and are distributed to the *muscles of mastication,* the *anterior belly of the digastric,* the *mylohyoid,* the *tensor palati,* and the *tensor tympani muscles,* i.e., those muscles which are derived from the mesenchyme in the mandibular process of the first pharyngeal arch.

The axons of the main sensory component arise from neurons derived from the cephalic extension of the neural crest cells. The neurons are of the unipolar type, and together form the large *trigeminal ganglion* (equivalent to the posterior root ganglion cells of spinal nerves). The peripheral axons conduct sensory impulses from the skin of the face. The central axons enter the ventral surface of the pons as a massive bundle and end in the *main sensory nucleus* or *spinal sensory nucleus*. The neurons of these sensory nuclei are derived from the primitive neurocytes in the alar plates in the developing hindbrain. The axons of the small sensory component are associated with the *mesencephalic nucleus*. This trigeminal nucleus is considered by some authorities to consist of sensory neurons derived from neural crest cells that have become included in the neural plate. The neurons of the mesencephalic nucleus are of the unipolar type, and the peripheral axons conduct proprioceptive impulses to the brain from the muscles of mastication and possibly also from the extrinsic muscles of the eyeball. It is important to note that these axons have no cell bodies in the trigeminal ganglion.

Abducent or Sixth Cranial Nerve

This motor nerve has a small somatic efferent component only. The neurons differentiate

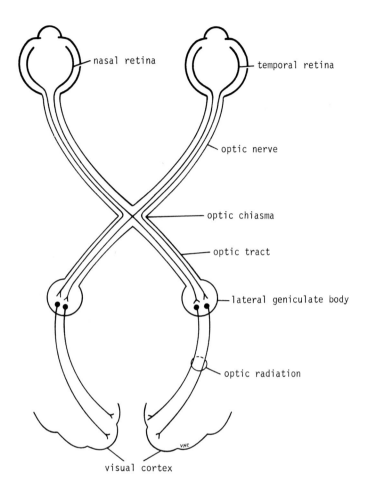

Fig. 20-2. The visual pathway.

from the primitive neurocytes in the basal plates in the developing pons. The axons emerge on the ventral surface of the brain in the groove between the pons and the medulla and eventually supply the *lateral rectus muscle* of the eye.

Facial or Seventh Cranial Nerve

This nerve has three components: (1) a large motor efferent component, (2) a small parasympathetic efferent component, and (3) a sensory afferent component.

The neurons of the efferent components differentiate from the primitive neurocytes in the basal plates of the developing pons. Once the axons of the large efferent component have arisen, the cells of origin undergo migration. This results in the motor axons being pulled dorsally over the abducens nucleus as shown in Figure 20-3. The cells of origin of the small parasympathetic efferent component remain stationary and form the *superior salivatory nucleus*. The axons of the motor efferent component supply the *muscles of facial expression,* the *stylohyoid,* the *posterior belly of the digastric,* and the *stapedius muscle,* i.e., the muscles derived from the mesenchyme of the second

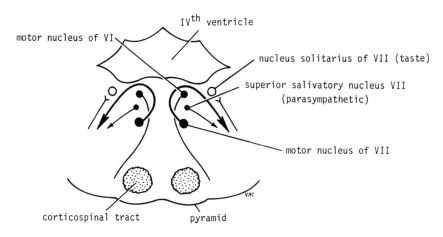

Transverse section of pons

Fig. 20-3. The development of the nuclei of the seventh cranial nerve and their relationship to the nucleus of the sixth cranial nerve.

pharyngeal arch. The axons of the small, efferent component are ultimately distributed as parasympathetic fibers to the *submandibular, sublingual, nasal, palatal,* and *lacrimal glands.*

The sensory afferent component is composed of axons that arise from neurons derived from the cephalic extension of the neural crest. The neurons are of the unipolar type and together form the *geniculate ganglion.* The peripheral axons conduct impulses of taste from the anterior two-thirds of the tongue and the floor of the mouth via the *chorda tympani nerve.* The central axons terminate on neurons derived from the alar plates, which together form part of the *nucleus solitarius.*

Vestibulocochlear or Eighth Cranial Nerve

This is a large sensory nerve having two components serving the vestibular and auditory systems.

The axons of the vestibular component arise from neurons derived from the cephalic extension of the neural crest. The neurons are bipolar in type, and collectively they form the *vestibular ganglion.* The peripheral axons

conduct sensory impulses concerned with balance from the *maculae* and *cristae* of the membranous labyrinth of the internal ear. The central axons enter the ventral surface of the brain in the groove between the pons and the medulla and end in the *vestibular nuclei.* The neurons of these sensory nuclei are derived from primitive neurocytes in the alar plates in the developing hindbrain.

The axons of the cochlear component also arise from neurons derived from the neural crest. The neurons are bipolar and collectively form the *spiral ganglion.* Their peripheral axons spread around the hair cells of the *organ of Corti,* and their central axons enter the ventral surface of the brain in company with the vestibular component of the eighth nerve. The axons end in the *cochlear nuclei.* The neurons of these nuclei are derived from primitive neurocytes in the alar plates in the developing hindbrain.

Glossopharyngeal or Ninth Cranial Nerve

This nerve has four components: (1) motor efferent fibers, (2) parasympathetic efferent fibers, (3) general sensory afferent fibers, and (4) taste afferent fibers.

The neurons of the efferent components differentiate from the primitive neurocytes in the basal plates of the developing medulla. The axons emerge from the ventral aspect of the medulla between the olives and the inferior cerebellar peduncles, and the motor efferent fibers eventually supply the *stylopharyngeus muscle* and probably some of the *upper pharyngeal muscles,* i.e., the muscles formed from the mesenchyme of the third pharyngeal arch. The nerve cells of the parasympathetic axons are collectively known as the *inferior salivatory nucleus.* Their axons eventually supply the *parotid salivary gland.*

The sensory afferent components of the ninth cranial nerve are composed of axons which arise from neurons derived from the cephalic extension of the neural crest. The neurons are of the unipolar type and collectively form the *superior* and *inferior glossopharyngeal ganglia.* The peripheral axons conduct impulses of general sensation and taste from the region of the posterior third of the tongue. The central axons terminate on neurons derived from the alar plates. The neurons that receive information of taste are collectively known as the *nucleus solitarius.*

Vagus or Tenth Cranial Nerve

This nerve has four components: (1) motor efferent fibers, (2) parasympathetic efferent fibers, (3) general sensory afferent fibers, and (4) taste afferent fibers.

The neurons of the efferent components differentiate from the primitive neurocytes in the basal plates of the developing medulla. The nerve cells of the motor efferent fibers collectively form part of the *nucleus ambiguus.* The axons emerge from the ventral aspect of the medulla between the olives and the inferior cerebellar peduncles and eventually supply the *muscles of the pharynx and larynx,* i.e., muscles derived from mesenchyme of the fourth, fifth, and sixth pharyngeal arches. The nerve cells of the parasympathetic efferent fibers collectively form the dorsal *parasympathetic motor nucleus.* Their axons eventually supply the *heart, lungs,* and the whole of the *foregut* and its derivatives, as well as the major part of the *midgut.*

The sensory afferent components of the vagus are composed of axons that arise from neurons derived from the cephalic extension of the neural crest. The neurons are of the unipolar type and collectively form the *superior* and *inferior ganglia* of the vagus. The peripheral axons conduct sensory impulses from the heart, lungs, foregut, and midgut regions. The peripheral axons carrying information of taste come from the mucous membrane of the *valleculae* and *pyriform fossae,* i.e., from the region around the aditus into the larynx. The central axons terminate on neurons derived from the alar plates. The cells which receive information of general sensation are collectively known as the *dorsal sensory nucleus;* the cells concerned with information of taste form part of the *nucleus solitarius.*

Accessory or Eleventh Cranial Nerve

This is a pure motor nerve and consists of two parts: (1) a cranial part and (2) a spinal part.

The cell bodies of the axons differentiate from the primitive neurocytes in the basal plates of the medullary and upper cervical regions of the neural tube. The nerve cells of the cranial fibers collectively form the lowermost part of the *nucleus ambiguus.* The axons emerge on each side from the ventral aspect of the medulla between the olive and the inferior cerebellar peduncle and join the vagus nerve, where they are distributed via the *recurrent laryngeal nerve,* a branch of the vagus, to most of the muscles of the larynx.

The nerve cells of the spinal fibers collectively form a group of motor cells in the lateral part of the anterior gray horn of the upper five cervical segments of the spinal cord. These cells are in line with the cells of the nucleus ambiguus, and it is believed that during development they are drawn caudally. The axons emerge from the lateral surface of the spinal cord between the anterior and posterior nerve roots of the cervical nerves. They pass superiorly into the developing skull through the foramen magnum and finally emerge from the skull through the jugular foramen to supply the *sternocleido-mastoid* and the *trapezius muscles.*

Hypoglossal or Twelfth Cranial Nerve

This is a somatic efferent nerve, the cells of which differentiate from primitive neurocytes in the basal plates of the developing medulla. The axons emerge on each side from the ventral aspect of the medulla between the olive and the pyramid (Fig. 19-8), and are distributed to the occipital myotomes, which later become the *muscles of the tongue.* With the development of the neck and the migration of the occipital myotomes into the developing tongue, the nerve is pulled caudally and then superiorly lateral to the neurovascular bundle (carotid sheath) of the neck.

Spinal Nerves

The thirty-one pairs of spinal nerves are named and numbered according to the regions of the vertebral column with which they are associated. Each spinal nerve is attached to the spinal cord by an *anterior* and a *posterior root.*

The *anterior root* of each spinal nerve is a collective name for the axons of the large multipolar motor neurons in the anterior gray horn. Between the first thoracic and second or third lumbar segments of the mature spinal cord, the neurons of the lateral gray horn also send their preganglionic sympathetic axons in the anterior root (*sympathetic outflow*). In a similar manner, the neurons of the sacral portion of the *parasympathetic outflow* send their preganglionic axons in the anterior roots of spinal

nerves S_2, $_3$, $_4$. All the neurons mentioned develop from the primitive neurocytes in the basal plates of the developing spinal cord.

The *posterior root* of each spinal nerve is a collective name for the central axons of sensory neurons in the posterior root ganglion. These neurons are unipolar and are derived from neural crest cells.

Ganglia

These may be divided into (1) sensory ganglia of spinal nerves (posterior root ganglia) and cranial nerves and (2) autonomic ganglia.

Sensory Ganglia

The neurons are derived from neural crest cells. These differentiate into primitive neurocytes that develop axons and become unipolar neurons. The central axons enter the central nervous system in the posterior roots or in the cranial nerves and establish connections within the spinal cord or brain, respectively. The peripheral axons grow laterally and become the axons of sensory nerves; the dendritic region of these neurons is the receptive area at the periphery. Some of the neural crest cells do not differentiate into neurons but form cells that surround the neurons and are known as *capsule cells* (Figs. 20-4 & 20-5). The clusters of sensory neurons with their associated capsule cells are collectively called *posterior root ganglia.* Those sensory neurons and capsule cells that are found along the course of cranial nerves V, VII, VIII, IX, and X are called simply *sensory ganglia* of these nerves.

Autonomic Ganglia

The neurons are derived from neural crest cells. They differentiate into primitive neurocytes, which in many instances migrate long distances to take up their final positions in different parts of the body. These cells differentiate into multipolar neurons, and each de-

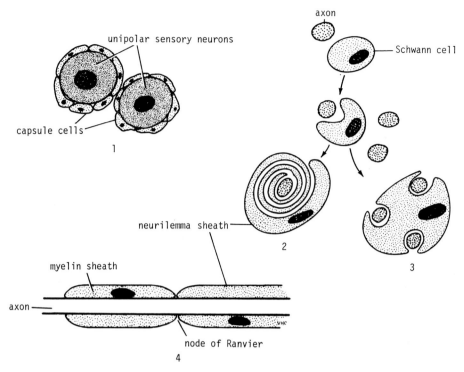

Fig. 20-4. (1) Capsule cells that surround unipolar sensory neurons in sensory ganglia, (2) the process of myelination of an axon, (3) the relationship of nonmyelinated axons to a Schwann cell, and (4) a longitudinal section of a myelinated axon.

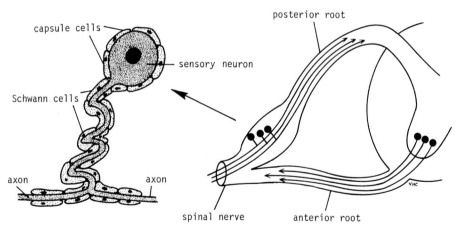

Fig. 20-5   The structure of a posterior root ganglion.

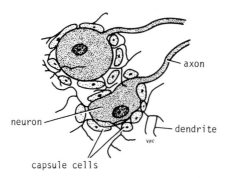

Fig. 20-6. Two multipolar sympathetic neurons in a sympathetic ganglion.

velops dendrites and an axon. The axons of autonomic ganglion cells are called *postganglionic fibers*. Some of the neural crest cells form *capsule cells* around the neurons (Fig. 20-6).

The *sympathetic trunks* are paired, each trunk consisting of a series of autonomic ganglia connected by intervening fibers. The neurons of the ganglia first appear in the thoracic region of the embryo and later extend cranially into the cervical region and caudally into the lumbosacral region. The *preaortic* and *visceral sympathetic ganglia* are formed from primitive neurocytes that migrate beyond the sympathetic trunks. The preganglionic myelinated axons passing from the spinal nerves to the sympathetic trunks are known as *white rami communicans,* and the nonmyelinated axons passing from the sympathetic ganglion cells to the spinal nerves are called *gray rami communicans* (Fig. 20-7).

Myelination of Peripheral Nerves

This is brought about by the *neurilemma cells of Schwann,* which are derived from

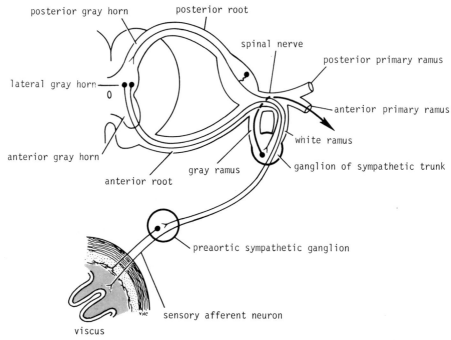

Fig. 20-7. Transverse section of spinal cord in the thoracic region, showing two examples of efferent sympathetic fibers leaving the lateral gray horn. The afferent sensory neuron is passing from a viscus into the spinal cord.

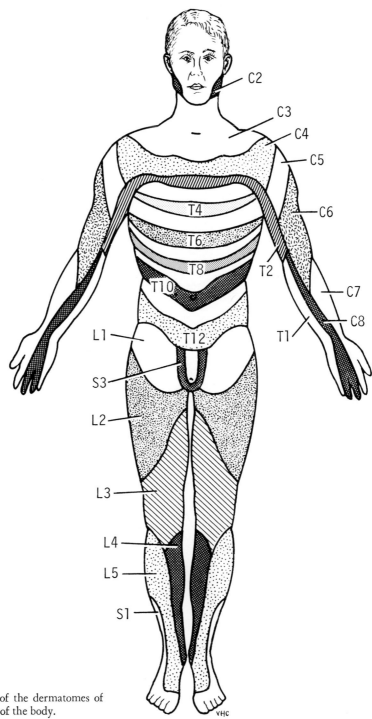

Fig. 20-8. The arrangement of the dermatomes of the skin on the anterior aspect of the body.

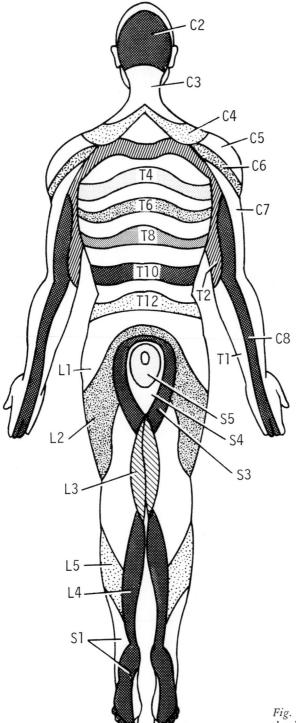

Fig. 20-9. The arrangement of the dermatomes of the skin on the posterior aspect of the body.

cells of the neural crest. As the axons grow out of the developing motor and sensory neurons, they are accompanied by neurilemma cells that wrap themselves around the axons, forming the *neurilemma sheath* (Fig. 20-4). One neurilemma cell may have from one to twenty axons indenting the surface membrane. As development continues, the surface membrane of the neurilemma cell becomes spirally wrapped around the axon, and it is the spiral layers of the surface membrane of the neurilemma cell which constitute the *myelin sheath*. The neurilemma cells become arranged in series along the axons and their branches, and the site at which two neurilemma cells abut against one another is known as a *node of Ranvier*. Each internodal segment of a nerve fiber between two consecutive nodes of Ranvier is composed of a centrally placed axon and a single neurilemma cell with its contained myelin lamellae. The neurilemma sheath may now be defined as the outer membrane of the neurilemma cell and its immediately adjacent cytoplasm (Fig. 20-4).

Distribution of Spinal Nerves and the Formation of Nerve Plexuses

Once the spinal nerve is formed, it divides into a *posterior* and an *anterior primary ramus*. The posterior primary ramus supplies the myotomes and the dermatomes of the posterior body wall, and the anterior ramus supplies the anterior part of the myotomes, the mesenchyme, and the dermatomes of the anterior and lateral surfaces of the body.

The growth of the nerves into the developing limb buds complicates the picture. Each anterior primary ramus, instead of passing directly into a limb, tends to join its fellows, thus forming a plexus of nerves; the *brachial plexus* is formed at the root of the upper limb and the *lumbosacral plexus* at the root of the lower limb.

It is important that a physician have a sound knowledge of the *segmental innervation of the skin*. This is shown diagrammatically in Figures 20-8 & 20-9. It is also important to realize that there is considerable overlap of adjacent dermatomes, so that if, for example, one wished to denervate the skin in the region of the dermatome supplied by the sixth thoracic segment of the spinal cord, it would be necessary to cut the spinal nerves of the fifth, sixth, and seventh thoracic segments to produce total anesthesia.

Limb muscles are also innervated segmentally. However, as in dermatomes, there is considerable overlap of muscle boundaries, so that if one spinal nerve is cut, more than one muscle will show weakness rather than there being complete paralysis of one muscle. The segmental innervation of the *biceps, triceps,* and *brachioradialis muscles* of the upper limb and the *quadriceps* and *gastrocnemius muscles* of the lower limb should be remembered (Fig. 20-10).

CONGENITAL ANOMALIES

Spinal Nerves

Great variations occur in the arrangement and distribution of the peripheral nerves. This can be most easily seen in the variations commonly found in the arrangement of the brachial plexus.

Autonomic Ganglia

Accessory Ganglion Cells

Sympathetic ganglion cells may occur singly or in clusters along anterior nerve roots, spinal nerves, or communicating rami, and are called *intermediate ganglia*. These neurons receive preganglionic nerve fibers and give origin to postganglionic fibers in the usual manner.

Absence of Ganglion Cells

Parasympathetic ganglion cells may fail to migrate into the wall of the colon and rectum

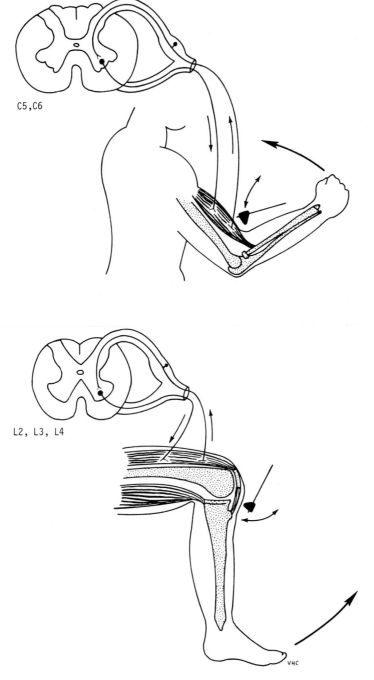

C5,C6

L2, L3, L4

VHC

Fig. 20-10. The nervous pathways involved in the production of the biceps and knee jerks.

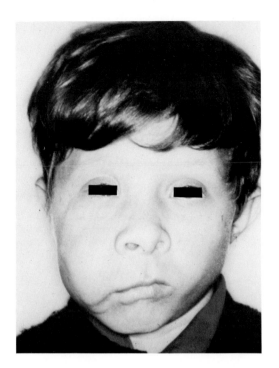

Fig. 20-11. Neurofibromatosis. The tumor involves a branch of the right trigeminal nerve. (Courtesy of Dr. L. Thompson.)

so that Auerbach's plexus does not develop between the longitudinal and circular layers of smooth muscle. This condition results in the development of *primary megacolon* (Hirschsprung's disease) (see Chap. 12).

Neurofibromatosis (Von Recklinghausen's Disease)

This condition is inherited as an autosomal dominant trait, and consists of "café au lait" pigmented lesions of the skin; these are irregular areas of light brown discoloration. Multiple connective tissue tumors called *neurofibromas* occur in the spinal and cranial nerves (Fig. 20-11) and in parts of the central nervous system and autonomic system. Treatment is removal of the neurofibromas, particularly those situated on nerve roots or those producing pressure on the brain stem or spinal cord.

Clinical Problems
Answers on page 452

1. A medical student, who had carefully dissected the brachial plexus of nerves in the neck and the axilla of his cadaver, was surprised to find that there was no contribution from C4 and a large contribution from T2. He told his anatomy instructor about his finding and was informed that this condition is not uncommon and is referred to as a *postfixed plexus*. Can you explain embryologically a postfixed brachial plexus? Is there such a condition as a prefixed brachial plexus?

2. A surgeon, while carefully dissecting out the axilla in the performance of a radical mastectomy operation, noted that a branch from the musculocutaneous nerve joined the median nerve. Is this a common occurrence?

3. A 12-year-old boy was seen by a pediatrician because he had developed "brown patches" on his skin. On examination the skin showed numerous scattered pigmented areas on the arms, legs, and trunk. The areas varied in size from a few millimeters to several centimeters in diameter. Many small pedunculated and sessile pigmented fibromata of the skin were also present. On questioning, the mother said she had another son with similar brown patches on the skin of the arms. A neuro-

logical examination revealed nothing abnormal. What is the diagnosis? Why is it necessary to perform a careful neurological examination in this case? Is this condition hereditary?

REFERENCES

Bardeen, C. R. The Growth and Histogenesis of the Cerebrospinal Nerves in Mammals. *Amer. J. Anat.* 2:231, 1903.

Barron, D. H. The Functional Development of Some Mammalian Neuromuscular Mechanisms. *Biol. Rev.* 16:1, 1941.

Barry, A. A Quantitative Study of the Prenatal Changes in Angulation of the Spinal Nerves. *Anat. Rec.* 126:97, 1956.

Boyd, J. D., and Hughes, A. F. W. Aberrant Nerve Fibres in Human Development. *J. Embryol. Exp. Morph.* 8:119, 1960.

Bremer, J. L. Aberrant Roots and Branches of the Abducent and Hypoglossal Nerves. *J. Comp. Neurol. Psychol.* 18:619, 1908.

Campenhout, E. Historical Survey of the Development of the Sympathetic Nervous System. *Quart. Rev. Biol.* 5:23, 1930.

Detwiler, S. R., and Kehoe, K. Further Observations on the Origin of the Sheath Cells of Schwann. *J. Exp. Zool.* 81:415, 1939.

Gasser, R. F. The Development of the Facial Nerve in Man. *Ann. Otol.* 76:37, 1967.

Harrison, R. G. Neuroblast Versus Sheath Cell in the Development of Peripheral Nerves. *J. Comp. Neurol.* 37:123, 1924.

Hewer, E. E. The Development of Nerve Endings in the Human Foetus. *J. Anat.* 69:369, 1935.

Hogg, I. D. Sensory Nerves and Associated Structures in the Skin of Human Fetuses of 8 to 14 Weeks of Menstrual Age Correlated with Functional Capability. *J. Comp. Neurol.* 75:371, 1941.

Hooker, D. Early Fetal Activity in Mammals. *Yale J. Biol. Med.* 8:579, 1936.

Horstadius, S. *The Neural Crest.* Oxford University Press, London, 1950.

Humphrey, T. The Development of the Olfactory and Accessory Olfactory Formations in Human Embryos and Fetuses. *J. Comp. Neurol.* 73:431, 1940.

Humphrey, T. Sensory Ganglion Cells Within the Central Canal of the Embryonic Human Spinal Cord. *J. Comp. Neurol.* 86:1, 1947.

Humphrey, T. Intramedullary Sensory Ganglion Cells in the Root Plate Area of the Embryonic Human Spinal Cord. *J. Comp. Neurol.* 92:333, 1950.

Humphrey, T. The Spinal Tract of the Trigeminal Nerve in Human Embryos Between 7½ and 8½ Weeks of Menstrual Age and Its Relation to Early Fetal Behavior. *J. Comp. Neurol.* 97:143, 1952.

Humphrey, T. The Development of Trigeminal Nerve Fibers to the Oral Mucosa, Compared with Their Development to Cutaneous Surfaces. *J. Comp. Neurol.* 126:91, 1966.

Keegan, J. J., and Garrett, F. D. The Segmental Distribution of the Cutaneous Nerves in the Limbs of Man. *Anat. Rec.* 102:409, 1948.

Kimmel, D. L., and McCrea, E. The Development of the Pelvic Plexuses and the Distribution of the Pelvic Splanchnic Nerves in the Human Embryo and Fetus. *J. Comp. Neurol.* 110:271, 1958.

Kuntz, A. Origin and Early Development of the Pelvic Neural Plexuses. *J. Comp. Neurol.* 96:345, 1952.

Luse, S. A. The Fine Structure of the Morphogenesis of Myelin. In *The Biology of Myelin,* edited by S. R. Korey. Cassell, London, 1959.

Miller, R. A., and Detwiler, S. R. Comparative Studies upon the Origin and Development of the Brachial Plexus. *Anat. Rec.* 65:273, 1936.

Pearson, A. A. The Spinal Accessory Nerve in Human Embryos. *J. Comp. Neurol.* 68:243, 1938.

Pearson, A. A. The Hypoglossal Nerve in Human Embryos. *J. Comp. Neurol.* 71:21, 1939.

Pearson, A. A. The Development of the Olfactory Nerve in Man. *J. Comp. Neurol.* 75:199, 1941.

Pearson, A. A. The Trochlear Nerve in Human Fetuses. *J. Comp. Neurol.* 78:29, 1943.

Pearson, A. A. The Oculomotor Nucleus in the Human Fetus. *J. Comp. Neurol.* 80:47, 1944.

Pearson, A. A. The Development of the Motor Nuclei of the Facial Nerve in Man. *J. Comp. Neurol.* 85:461, 1946.

Pearson, A. A. The Roots of the Facial Nerve in Human Embryos and Fetuses. *J. Comp. Neurol.* 87:139, 1947.

Pearson, A. A. The Development and Connection

of the Mesencephalic Root of the Trigeminal Nerve in Man. *J. Comp. Neurol.* 90:1, 1949.

Pearson, A. A. Further Observations on the Mesencephalic Root of the Trigeminal Nerve. *J. Comp. Neurol.* 91:147, 1949.

Pearson, A. A., and Eckhardt, A. L. Observations on the Gray and White Rami Communicantes in Human Embryos. *Anat. Rec.* 138:115, 1960.

Streeter, G. L. The Development of the Cranial and Spinal Nerves in the Occipital Region of the Human Embryo. *Amer. J. Anat.* 4:83, 1904.

Windle, W. F., and Fitzgerald, J. E. Development of the Spinal Reflex Mechanism in Human Embryos. *J. Comp. Neurol.* 67:493, 1937.

Windle, W. F., and Fitzgerald, J. E. Development of the Human Mesencephalic Trigeminal Root and Related Neurons. *J. Comp. Neurol.* 77:597, 1942.

Yntema, C. L., and Hammond, W. S. The Development of the Autonomic Nervous System. *Biol. Rev.* 22:344, 1947.

DEVELOPMENT

The Eye

The eye develops as a diverticulum from the lateral aspect of the forebrain. The diverticulum grows out laterally toward the side of the head, and the end becomes slightly dilated to form the *optic vesicle,* while the proximal portion becomes constricted to form the optic stalk (Fig. 21-1). At the same time, a small area of surface ectoderm overlying the optic vesicle thickens to form the *lens placode.* The lens placode invaginates and sinks below the surface ectoderm to form the *lens vesicle.* Meanwhile the optic vesicle becomes invaginated to form a double-layered *optic cup.* The inferior edge of the optic cup is deficient, and this notch is continuous with a groove on the inferior aspect of the optic stalk called the *optic fissure* (Fig. 21-2). Vascular mesenchyme now grows into the optic fissure and takes with it the *hyaloid artery.* Later the fissure becomes narrowed by growth of its margins around the artery, and by the seventh week the fissure closes, forming a narrow tube, the *optic canal,* inside the optic stalk (Fig. 21-3). By the fifth week, the lens vesicle loses contact with the surface ectoderm and lies within the mouth of the optic cup, the edges of which form the future *pupil.*

Retina

For purposes of description, the retina may be divided into two developmental layers: (1) the pigment layer and (2) the neural layer.

THE PIGMENT LAYER. This is formed from the outer thinner layer of the optic cup, as a result of the development of pigment granules in the cells (Figs. 21-4 & 21-5).

THE NEURAL LAYER. This is formed from the inner thicker layer of the optic cup. By the sixth month of development, all the layers of the nervous portion of the retina have developed, including the *rod* and *cone cells, bipolar cells, ganglionic cells,* and supporting elements (Fig. 21-5).

Anteriorly, the edge of the cup continues as a two-layered epithelium onto the posterior surface of the developing ciliary body and iris (Fig. 21-6). It is thus seen that the inner layer of the optic cup may be divided into a small nonnervous portion near the edge of the cup and a large photosensitive portion, and the two are separated by a wavy line, the *ora serrata.*

Optic Nerve

The ganglion cells of the retina develop axons which converge to a point where the optic stalk leaves the posterior surface of the

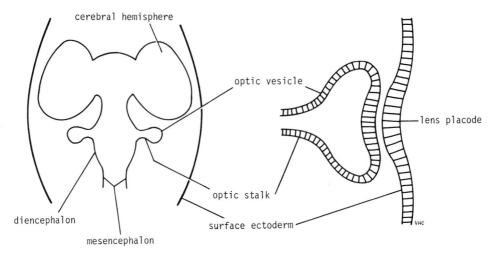

Fig. 21-1. The formation of the optic vesicle, which grows out as a diverticulum from the lateral aspect of the forebrain.

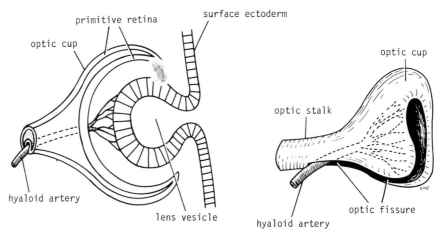

Fig. 21-2. The invagination of the optic vesicle to form the optic cup and the depression of the lens placode to form the lens vesicle. The deficiency in the inferior edge of the optic cup, which is continuous with the optic fissure, is shown.

optic cup. The axons now pass among the cells which form the inner layer of the stalk (Fig. 21-3). Gradually the inner layer encroaches on the cavity of the stalk until the inner and outer layers fuse. The cells of the optic stalk form neuroglial supporting cells to the axons, and the cavity of the stalk disappears. The stalk, together with the optic axons, forms the optic nerve; the hyaloid artery and vein become the *central artery* and *vein of the retina.*

Lens

As the lens vesicle sinks beneath the level of the surface ectoderm, the cells forming the posterior wall rapidly elongate, lose their

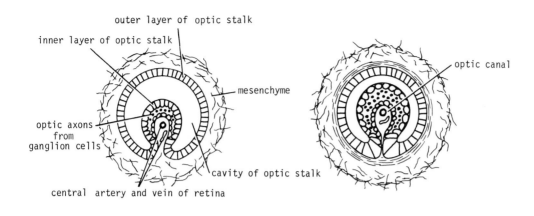

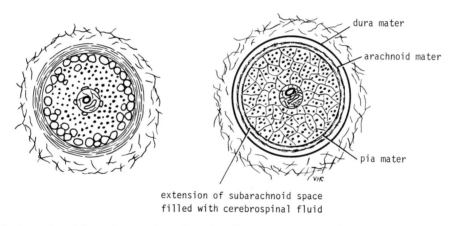

Fig. 21-3. The formation of the optic nerve from the optic stalk as seen on cross section.

nuclei, and form transparent lens fibers (Figs. 21-2 & 21-4). With the increase in length of these cells, the cavity of the lens vesicle gradually becomes obliterated. The laminated arrangement of the lens fibers occurs as the result of additional fibers being produced and added to the outer surface of the lens by the division of cells in the equatorial region of the lens. The cells forming the anterior wall of the lens remain as low columnar cells, and these form the *lens epithelium.*

Meanwhile vascular mesenchyme is growing into the optic cup and surrounds the developing lens (Fig. 21-4). The mesenchyme immediately adjacent to the lens becomes the *lens capsule,* which in the earliest stages receives an abundant arterial supply from the hyaloid artery. Later this blood supply regresses, and it disappears before birth.

Ciliary Body and Suspensory Ligaments of the Lens

The mesenchyme situated at the edge of the optic cup differentiates to form: (1) the connective tissue of the *ciliary body,* (2) the

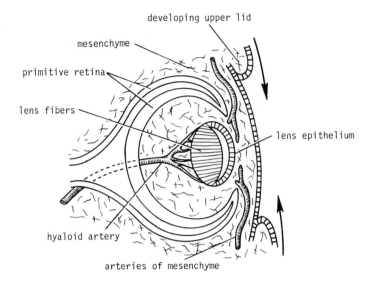

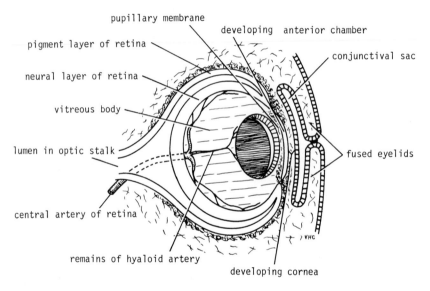

Fig. 21-4. The eye at different stages of development. The formation of the lens and the reduction in size of the hyaloid artery are shown. The eyelids remain fused until the seventh month.

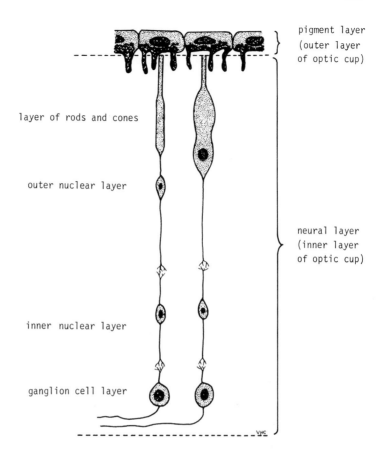

pigment layer (outer layer of optic cup)

layer of rods and cones

outer nuclear layer

neural layer (inner layer of optic cup)

inner nuclear layer

ganglion cell layer

Fig. 21-5. The retina, showing the fate of the outer and inner layers of the optic cup.

smooth muscle fibers of the *ciliary muscle,* and (3) the *suspensory ligaments* of the lens. The two layers of ectoderm forming the edge of the optic cup grow onto the posterior surface of the ciliary muscle and become folded to form the *ciliary processes* (Fig. 21-6). The suspensory ligaments extend between the ciliary processes and the lens capsule.

Iris and Aqueous Chamber

The mesenchyme situated on the anterior surface of the lens condenses to form the *pupillary membrane* (Figs. 21-4 & 21-6). The two layers of ectoderm forming the edge of the optic cup, having covered the ciliary muscle, now extend onto the posterior surface of the pupillary membrane. These structures fuse and form the iris. The *sphincter* and

dilator pupillae muscles develop within the iris, and before birth the central part of the pupillary membrane degenerates so that the *pupil* is formed.

The aqueous chamber arises as a cavity in the mesenchyme between the surface ectoderm and the developing iris. This constitutes the *anterior chamber* (Figs. 21-6 & 21-7). The *posterior chamber* develops as a split in the mesenchyme posterior to the developing iris and anterior to the developing lens (Fig. 21-7). The anterior and posterior chambers communicate when the pupil is formed.

Vitreous Body

The mesenchyme that invades the optic cup and occupies the space between the developing retina and the lens differentiates into a

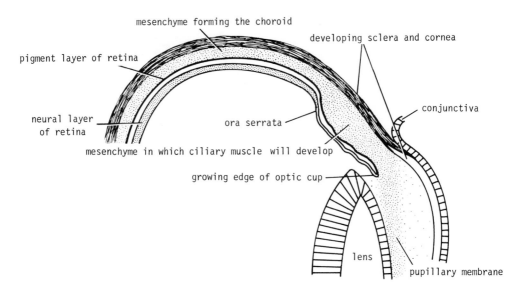

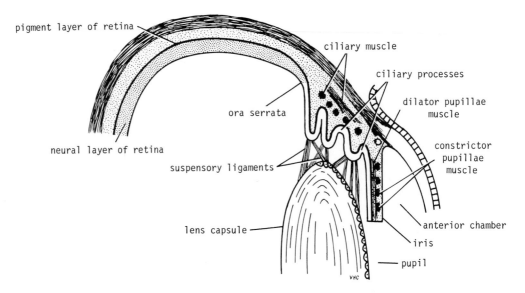

Fig. 21-6. The development of the ciliary body and iris. The two layers of ectoderm forming the edge of the optic cup cover the ciliary muscle and then extend onto the posterior surface of the pupillary membrane.

delicate network of fibers embedded in jelly-like material called the *vitreous body.* The vitreous body is surrounded by a thin membrane, the *hyaloid membrane,* which is pierced by a channel that allows the hyaloid artery to pass through it to the posterior surface of the lens (Figs. 21-4 & 21-7).

Cornea, Sclera, and Choroid

The *cornea* of the eye is formed from two sources: (1) the surface ectoderm, which forms the *corneal epithelium,* and (2) the underlying mesenchyme which differentiates to form dense connective tissue, the *substantia propria* of the cornea (Figs. 21-4 & 21-7).

The *sclera,* the outer tough fibrous coat of the eyeball, is formed from surrounding mesenchyme. At the attachment of the optic nerve to the eyeball, the sclera becomes continuous with the dura mater of the brain, which forms a fibrous sheath around the optic nerve.

The *choroid,* the inner vascular coat of the eyeball situated between the sclera and the pigment layer of the retina, is also formed from surrounding mesenchyme. At the attachment of the optic nerve to the eyeball, the choroid becomes continuous with the pia-arachnoid of the brain, which forms a sheath around the optic nerve. It is important to note that the *subarachnoid space,* with its contained cerebrospinal fluid, extends as a tubular space around the optic nerve through the optic foramen in the skull into the orbital cavity as far anteriorly as the attachment of the optic nerve to the eyeball (Fig. 21-7).

Extra-ocular Muscles

The four *rectus muscles* and the *superior* and *inferior oblique muscles* are formed from the mesenchyme in the region of the developing

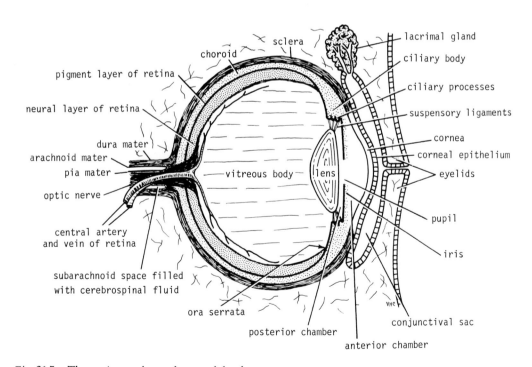

Fig. 21-7. The eye in an advanced stage of development.

eyeball (preotic myotomes). They are innervated by the third, fourth, and sixth cranial nerves.

Accessory Eye Structures

The *eyelids* develop as ectodermal folds superiorly and inferiorly to the cornea (Fig. 21-4). As they grow, they become united with each other at about the third month of intrauterine life. The lids remain fused until the seventh month. While the lids are fused, a closed space exists in front of the cornea called the *conjunctival sac*. The mesenchymal core of the lids forms the connective tissue and tarsal plates. The *orbicularis oculi muscle* is formed from the mesenchyme of the second pharyngeal arch, which invades the eyelids and is supplied by the seventh cranial nerve.

The *lacrimal gland* is formed as a series of ectodermal buds that grow superlaterally from the superior fornix of the conjunctiva into the underlying mesenchyme. These later canalize, forming the secretory units and multiple ducts of the gland (Fig. 21-7).

Lacrimal Sac and Nasolacrimal Duct

These have been seen to develop as a solid cord of ectodermal cells between the lateral nasal process and the maxillary process of the developing face (see Chap. 9). Later the cord becomes canalized to form the *nasolacrimal duct,* and the superior end becomes dilated to form the *lacrimal sac*. Further cellular proliferation results in the formation of *lacrimal ducts,* which enter each eyelid.

The Ear

For purposes of description, the ear may be divided into three parts: (1) the external ear, (2) the middle ear, and (3) the internal ear.

External Ear

The *pinna* or *auricle* is formed from three mesenchymal proliferations derived from the first pharyngeal arch and three similar proliferations from the second pharyngeal arch. These produce six surface elevations that surround the developing external auditory meatus and later fuse to form the auricle.

The *external auditory meatus* is formed from the first pharyngeal cleft. This ectodermal depression grows medially until it reaches the region of the entodermal lining of the first pharyngeal pouch (Fig. 21-8). The lining cells proliferate to form a temporary epithelial plug that disappears before birth.

The *tympanic membrane* is a fibrous sheet formed from mesenchyme. It is covered on its lateral surface by epithelium that is derived from the ectoderm forming the floor of the first pharyngeal cleft. It is covered on its medial surface by epithelium that is derived from the entoderm of the first pharyngeal pouch (Fig. 21-8).

Middle Ear

A diverticulum of entoderm called the *tubotympanic recess* grows laterally from the first pharyngeal pouch and extends laterally to meet the floor of the first pharyngeal cleft. On reaching the base of the skull, it comes into close contact with the developing internal ear and the dorsal ends of the first and second pharyngeal arches; these arches will form the bony ossicles, the *malleus, incus,* and *stapes*. The recess now expands and wraps itself around these small bones at that level and forms the tympanic cavity (Fig. 21-8). The neck of the recess narrows and becomes the *pharyngotympanic tube*. The entoderm lining the tympanic cavity forms the inner epithelial covering of the tympanic membrane and also invests the ossicles and the chorda tympani nerve. The *epitympanic recess* and the *antrum* develop as extensions from the tympanic cavity. After birth the *mastoid process of the temporal bone* develops, and the *mastoid air cells* form from entodermal diverticula that grow from the antrum into the developing bone.

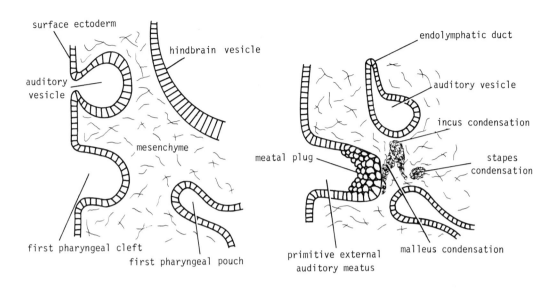

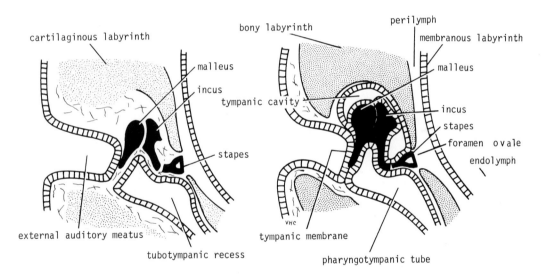

Fig. 21-8. Four stages in the development of the ear. The formation of the auditory vesicle from the surface ectoderm is shown. Shown also is the manner in which the tubotympanis recess expands to form the tympanic cavity and its epithelium envelops the ossicles.

The ossicles in the early stages are condensations of mesenchyme that become cartilaginous precursors of the *malleus, the incus,* and the *stapes.* The malleus and incus are formed from the first pharyngeal arch and the stapes from the second pharyngeal arch. The muscle attached to the malleus, the *tensor tympani,* is also derived from the first arch and is therefore innervated by the mandibular division of the trigeminal nerve. The muscle attached to the stapes, the *stapedius,* is derived from the second arch and is therefore innervated by the facial nerve.

Internal Ear

The internal ear begins as a thickening of the surface ectoderm opposite the hindbrain (Fig. 21-9). The thickened ectodermal plate is called the *auditory placode,* and this invaginates the surface to form the *auditory pit.* Later the mouth of the pit closes to form the *auditory vesicle.* The vesicle now sinks below the surface and will form the *membranous labyrinth.* This will become filled with fluid called *endolymph.*

As growth continues, a hollow diverticulum grows out from the medial side of the auditory vesicle; this elongates to form the *endolymphatic sac* (Fig. 21-9). The auditory vesicle may now be subdivided into a superior *vestibular part* and an inferior *cochlear part.* The semicircular canals develop during the sixth week as flattened diverticula from the vestibular part of the auditory vesicle. In the central portion of each diverticulum, the walls fuse and disappear, leaving the rims as the *semicircular canals* (Fig. 21-9). The superior, posterior, and lateral semicircular canals now become arranged at right angles to each other. The inferior portion of the vestibular part of the auditory vesicle is called the *utricle* (Fig. 21-9).

The cochlear part of the auditory vesicle is now divided into a superior portion, known as the *saccule,* and an inferior portion, which grows rapidly and becomes spirally arranged,

the *cochlear duct* (Fig. 21-9). Later, the connection between the saccule and cochlear duct becomes constricted to form the *ductus reuniens.*

Meanwhile the mesenchyme surrounding the membranous labyrinth differentiates into a fibrous membrane that lies outside the epithelium and into cartilage that encloses the entire labyrinth. Later the cartilage that lies immediately adjacent to the membranous labyrinth dedifferentiates to form loose tissue that subsequently becomes the *perilymphatic space.* The membranous labyrinth is now seen to be suspended in fluid, the *perilymph,* in the perilymphatic space. Eventually the perilymphatic space communicates with the subarachnoid space through the *aqueduct of the cochlea.* During the fifth month, the cartilage surrounding the membranous labyrinth is replaced by bone, which is now called the *bony labyrinth.*

The development of the perilymphatic space in relation to the cochlear duct differs from elsewhere in that the space does not surround the duct but occurs as two distinct spaces that lie in contact with two surfaces of the cochlear duct. The spaces are known as the *scala vestibuli* and *scala tympani,* and they run the whole length of the cochlear duct, communicating with each other at the apex of the cochlea (Fig. 21-10). The wall of the cochlear duct, which lies in contact with the scala vestibuli, becomes known as the *vestibular membrane,* and the wall in contact with the scala tympani forms the *basilar membrane* (Fig. 21-10). The lateral wall of the cochlear duct remains attached to the bony labyrinth, and its inner edge is attached to the bony *modiolus* of the cochlea (Fig. 21-10). The scala tympani and scala vestibuli now grow toward the tympanic cavity; they abut onto this cavity at the round and oval windows.

The cells lining the membranous labyrinth are at first of the low columnar type, and they form a single layer of epithelium. As

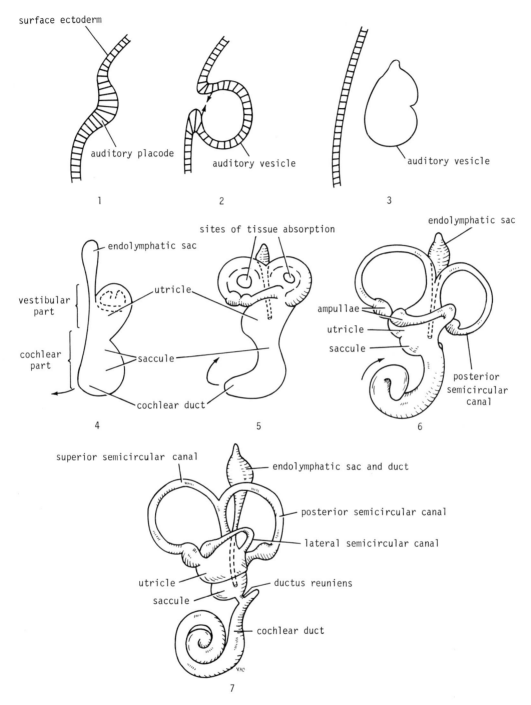

Fig. 21-9. The formation of the auditory vesicle from the surface ectoderm and its progressive development into the membranous labyrinth.

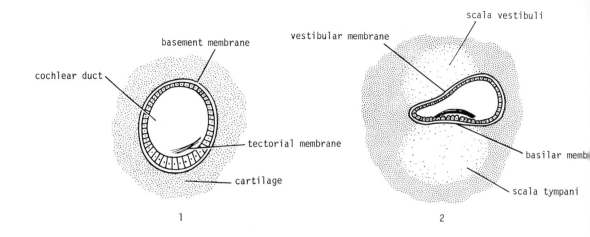

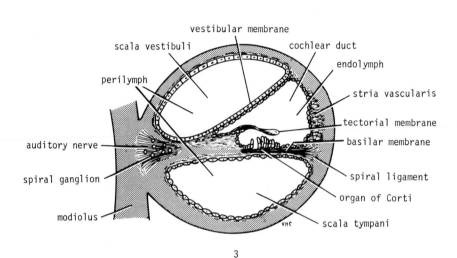

Fig. 21-10. The different stages in the formation of the cochlea: (1) A cross section of the cochlear duct surrounded by a fibrous basement membrane and cartilage. (2) A cross section of the cochlear duct at a later stage. The cartilage is becoming dedifferentiated to form loose periotic tissue, and two spaces are forming, called the *scala vestibuli* and *scala tympani*. (3) At a still later stage the organ of Corti has differentiated.

development continues, the epithelium becomes thickened in certain areas to form sense organs. In the dilated end (ampulla) of each semicircular canal (Fig. 21-9), the *crista ampullaris* appears (Fig. 21-11); the *saccular macula* of the saccule and the *utricular macula* of the utricle also develop. The cells of these sensory areas become associated with the peripheral processes of the neurons of the vestibular ganglion. Impulses concerned with balance will be carried to the brain by the vestibular fibers of the eighth cranial nerve.

At the same time the *spiral organ of Corti* develops as an epithelial thickening in the coiled cochlear duct (Fig. 21-10). The *hair cells* and *supporting cells* appear, and the *tectorial membrane,* which is a gelatinous substance, is secreted by the epithelium. The peripheral nerve fibers of neurons in the *spiral ganglion* branch around the bases of the hair cells, and the nervous impulses concerned with hearing are carried to the brain by the auditory fibers of the eighth cranial nerve.

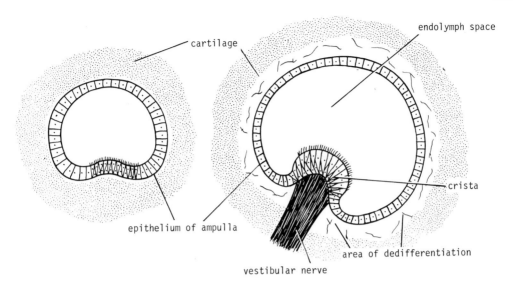

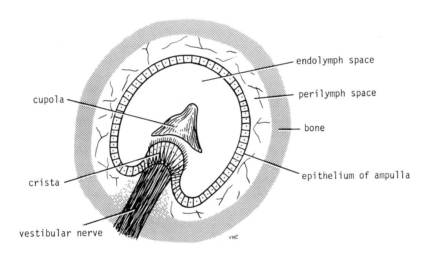

Fig. 21-11. The different stages in the development of the ampullae and cristae of the semicircular canals.

CONGENITAL ANOMALIES

Eye

STRABISMUS (SQUINT). Normal binocular vision occurs when a baby is about 1 month old. If a squint is present after the third month, it is probably caused by muscle imbalance, and if allowed to continue without treatment, blindness of the affected eye occurs because of cortical suppression of the extra image. There is a strong familial tendency to squints. Once the diagnosis has been made, ophthalmic treatment must be instituted.

CATARACT. In this condition, the lens becomes opaque (Fig. 21-12) during intra-uterine life. The principal causes appear to be infection and malnutrition. If the mother should suffer from the rubella virus between

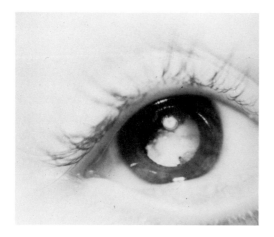

Fig. 21-12. Congenital cataract. (Courtesy of Dr. D. Friendly.)

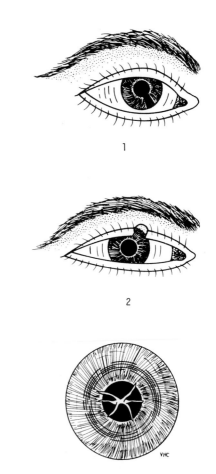

Fig. 21-13. Some congenital anomalies of the eye: (1) coloboma of the iris, (2) cleft of the upper eyelid, and (3) remnants of pupillary membrane stretching across the pupil.

the fourth and seventh weeks of pregnancy, a time when the lens is actively developing, congenital cataract may appear in the child. If the mother is infected with rubella after the seventh week, the lens is not affected. Many of the children with congenital cataract are of low birth weight and may have suffered from intra-uterine malnutrition resulting from poor diet during the mother's pregnancy, maternal toxemia, or multiple pregnancy. A chromosomal anomaly may be another factor; mongoloid children, for example, have a higher incidence of congenital cataract than others. In severe cases, it will be necessary for an ophthalmic surgeon to needle the lens.

GLAUCOMA. In this condition, there is a raised intraocular tension resulting from a developmental anomaly of the absorption mechanism of aqueous humor from the anterior chamber of the eye. Eighty percent of cases are bilateral, and the condition is responsible for 5 to 10 percent of cases of blindness in children. The eye is enlarged. Surgical removal of the abnormal tissues in the region of the filtration angle is required.

PERSISTENT PUPILLARY MEMBRANE. Normally the central part of pupillary membrane dis-appears before birth. Very occasionally this part of the membrane persists as strands of connective tissue which stretch across the pupil (Figs. 21-13 & 21-14). It is a simple matter to remove the connective tissue surgically.

COLOBOMA. This is a notched defect of a sector of the iris, ciliary body, retina, or choroid and is caused by a failure of closure of the optic fissure (Figs. 21-13 & 21-15). This

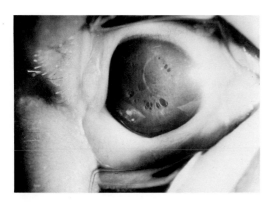

Fig. 21-14. Persistent pupillary membrane. (Courtesy of Dr. D. Friendly.)

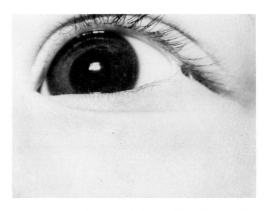

Fig. 21-16. Adhesion of the eyelids. The eyelids have failed to separate completely at the seventh month. (Courtesy of Dr. D. Friendly.)

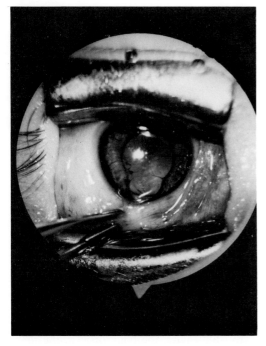

Fig. 21-15. Coloboma of iris. (Courtesy of Dr. D. Friendly.)

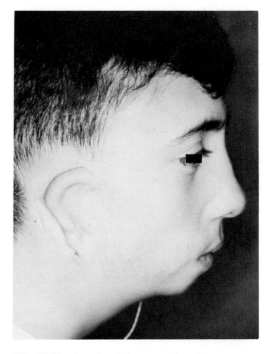

Fig. 21-17. Atresia of the external auditory meatus. (Courtesy of Dr. L. Thompson.)

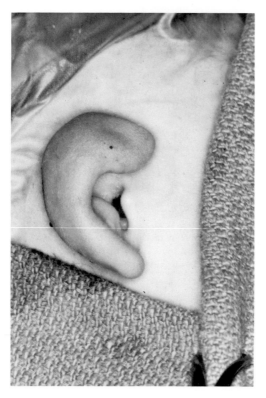

Fig. 21-18. Congenital cup-shaped ear. (Courtesy of Dr. L. Thompson.)

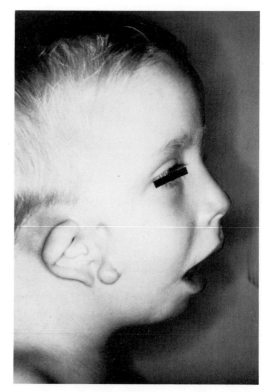

Fig. 21-19. Multiple auricular appendages. (Courtesy of Dr. L. Thompson.)

condition may occur as an isolated lesion or in association with other malformations, especially cleft lip or palate.

ABSENCE OF PIGMENT IN THE RETINA AND IRIS. This lack is part of the syndrome of albinism, which is discussed in detail in Chapter 22.

CLEFT EYELID. This defect usually occurs in the upper lid (Fig. 21-13). If the cornea is left exposed when the eyes are closed, the defect must be closed surgically at once.

ADHESION OF EYELID MARGINS. In this rare condition the eyelid margins are connected by bands of tissue which reduce the palpebral fissure and impair the mobility of the eyelids (Fig. 21-16). Microscopically, the bands have a core of connective tissue and are covered on the outside with epithelium.

ATRESIA OF THE NASOLACRIMAL DUCT. Atresia causes watering from the affected eye and liability to infection of the lacrimal duct and sac. For details, see Chapter 9.

Ear

Imperfect development of the external auditory meatus, the tympanic membrane, the tympanic cavity, the bony ossicles, the membranous labyrinth, and the eighth cranial nerve do occur and are a cause of congenital deafness.

ATRESIA OF THE EXTERNAL AUDITORY MEATUS. Children born with this condition (Fig. 21-17) and with the ossicles present should have an artificial meatus created surgically, since this will permit the use of an air-conducting

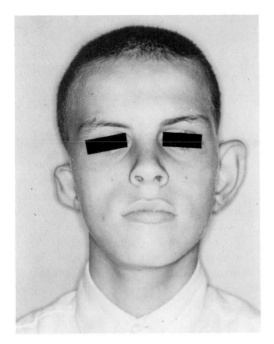

Fig. 21-20. Right-sided microtia. (Courtesy of Dr. L. Thompson.)

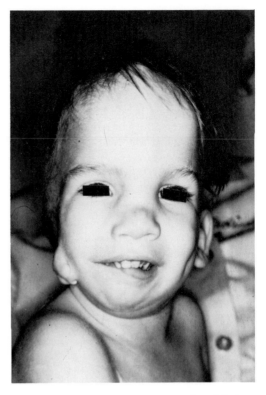

Fig. 21-21. Right-sided ear which has failed to ascend adequately. (Courtesy of Dr. L. Thompson.)

hearing aid, which is more efficient than a bone-conducting aid.

INTRA-UTERINE DAMAGE TO THE COCHLEA. Maternal rubella occurring during the first 3 months of pregnancy is liable to cause damage to the organ of Corti with consequent deafness in about 30 percent of cases. In one-third of the cases, the condition is unilateral. Erythroblastosis fetalis with hyperbilirubinemia may damage the cochlear nuclei, and this may produce high-tone deafness. Intracranial injury and asphyxia associated with a difficult labor may also cause deafness.

ANOMALIES OF THE AURICLE. Abnormal fusion of the surface elevations which surround the opening of the external auditory meatus may occur, producing malformed auricles (Fig. 21-18) or accessory auricular appendages (Fig. 21-19). Occasionally the auricle fails to develop adequately, producing *microtia* (Fig. 21-20) or is low set in position (Fig. 21-21). For preauricular and auricular sinuses, see Chapter 10.

Clinical Problems

Answers on page 453

1. A 4-year-old girl was taken to an ophthalmologist because her right eye "turned inward" when she was tired or excited and especially when she was looking at an object intently. On physical examination it was noted that she had a medial strabismus of the right eye. On questioning the child it was apparent that she did not have double vision. Examination of the fundus showed it to be normal in both the right and left eyes. Covering the nonstrabismic eye showed that the child had severe impairment of vision in the strabismic eye. What is strabismus? Can it be a congenital anomaly? Is this condition hereditary? Does this condition cure itself spontaneously?

2. A 3-month-old boy was taken to an ophthalmologist because the mother had noticed an opacity of the left eye since birth. The mother gave a history of rubella infection during the first trimester of the pregnancy. On physical examination a pearly nuclear cataract of the left eye was found. The child also had impaired hearing of the right ear and evidence of a ventricular septal defect. Is there any connection between the rubella infection of the mother and the congenital defects noted in the child?

3. A 6-year-old boy was routinely examined by an ophthalmologist and was found to have a small notch on the inferior nasal sector of his left iris. The notch measured about 0.5 mm in length and involved the pupillary margin. The boy's mother stated that he had had the notch since birth. What is your diagnosis? How would you explain this condition embryologically?

4. A 5-year-old boy was seen by a pediatrician because of deafness in the left ear. On examination the right ear was found to be normal. The left auricle was normal but there was a small swelling anterior to the tragus. The swelling was sessile, and on palpation a firm structure could be identified within it. Examination of the external auditory meatus revealed that it ended blindly about 5 mm from the surface. The inner ear appeared to be intact, since the child could hear a vibrating tuning fork placed on the mastoid process. The air conduction test, of course, showed no hearing. What is the diagnosis?

REFERENCES

Altmann, F. Malformations, Anomalies and Vestigial Structures of the Inner Ear. *A.M.A. Arch. Otolaryng.* 57:591, 1953.

Anson, B. J., and Bast, T. H. Development of the Incus of the Human Ear. *Quart. Bull. Northw. Univ. Med. Sch.* 33:110, 1959.

Anson, B. J., and Bast, T. H. Development of the Stapes of the Human Ear. *Quart. Bull. Northw. Univ. Med. Sch.* 33:44, 1959.

Anson, B. J., Bast, T. H., and Cauldwell, E. The Development of the Auditory Ossicles, the Otic Capsule and the Extracapsular Tissues. *Ann. Otol.* 57:603, 1948.

Anson, B. J., and Black, W. T. The Early Relation of the Auditory Vesicle to the Ectoderm in Human Embryos. *Anat. Rec.* 58:127, 1934.

Bach, L., and Seefelder, R. *Atlas Zur Entwicklungs Geschichte des Menschlichen Auges.* W. Englemann, Leipzig, 148 S., 50 pl., 1911.

Barber, A. N. *Embryology of the Human Eye.* Mosby, St. Louis, 1955.

Bartelmez, G. W. The Origin of the Otic and

Optic Primordia in Man. *J. Comp. Neurol.* 34: 201, 1922.

Bast, T. H., and Anson, B. J. *The Temporal Bone and the Ear.* Thomas, Springfield, Ill., 1949.

Beard, C. Congenital and Hereditary Abnormalities of the Eyelids, Lacrimal System, and Orbit. In *Congenital Anomalies of the Eye,* edited by C. Beard et al. Mosby, St. Louis, 1968.

Brown, C. A. Congenital Abnormalities of the Eye with Particular Reference to Prematurity. *Proc. Roy. Soc. Med.* 53:189, 1960.

Coulombre, A. J. Cytology of Developing Eye. *Int. Rev. Cytol.* 11:161, 1961.

Coulombre, A. J., and Coulombre, J. L. Corneal Development. I. Corneal Transparency. *J. Cell. Comp. Physiol.* 51:1, 1958.

Gilbert, P. W. The Origin and Development of the Human Extrinsic Ocular Muscles. *Contrib. Embryol.* 36:59, 1957.

Gray, J. E. Rubella in Pregnancy: Fetal Pathology in the Internal Ear. *Ann. Otol.* 68:170, 1959.

Gregg, N. M. Congenital Cataract Following German Measles in the Mother. *Trans. Ophthal. Soc. Aust.* 3:35, 1941.

Mall, F. P. Cyclopia in the Human Embryo. *Contrib. Embryol.* 6:5, 1917.

Mann, I. C. *The Development of the Human Eye.* Grune & Stratton, New York, 1949.

Mann, I. C. *Developmental Abnormalities of the Eye.* Lippincott, Philadelphia, 1957.

O'Rahilly, R. The Early Development of the Otic Vesicle in Staged Human Embryos. *J. Embryol. Exp. Morph.* 11:741, 1963.

O'Rahilly, R. The Early Development of the Eye in Staged Human Embryos. *Contrib. Embryol.* 38:1, 1966.

Prentiss, C. W. On the Development of the Membrana Tectoria with Reference to Its Structure and Attachments. *Amer. J. Anat.* 14:425, 1913.

Proctor, B. Development of Middle Ear Spaces. *J. Laryng.* 78:631, 1964.

Rones, B. Development of the Human Cornea. *Arch. Ophthal.* (Chicago) 8:568, 1932.

Scammon, R. E., and Armstrong, E. L. On the Growth of the Human Eyeball and Optic Nerve. *J. Comp. Neurol.* 38:165, 1925.

Scheie, H. G., and Albert, D. M. *Adler's Textbook of Ophthalmology,* 8th ed. Saunders, Philadelphia, 1969. P. 140.

Streeter, G. L. On the Development of the Membranous Labyrinth and the Acoustic and Facial Nerves in the Human Embryo. *Amer. J. Anat.* 6:139, 1906.

Streeter, G. L. The Histogenesis and Growth of the Otic Capsule and Its Contained Periotic Tissue Spaces in the Human Embryo. *Contrib. Embryol.* 7:5, 1918.

Streeter, G. L. Development of the Auricle in the Human Embryo. *Contrib. Embryol.* 14:111, 1922.

Van der Stricht, O. The Arrangement and Structure of Sustentacular Cells and Hair Cells in the Developing Organ of Corti. *Contrib. Embryol.* 9:109, 1920.

Watzke, D., and Bast, T. H. The Development and Structure of the Otic (Endolymphatic) Sac. *Anat. Rec.* 106:361, 1950.

Wood-Jones, F., and Wen, J. C. The Development of the External Ear. *J. Anat.* 68:525, 1934.

Zimmermann, A. A., Armstrong, E. L., and Scammon, R. E. The Change in Position of the Eyeballs During Fetal Life. *Anat. Rec.* 59:109, 1934.

DEVELOPMENT

Skin

The skin is composed of two distinct parts, the epidermis and the dermis, the *epidermis* being derived from ectoderm and the *dermis* from mesenchyme. The ectoderm covering the surface of the embryo is at first a single layer of cuboid cells; later these multiply and become arranged in two layers (Fig. 22-1), an outer layer, the *epitrichium,* and an inner layer, the epidermis. The epitrichium soon degenerates and is shed at about the sixth month, when it becomes mixed with the secretion of the sebaceous glands to form a white cheesy material, the *vernix caseosa.* The vernix covers the fetus until birth and protects it from maceration as it floats in the amniotic fluid. Meanwhile the epidermis proliferates and becomes differentiated into several layers. The deepest layer is the *stratum germinativum;* superficial to this are the *stratum spinosum,* the *stratum granulosum,* the *stratum lucidum,* and the *stratum corneum.* While the proliferation of cells is proceeding, the epidermis sends down blunt ridges into the underlying mesenchyme so that the *epidermal ridges* and *dermal papillae* are formed.

At about the thirteenth week, the epidermis is invaded by cells of neural crest origin (Fig. 22-2). These cells have long processes, or dendrites, and are known as *melanoblasts.* Once they enter the epidermis and take up their final position between adjacent keratinocytes in the stratum germinativum, *tyrosinase* appears in their cytoplasm and they start to form the pigment *melanin.* These cells are now known as *melanocytes.* The melanocytes donate their melanin to adjacent keratinocytes by a process called *cytocrine activity.* The amount and color of the melanin present in the epidermis are responsible for the differences in skin color of those of different races. In the Caucasian and Negro the epidermis possesses the same number of melanocytes, but in the Negro the production of melanin by the melanocytes is greater than in the Caucasian.

The dermis is formed from a condensation of the underlying mesenchyme. The mesenchyme in this region is derived from two sources (Fig. 22-3): the cells of the somatopleuric mesoderm of the body wall and limbs and the cells of the dermatome, which migrate from each somite. Fibroblasts are soon formed, and a feltwork of collagen and elastic fibers is laid down. Blood capillaries and lymphatic vessels are also formed. Adipose tissue appears in the deeper parts of the

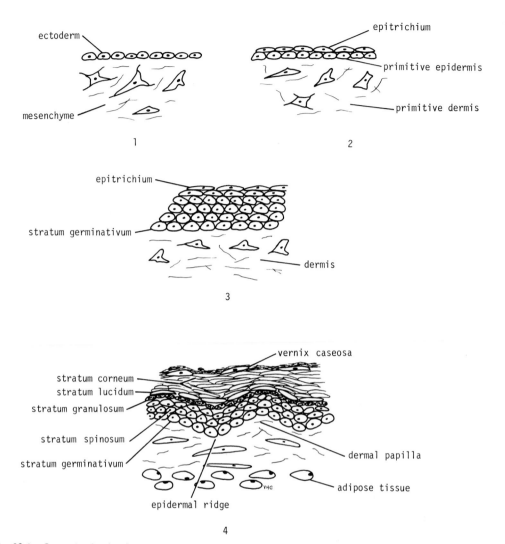

Fig. 22-1. Stages in the development of the skin.

dermis and the subcutaneous tissue, and this increases in amount during the later months of pregnancy and is responsible for the rounded contours of the newborn child.

Hair

During the third month the hairs begin to develop as cylindrical downgrowths of epidermis into the underlying mesenchyme

(Fig. 22-4). The terminal end of each *hair bud* expands to form a *hair bulb*. The hair bulb becomes invaginated from below by a condensation of mesoderm called the *hair papilla*. The central cells of each hair bud now elongate and become keratinized and form the *hair shaft*. The peripheral cells of the hair bud become cuboid and form the root sheath of the *hair follicle*. Proliferation of the hair bulb cells continues and pushes

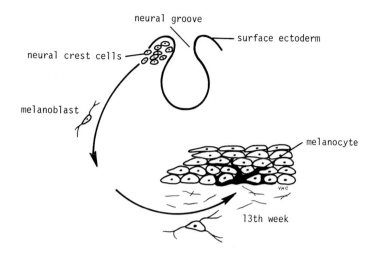

Fig. 22-2. Migration of the neural crest cells to the epidermis.

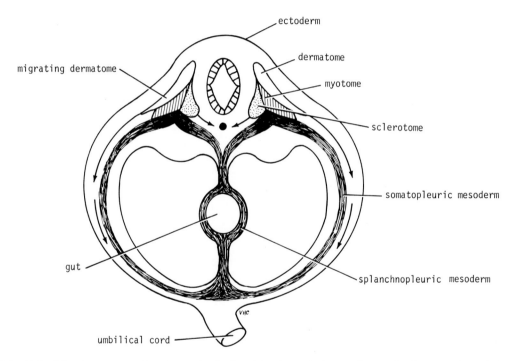

Fig. 22-3. The dermatome migrating to its final position beneath the ectoderm. The dermis is formed from a mixture of the dermatome and the local somatopleuric mesoderm.

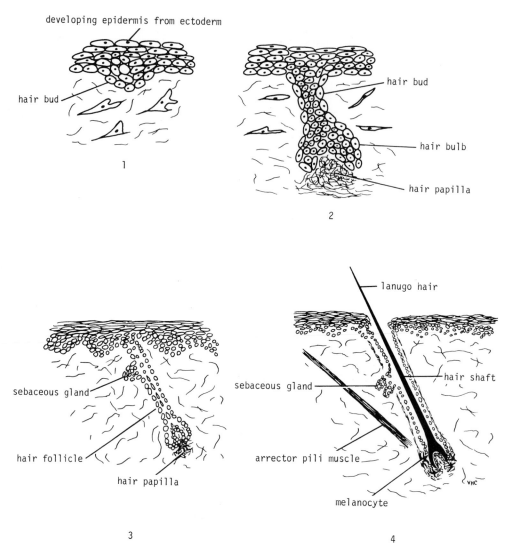

Fig. 22-4. Development of a hair follicle.

the hair shaft upward until it emerges on the skin surface. Meanwhile melanoblasts from the neural crest invade the hair bulb, tyrosinase appears in their cytoplasm, and they differentiate into *melanocytes*. The melanin pigment is then donated to the cells forming the hair shaft. By this means, the hair becomes pigmented. The first hairs to appear on the skin surface are of fine texture and are known as *lanugo*. Later these are cast off at about the time of birth and are replaced by coarser hairs.

The *sebaceous glands* develop as solid outgrowths of ectodermal cells in the region of the neck of the hair follicles (Fig. 22-4). The outgrowths extend into the mesenchyme, and the central cells degenerate and form a fatty secretion that passes out into the hair follicle as *sebum*. Some of the surrounding mesenchymal cells differentiate to form the smooth muscle called the *arrector pili muscle*.

Sweat Glands

These appear at about the fifth month as a solid downgrowth of ectodermal cells into the mesenchyme (Fig. 22-5). The terminal part of the downgrowth becomes convoluted and forms the body of the gland. Later the central cells degenerate to form the lumen of the gland. The peripheral cells differentiate into secretory cells and outer contractile *myoepithelial cells*.

Nails

These commence as thickened fields of ectoderm at the tip of each digit. Later they migrate onto the dorsal aspect of each digit but retain their innervation from the ventral surface.

At the proximal end of the nail field, ectodermal proliferation occurs, forming the *proximal nail fold*. The nail is formed from a proliferation of cells in the nail fold (Fig. 22-5). The cells become flattened and keratinized, and consolidate to form the *nail plate*. As growth continues, the nail plate gradually moves distally over the *nail bed* and reaches the tip of the digit 1 month before birth. The development of the fingernails is slightly ahead of that of the toenails.

The ectoderm on either side of the nail field tends to overgrow the field to form the *lateral nail folds*. At first the developing nail is covered by superficial layers of the epidermis and the epitrichium, which are collectively called the *eponychium*. The

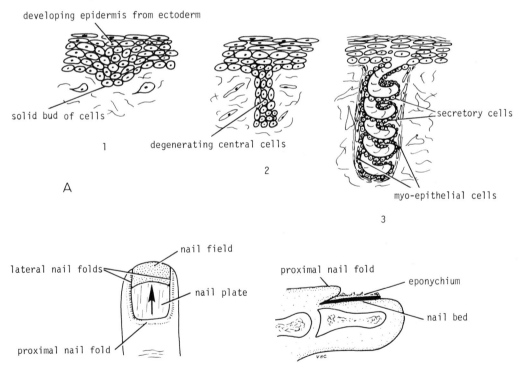

Fig. 22-5. Development of (A) the sweat gland and (B) the nail.

eponychium is later discarded, and the underlying nail is exposed.

The Mammary Glands

In the young embryo a linear thickening of ectoderm appears called the *milk ridge,* which extends from the region of the axilla obliquely to the inguinal region (Fig. 22-6).

In lower animals several mammary glands are formed along it. In the human subject the ridge disappears except for a small part in the pectoral region. This localized area now thickens, becomes slightly depressed, and sends off 15 to 20 solid cords that grow into the underlying mesenchyme. Each cord represents a future milk duct and a lobe of the mammary gland. The cords continue to grow

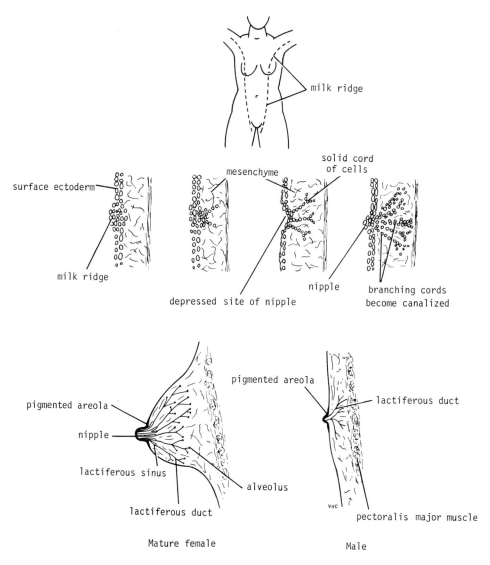

Fig. 22-6. Development of the mammary gland in the female and male.

and branch throughout fetal life, and by the time of birth they are canalized and form the *lactiferous sinuses, lactiferous ducts,* and *secretory alveoli.* Meanwhile the depressed ectodermal thickening becomes raised to form the *nipple* as the result of proliferation of the underlying mesenchyme. At the fifth month, the *areola* is recognized as a circular pigmented area of skin around the future nipple.

At birth the rudimentary mammary glands in both sexes are identical. Sometimes a milky secretion is produced in both sexes during the first few days after birth. This glandular activity is probably a result of stimulation by the maternal sex hormones that have crossed the placental barrier prior to delivery. At puberty, in the female estrogen will stimulate further duct growth and the breast will become hemispherical in shape, largely as the result of the deposition of fat. During pregnancy, a great development of the duct system occurs and considerable alveolar development takes place in response to hormonal stimulation. Following childbirth, lactation begins in response to *prolactin* secretion from the anterior lobe of the pituitary. In the male the mammary gland remains as a rudimentary duct system throughout life.

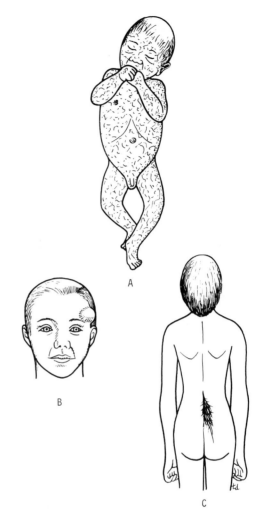

Fig. 22-7. (A) A baby with severe ichthyosis, (B) a young boy with an external angular dermoid cyst, and (C) a girl with localized hypertrichosis in the lumbar region of the back.

CONGENITAL ANOMALIES

Skin

ICHTHYOSIS. This is a congenital abnormality of cornification, associated with dryness and scaliness (Figs. 22-7 & 22-8). The disease is often familial and has a genetic background. The increased thickness of the epidermis is caused by retardation of the process of exfoliation of the cells of the stratum corneum, so that the cells are retained for a longer period than normal.

SEQUESTRATION DERMOID. This is a congenital cyst caused by the burying by skin fusion of ectodermal cells along the lines of closure of embryonic clefts and sinuses. The cyst is lined by epidermis and contains desquamated material. The cysts are commonly found in the midline of the body, particularly the neck, superior to the lateral canthus of the eye (Fig. 22-7), and in the anterior triangle of the neck (see branchial cyst, p. 135).

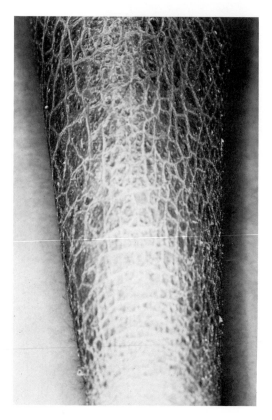

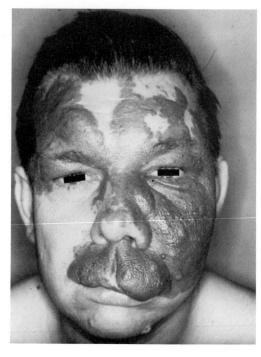

Fig. 22-9. Diffuse capillary hemangioma of the face. (Courtesy of Dr. L. Thompson.)

Fig. 22-8. Ichthyosis simplex of the leg. (Courtesy of Dr. M. Elgart.)

HEMANGIOMAS. These are very common and occur in the dermis as local malformations of blood vessels. There are two types. (1) *The capillary hemangioma* is a sharply demarcated erythematous swelling which is present at birth or appears shortly afterward. It is composed of collections of capillaries filled with blood. These tumors usually regress and require no treatment. Sometimes they occupy large areas of the face or upper part of the body and are then referred to as *port-wine stains* (Figs. 22-9 & 22-10). (2) The *cavernous hemangioma* is a reddish-blue spongy swelling composed of vascular channels, considerably larger than capillaries, which are filled with blood (Figs. 22-11 & 22-

12). Although these tumors tend to regress, they usually require surgical removal.

Hair

Gray hair occurs in albinism and is associated with lack of pigmentation in the skin and irides.

PILI TORTI. The hairs are twisted and bent. This is a congenital familial disorder of hair growth. Other ectodermal defects such as distorted nails may be associated with this disorder.

HYPERTRICHOSIS. The presence of excessive hair production may be localized or diffuse. The localized form may occur in the lumbar or sacral area (Fig. 22-7) and may be associated with spina bifida (see Chap. 19). The diffuse form may involve large areas of the body, even the face.

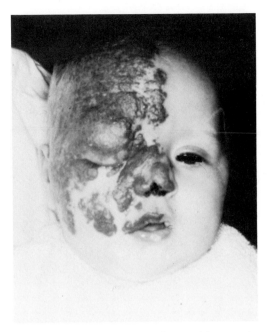

Fig. 22-10. Sturge-Weber syndrome. The association of a facial capillary hemangioma with epileptiform seizures due to hemangioma of the intracranial meninges. (Courtesy of Dr. M. Platt.)

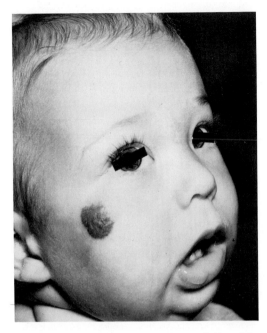

Fig. 22-11. Cavernous hemangioma of the right cheek. (Courtesy of Dr. R. Chase.)

ALOPECIA, or loss of hair. Total and localized forms of this condition occur. It is a result of congenital absence or lack of development of the hair follicles.

Nails

ANONYCHIA, or absence of nails, is a rare anomaly. This may be restricted to one or more nails of the fingers and toes, and their development may never take place. *Deformed nails* may occasionally occur.

Mammary Glands

ATHELIA. The absence of the nipple is very rare and it usually occurs only with amastia.

POLYTHELIA. Occasionally, supernumerary nipples occur along a line corresponding to the position of the milk ridge (Figs. 22-13 &

22-14). They are liable to be mistaken for moles.

RETRACTED NIPPLE OR INVERTED NIPPLE. This is a failure in the development of the nipple during its later stages (Fig. 22-15). In about one-quarter of the cases it is bilateral. Clinically it is important, since normal suckling of an infant cannot take place and the nipple is prone to infection. This condition must not be confused with a nipple that recently has become retracted from an underlying scirrhous carcinoma (Fig. 22-16).

AMASTIA. Absence of the breast may occur very rarely on one or both sides.

POLYMASTIA. Supernumerary breasts may rarely occur along a line corresponding to the milk ridges (Fig. 22-13). Very rarely they may occur elsewhere, such as on the arm or thigh.

MICROMASTIA. An excessively small breast on one side occasionally occurs, resulting from lack of development (Fig. 22-17).

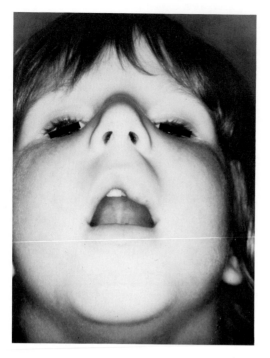

Fig. 22-12. Hemangioma of the upper lip. (Courtesy of Dr. L. Thompson.)

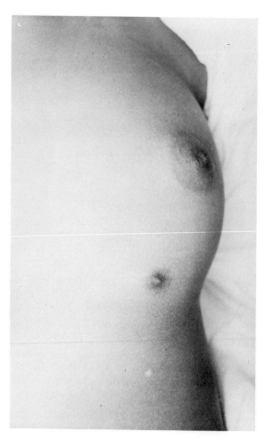

Fig. 22-14. Polythelia. (Courtesy of Dr. J. Randolph.)

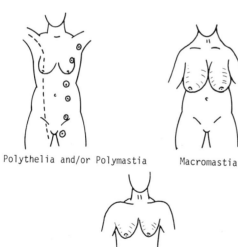

Polythelia and/or Polymastia   Macromastia

Gynecomastia

Fig. 22-13. Anomalies of the mammary glands.

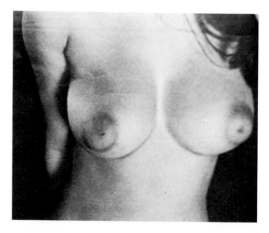

Fig. 22-15. Bilateral inverted nipples. (Courtesy of Dr. G. Avery.)

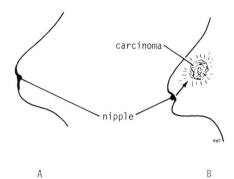

Fig. 22-16. (A) Congenitally retracted nipple of long standing and (B) retracted nipple of short duration, caused by underlying carcinoma of breast.

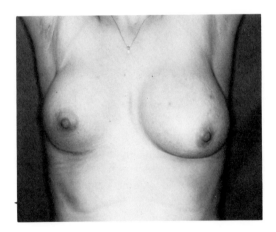

Fig. 22-17. Right-sided micromastia. (Courtesy of Dr. L. Thompson.)

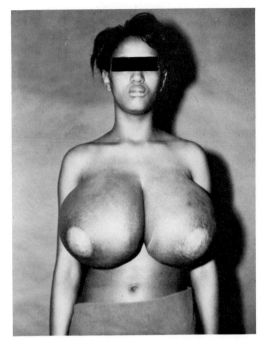

Fig. 22-18. Macromastia. (Courtesy of Dr. L. Thompson.)

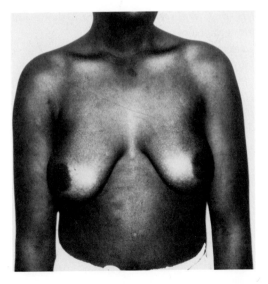

Fig. 22-19. Gynecomastia. (Courtesy of Dr. L. Thompson.)

MACROMASTIA. Diffuse hypertrophy of one or both breasts occasionally occurs in otherwise normal girls at puberty (Figs. 22-13 & 22-18). Plastic surgery may be indicated in extreme cases.

GYNECOMASTIA. Unilateral or bilateral enlargement of the male breast occasionally occurs (Figs. 22-13 & 22-19), usually at puberty. The cause is unknown, but it is probably because of some form of hormonal imbalance.

Anomalies of Pigmentation

SACRAL SPOTS. These are blue to slate gray in color and are found most commonly in the skin of the sacral region. The spots are due to the presence of diffuse collections of melanocytes in the dermis. It is assumed that these cells failed to reach the epidermal-dermal junction when they migrated from the neural crest. They are seen most frequently in Negro children, probably because the melanocytes contain more melanin in the Negro and the spots are more easily recognized.

NEVI. Pigmented lesions are often present at birth, but they rarely cover a large area of the body.

NEUROFIBROMATOSIS (VON RECKLINGHAUSEN'S DISEASE). This consists of areas of light brown pigmentation associated with multiple connective tissue tumors (Fig. 22-20) called *neurofibromas* (see Chap. 20).

ALBINISM. This is transmitted as a non-sex-linked simple mendelian recessive trait. In this condition, there is a genetic absence of the enzyme *tyrosinase* in the melanocytes. It is unusual to find total albinism in man; the eyes may not remain pink throughout life and some hairs may darken.

PARTIAL ALBINISM. This is transmitted as a dominant trait and is usually diagnosed by

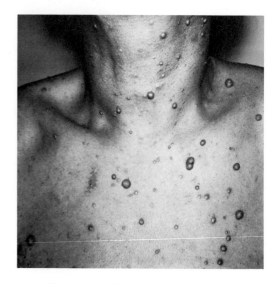

Fig. 22-20. Neurofibromatosis. (Courtesy of Dr. M. Elgart.)

the presence of a white forelock and patches of skin that are devoid of melanin pigment. The affected areas remain the same throughout life.

PHENYLKETONURIA. This is transmitted as a recessive trait. Light-colored skin, hair, and eyes are found in this condition. These subjects are unable to oxidize phenylalanine to tyrosine, and it is the relative absence of the latter substance that is responsible for the lack of melanin pigmentation.

Clinical Problems

Answers on page 453

1. An 18-month-old girl was taken to a dermatologist because of the dryness and scaliness of her skin. On physical examination the scales were noted to be quadrilateral or polygonal in shape, with upturned edges. The extensor surfaces of the arms and legs were more severely affected than the flexor surfaces, and the skin of the back was more severely affected than the anterior surface of the trunk. The face was only slightly affected. The mother said that the "fish scales" had first made their appearance when her daughter was 8 months old. The condition improved during the summer months but became worse in winter. The child

was otherwise perfectly healthy. On questioning, the mother said that she had suffered from the same condition and that her two older daughters had a milder form of the disturbance. What is your diagnosis?

2. A 15-year-old boy was examined by a dermatologist because of the presence of a painless soft swelling superior to the lateral margin of the right orbit. The swelling had first been noticed 5 years previously, and since that time it had gradually increased in size. On examination a soft fluctuant swelling about the size of a pea was found to be situated over the zygomatic process of the frontal bone. The skin was freely movable over it, but it was adherent to the underlying bone. What is your diagnosis? How would you treat this patient?

3. A 4-year-old boy was taken to a dermatologist because of a lack of hair on his head. At birth the child had a good head of hair; however, after the first year the mother noticed that the hair was slow in growing and began to fall out. On examination the child was found to be nearly bald. The eyebrows were absent, and the eyelashes were very fine and scanty. A biopsy of the scalp revealed absence of hair follicles, and the sebaceous glands and arrectores pilorum muscles were hypoplastic. What is the diagnosis?

4. An 8-year-old girl was taken by her mother to a pediatrician because of the presence of conspicuous hair growth on her arms and legs. Fine hairs were first noticed on the child's limbs soon after birth, and since then they had become longer and coarser. On physical examination excessive hair growth was found on the arms and legs; the palms and soles were spared. What is the diagnosis?

5. A 19-year-old woman visited her physician because she had noticed a small brown spot below her right breast. She had first noticed the spot when she was 7 years old. When she was 12 years old the spot had become darker in color. On examination a small circular pigmented area was seen over the right ninth costal cartilage in the midclavicular line. The skin was slightly elevated in its center. Nothing else abnormal was discovered. What congenital anomaly is likely to be responsible for this condition?

6. A 24-year-old woman was expecting her first child in 6 months' time. At the prenatal clinic her physician examined her breasts and found inverted nipples on both sides. The physician asked her if she had had this condition all her life. She replied that her nipples had always been "small" and she was worried in case she could not breast-feed her child. What is the embryological explanation for the condition of inverted nipples? May this congenital condition, if occurring unilaterally, be secondary to a more serious condition? What advice would you give this woman?

7. An 18-year-old pregnant woman visited her obstetrician because she had noticed a swelling in her left groin. She first became aware of the swelling at the end of the first month of her pregnancy. She was now 7 months pregnant and the swelling was much larger. On physical examination a firm swelling measuring about 3 in. (7.5 mm) in diameter was found on the left side of the anterior abdominal wall just above the medial end of the left inguinal ligament. The swelling was situated just beneath the skin and was not tethered to deep structures. On the summit of the swelling a small pigmented mole appeared to be present. Nothing else abnormal was discovered. What is your diagnosis? What will happen to this swelling after parturition?

8. A 20-year-old woman who had a very attractive figure wished to take up model-

ing as a career. She had noticed, however, that her right breast was smaller than that on the left side. She decided to visit a plastic surgeon and see if anything could be done to make both her breasts of equal size. Is this a common condition?

9. A 14-year-old boy was taken to a pediatrician because he was embarrassed by the size of his left breast. He said that he had experienced a tingling sensation in both breasts a year previously. Since that time both his breasts had enlarged, but the enlargement was greater on the left side. Apart from a moderately severe facial acne, nothing else abnormal was found on physical examination. Special tests showed that he had a normal chromatin pattern and his urinary 17-ketosteroids

and gonadotropins were at normal levels. Both testes were normal. What is your diagnosis? How would you treat this patient?

10. A 6-year-old girl was seen by a dermatologist because her hair was white and her skin showed total absence of pigmentation. Examination of her eyes showed hypopigmented ocular fundi, translucent irides, and nystagmus. Bright light obviously upset the child and she tended to cover up her eyes. Her mother said that she was extremely sensitive to sunlight and her skin burned very easily. The mother also said she had an older daughter with exactly the same condition. What is your diagnosis? Is this condition inherited?

REFERENCES

Billingham, R. E., and Silvers, W. K.   Melanocytes of Mammals. *Quart. Rev. Biol.* 35:1, 1960.

Boyd, J. D.   The Embryology and Comparative Anatomy of the Melanocyte. In *Progress in the Biological Sciences in Relation to Dermatology,* edited by A. Rook. Cambridge University Press, London, 1960.

Breathnach, A. S., and Wyllie, L. M.   Electron Microscopy of Melanocytes and Langerhans Cells in Human Fetal Epidermis at Fourteen Weeks. *J. Invest. Derm.* 44:51, 1965.

Ebling, F. J. G.   The Embryology of Skin. In *An Introduction to the Biology of the Skin,* edited by R. H. Champion, T. Gillman, A. J. Rook, and R. T. Sims. Davis, Philadelphia, 1970.

Hale, A. R.   Morphogenesis of Volar Skin in the Human Fetus. *Amer. J. Anat.* 91:147, 1952.

Kissane, J. M., and Smith, M. G.   *Pathology of Infancy and Childhood.* Mosby, St. Louis, 1967.

Pinkus, H.   The Embryology of Hair. In *Biology of Hairgrowth,* edited by W. Montagna and R. A. Ellis. Academic, New York, 1958.

Rains, A. J. H., and Capper, W. M.   *Bailey and Love's Short Practice of Surgery,* 14th ed. Lippincott, Philadelphia, 1968.

Rawles, M. E.   Origin of Melanophores and Their Role in Development of Color Patterns in Vertebrates. *Physiol. Rev.* 28:383, 1948.

Snell, R. S.   An Electron Microscopic Study of the Dendritic Cells in the Basal Layer of Guinea-Pig Epidermis. *Z. Zellforsch.* 66:457, 1965.

Snell, R. S.   On Electron Microscopic Study of the Human Epidermal Keratinocyte. *Z. Zellforsch.* 79:492, 1967.

Snell, R. S.   Hormonal Control of Pigmentation in Man and Other Mammals. In *Advances in Biology of Skin: The Pigmentary System.* Pergamon, New York, 1967. Vol. 8, p. 447.

Snell, R. S., and Bischitz, P. G.   The Melanocytes and Melanin in Human Abdominal Wall Skin: A Survey Made at Different Ages in Both Sexes and During Pregnancy. *J. Anat.* 97:361, 1963.

Zelickson, A. S.   The Langerhans Cell. *J. Invest. Derm.* 44:201, 1965.

DEVELOPMENT

Muscle

Voluntary Muscle

Early in development the embryonic mesoderm becomes differentiated into three distinct regions: *paraxial mesoderm, intermediate mesoderm,* and *lateral mesoderm* (see Chap. 3). The paraxial mesoderm is a column of tissue situated on either side of the midline of the embryo, and at about the fourth week it becomes divided into blocks of tissue called *somites.* Each somite becomes differentiated into a ventromedial part called the *sclerotome* and a dorsolateral part, the *dermomyotome* (Fig. 23-1). The dermomyotome now further differentiates into the *myotome* and *dermatome.* The myotomes increase in thickness and their mesenchymal cells differentiate into *myoblasts.* Meanwhile myoblasts are also being formed locally from mesenchyme in the anterolateral body walls and in the limb buds. The myoblasts now elongate and become spindle-shaped; they are multinucleated and the nuclei are centrally placed. Homogeneous *myofibrillae* appear in the cytoplasm, and by the third month these show cross striations. As development continues, the nuclei move to the periphery of the muscle fiber and the large numbers of myofibrillae occupy the center of the cell.

Gradually the muscle fiber increases in diameter as the result of multiplication of the myofibrillae. The growth of fetal muscle is brought about by the formation of additional myoblasts from mesenchyme and the division of immature myoblasts; individual muscle fibers also undergo hypertrophy. After birth, muscle growth is accomplished by the increase in size of existing muscle fibers. Voluntary muscle derived from mesenchyme of the pharyngeal arches is developed in a similar manner.

While the individual muscle fibers are developing, they become arranged in groups and surrounded by connective tissue derived from local mesenchyme; in this manner individual muscles are formed. The tendons of muscle are formed separately from mesenchyme and they connect the muscles to bones.

Muscles of the Head

The majority of the muscles of the head are derived from the mesenchyme of the pharyngeal arches, and their development has been considered in detail in Chapter 10.

Three pairs of *occipital myotomes* can be recognized (Fig. 23-2). It is believed that these migrate inferiorly and anteriorly to form the muscles of the tongue. The segmental nerves which grow out toward these myotomes are collectively known as the

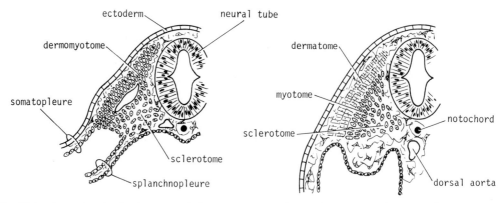

Fig. 23-1. Stages in the development of the paraxial mesoderm. The ventromedial part of the mesoderm forms the sclerotome and the dorsolateral part the dermomyotome. The dermomyotome differentiates into the dermatome and myotome.

hypoglossal nerve, which innervates the muscles of the tongue.

Three pairs of *preotic myotomes* are formed near the anterior aspect of the head (Fig. 23-2). These differentiate into the extrinsic muscles of the eye and are innervated by the third, fourth, and sixth cranial nerves.

Muscles of the Neck and Trunk

During the fifth week, the myotomes become divided into a small posterior part, the *epi-*

mere, and a larger anterior part, the *hypomere* (Fig. 23-3). Each segmental spinal nerve is also divided into a *posterior primary ramus* that innervates the epimere and an *anterior primary ramus* that supplies the hypomere. The epimeres gradually develop into the extensor muscles of the vertebral column, while the hypomeres form the prevertebral flexor muscles of the vertebral column. The mesenchyme of the somatopleure forms the anterior and lateral muscles of the

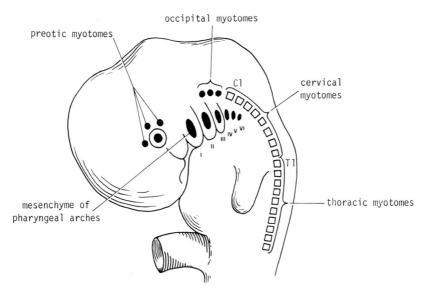

Fig. 23-2. Origin of the muscles of the head and neck.

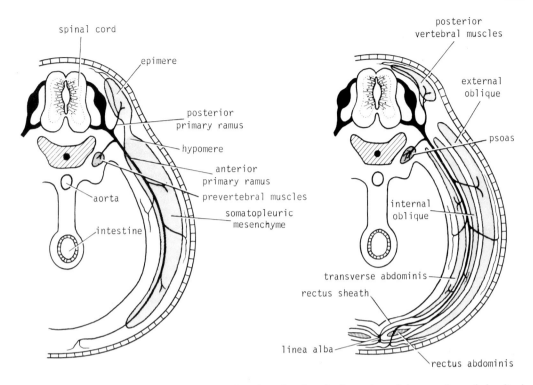

Fig. 23-3. Transverse sections of the abdominal region showing the formation of the muscles and the distribution of the spinal nerves to them.

neck and trunk, which are also supplied by the anterior primary rami.

In the neck the hypomeres fuse and form the scalenae muscles and the prevertebral muscles. In the thorax the muscles derived from the somatopleuric mesenchyme retain their segmental arrangement because of the presence of ribs, but in the abdomen, owing to the absence of ribs, the mesenchyme fuses to form large sheets of muscle. Two important events now take place in the somatopleuric mesenchyme. First, a narrow anterior portion becomes separated, which in the neck forms the *infrahyoid group of muscles,* in the thorax forms the *sternalis muscle,* and in the abdomen forms the *rectus abdominis* and *pyramidalis muscles* (Fig. 23-3). The sternalis muscle normally disappears. The rectus abdominis retains indications of its segmental character, as seen by the presence of the

tendinous intersections. Second, the antero-lateral parts of the somatopleuric mesenchyme become split tangentially into three layers, which in the thorax form the *external, internal,* and *transverse intercostal muscles* and in the abdomen form the *external oblique, internal oblique,* and *transversus abdominis muscles.*

The *quadratus lumborum* and *psoas muscles* are formed from the hypomeres of the second to the fifth lumbar segments.

The muscle of the diaphragm is developed from the third, fourth, and fifth cervical myotomes, which fuse and migrate caudally into the thorax as the septum transversum.

In the pelvis, the muscles of the pelvic diaphragm (the *levator ani* and the *coccygeus muscles*) and the voluntary muscle of the *external sphincter of the anal canal* and the *sphincter urethrae* and the muscles of the genital organs are formed from the hypomeres and local mesenchyme of the sacral and coccygeal regions.

The anterior body wall is finally closed in the midline at 3 months by the right and left sides meeting in the midline and fusing. In the abdomen the line of fusion of the mesenchyme forms the *linea alba,* and on either side of this the rectus muscles come to lie within their sheaths (Fig. 23-3).

Muscles of the Limbs

The muscles of the limb girdles are derived from the hypomeres and local body wall mesenchyme of the regions from which the limb buds develop. The muscles of the limbs are derived from the mesenchyme within the limb buds.

The limb buds appear during the sixth week of development as the result of a localized proliferation of somatopleuric mesenchyme. This causes the overlying ectoderm to bulge from the trunk as two pairs of flattened paddles (Fig. 23-4). The arm buds develop first and lie at the level of the lower six cervical and upper two thoracic segments. The leg buds arise at the level of the lower four lumbar and upper three sacral segments.

The flattened limb buds have a cephalic *preaxial border* and a caudal *postaxial border.* As the limb buds elongate, the anterior primary rami of the spinal nerves situated opposite the bases of the limb buds start to grow into the limbs. In the upper limb buds the mesenchyme situated along the preaxial border becomes associated and inner-

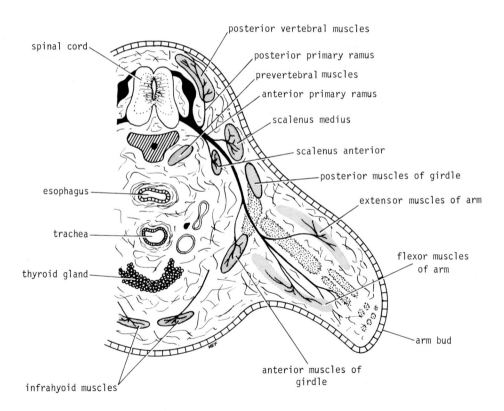

Fig. 23-4. Section through the lower cervical region showing the primordia of the muscle groups in the neck and upper limb. The muscles of the limb are derived from somatopleuric mesenchyme and the muscles of the girdle from the hypomeres and local mesenchyme.

vated with the lower five cervical nerves, while the mesenchyme of the postaxial border becomes associated with the eighth cervical and first thoracic nerves. In the lower limb buds the mesenchyme along the preaxial border becomes innervated by the second lumbar nerve to the first sacral nerve and that of the postaxial border becomes innervated by the first to the third sacral nerves. Later the mesenchymal masses divide into anterior and posterior groups, and the nerve trunks entering the base of each limb also divide into anterior and posterior divisions. As development continues and the limbs further elongate, their attachment to the trunk moves caudally. At the same time the mesenchyme within the limbs differentiates into individual muscles that migrate within each limb. As a consequence of these two factors, the anterior primary rami of the

spinal nerves become arranged in complicated plexuses that are found near the base of each limb, the *branchial plexus* for the upper limb and the *lumbosacral plexus* for the lower limb.

Involuntary Muscle

The development of involuntary muscle in different organs is described in the appropriate chapters.

Cardiac Muscle

The development of cardiac muscle is described in Chapter 7.

Cartilage

During the fifth week of development, local mesenchyme condenses in areas where cartilage will be formed (Fig. 23-5). The mesen-

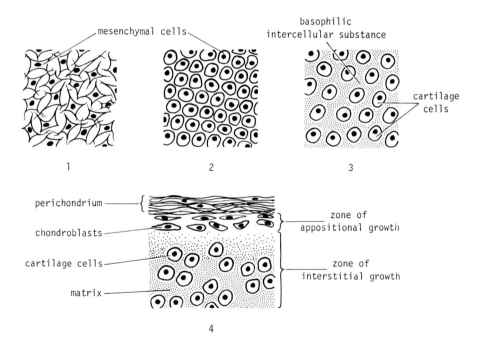

Fig. 23-5. Histogenesis of cartilage: (1) Loose mesenchyme with cells having long processes. (2) Compact mesenchyme; the cells have become rounded and have proliferated and now lie close together. (3) Cartilage cells secrete basophilic intercellular substance. (4) Mature cartilage; cells are surrounded by matrix in which are embedded collagenous fibers; the perichondrium is formed from surrounding mesenchyme.

chymal cells enlarge and proliferate to form a compact mass that assumes the shape of the future cartilage. The cells now become rounded in appearance and secrete a basophilic intercellular substance in which the collagenous fibers lying between them become embedded. The cells, now known as *cartilage cells,* continue to produce secretion or matrix and push themselves apart. The cartilage, except at the joint surfaces, is covered by a layer of fibrous tissue called *perichondrium* (Fig. 23-5).

Cartilage grows by *interstitial growth* and by *appositional growth.* Interstitial growth occurs as the result of division of cartilage cells within the interior of the cartilage and the secretion of more matrix. Appositional growth occurs as the result of differentiation of the inner cells of the perichondrium into *chondroblasts.* These cells develop into cartilage cells that secrete matrix. By these two methods new cartilage is formed in the interior and on the outer surface.

Three varieties of cartilage are formed: (1) *hyaline cartilage,* in which fine bundles of collagen fibers are obscured by the matrix; (2) *fibrocartilage,* in which large bundles of collagen fibers predominate in the matrix; and (3) *elastic cartilage,* in which large numbers of elastic fibers predominate in the matrix.

Bone

Bone is formed by two methods: (1) intramembranous ossification and (2) enchondral ossification.

Intramembranous Ossification

A condensation of mesenchyme occurs in the area where bone formation is to take place (Fig. 23-6). The cells are small and spindle-shaped, and they lie close and parallel to each other. The mesenchymal cells now lay down collagenous fibers so that the area closely resembles a fibrous membrane. Some of the cells now differentiate into *osteoblasts;* the amount of cytoplasm within the cells increases and the nuclei become eccentrically placed. The osteoblasts continue to produce large amounts of collagenous material and ground substance that fill up the intercellular spaces, known collectively as *osteoid* (Fig. 23-6). At this stage no calcium salts have been deposited in the matrix and the osteoid is still a pliable membrane. There is an increase in the number of capillaries in the region of the osteoblasts that is associated with the increased metabolic activity of these cells.

The osteoblasts now start to secrete *alkaline phosphatase,* which results in the deposition of calcium salts in the form of minute crystals of *apatite,* which are deposited on and obscure the fibrils of the matrix. In this manner the osteoid is converted into bone matrix. As more and more bone matrix is produced, some osteoblasts become trapped within it and are known as *osteocytes* (Fig. 23-6). The space within the bone matrix that is occupied by an osteocyte is known as a *lacuna.* Gradually the bone matrix grows in amount and extends in all directions within the membrane as *bone spicules.* A center of ossification has now been established.

Meanwhile a layer of vascular mesenchyme has condensed on the outside of the membrane to form the *periosteum.* This consists of an outer fibrous layer and an inner cellular layer composed of cells that differentiate into osteoblasts. These new osteoblasts now start to lay down bone in the form of parallel plates or *lamellae,* known as *compact bone,* just beneath the periosteum.

In a flat bone, such as that found in the vault of the skull, we now have the following situation: The original center of ossification in the middle of the membrane is laying down vascular *spongy* or *cancellous bone,* while the periosteal osteoblasts are laying down relatively avascular compact bone on the surface of the membrane (Fig. 23-7). The compact bone forms the *inner and outer*

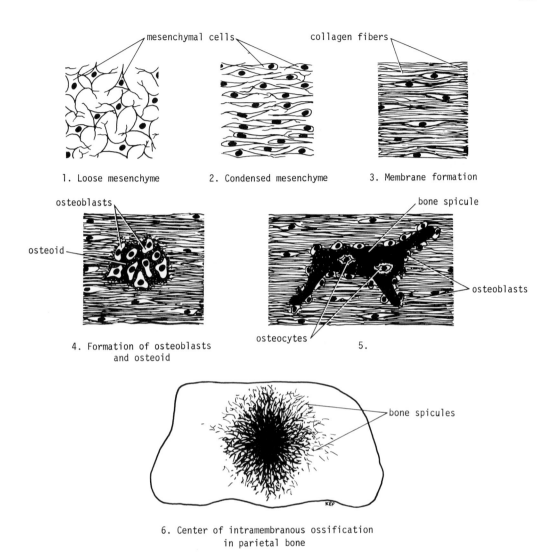

1. Loose mesenchyme   2. Condensed mesenchyme   3. Membrane formation

4. Formation of osteoblasts and osteoid

5.

6. Center of intramembranous ossification in parietal bone

Fig. 23-6. The stages in intramembranous ossification.

tables of the skull bone, while the central spongy bone is known as the *diploe*. The vascular tissue which fills the spaces of the cancellous bone differentiates into red *bone marrow* and becomes hematopoietic.

As development proceeds and the new bone grows, its shape is continually undergoing remodeling. Much of the original matrix laid down by the osteoblasts is resorbed by multinucleate giant cells called *osteoclasts*. These cells are thought to be formed either from osteoblasts or from undifferentiated mesenchymal cells. While bony resorption is taking place, new bone is being laid down by osteoblasts.

Enchondral Ossification

The long bones of the body are formed by this method of ossification. First the long bone is represented by a model of condensed

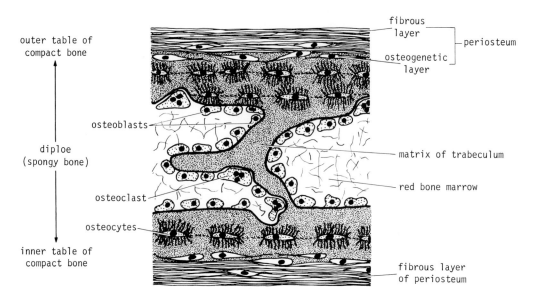

outer table of compact bone

diploe (spongy bone)

inner table of compact bone

osteoblasts

osteoclast

osteocytes

fibrous layer — periosteum

osteogenetic layer

matrix of trabeculum

red bone marrow

fibrous layer of periosteum

Fig. 23-7. Section of parietal bone of the vault of the skull, showing the inner and outer tables of compact bone and the central spongy bone.

mesenchyme that is soon replaced by a model of hyaline cartilage formed as described previously (Fig. 23-8). During the eighth week, ossification begins in the middle of the cartilaginous shaft. The cartilage cells in the region increase in size, and calcium salts are deposited in the intercellular matrix. The enlarged cartilage cells now degenerate and disappear, leaving empty cavities. Meanwhile the perichondrium becomes active and is now known as *periosteum*. The cells of its inner layer differentiate into osteoblasts, which start to lay down a collar of compact bone around the shaft. This formation of subperiosteal new bone may be regarded as a compensatory protective mechanism, since it will strengthen the developing bone at a time when the middle zone of the cartilage model is about to be broken down.

A bud of vascular tissue formed from the inner layer of the periosteum now grows inward. Accompanying the actively growing capillaries are osteoclasts and chondroclasts derived from mesenchymal cells. The osteo-

clasts break down areas in the newly formed periosteal bone and allow the vascular bud to invade the underlying calcified cartilaginous matrix. The chondroclasts break down the walls of lacunae previously occupied by the dead chondrocytes to form irregular spaces (Fig. 23-8). Osteoblasts which have accompanied the vascular bud now start to lay down bone on the walls of the spaces. Gradually, as the result of bone resorption by the osteoclasts and bone deposition by the osteoblasts, spongy bone is formed in the center of the shaft surrounded by compact bone. Later a large *marrow cavity* occupied by *red marrow* appears in the center of the bone.

The primary center of ossification has now been established in the center of the shaft of the cartilaginous model. This region of the developing bone is referred to as the *diaphysis*. Growth of the cartilaginous model continues by the proliferation of the chondrocytes and the deposition of further cartilaginous matrix. An examination of the cartilage in the region of the primary center of ossifica-

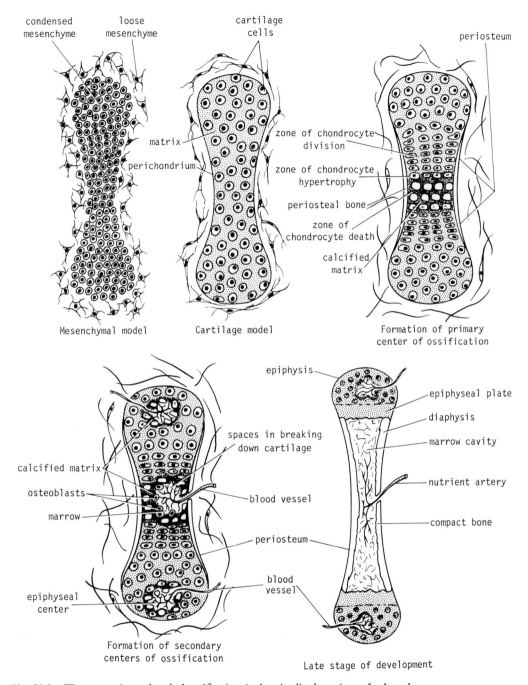

Fig. 23-8.   The stages in enchondral ossification in longitudinal sections of a long bone.

tion shows three regions of differentiation (Fig. 23-8). In the region close to the center, the chondrocytes are enlarged and degenerating, and calcium salts are being deposited in the matrix. In the second region, farther away from the center, the chondrocytes are enlarged but otherwise they appear normal. In the third region, which extends toward the ends of the cartilage model, the chondrocytes are actively dividing and becoming arranged in parallel rows. At the same time new cartilage is being formed, the center of ossification extends toward each end of the model.

At birth the long bone has a bony shaft, the *diaphysis,* with two cartilaginous ends, the *epiphyses* (Fig. 23-8). Later one or more secondary centers of ossification appear in each epiphysis. Now bone formation is taking place in three areas, the center of the shaft and in each extremity. The continuous growth in length of the cartilage model occurs as the result of division of the chondrocytes in the epiphyseal cartilage which, as development continues, is reduced to a thin plate, the *epiphyseal plate.* Growth in length of a long bone ceases when the chondrocytes in the epiphyseal cartilage cease to divide and form new cartilage. The epiphyseal plates now disappear and the epiphyses fuse with the diaphysis.

Meanwhile the diameter of the long bone has been increasing as the result of continued deposition of new compact bone under the periosteum and the resorption of old bone in the center of the shaft. The marrow cavity in this way also increases in size. In the epiphyseal region the transverse diameter increases as the result of growth of the epiphyseal ossification center.

In the long bones, at least one epiphyseal center is found at each end; in the smaller bones, such as the phalanges or metacarpals, one epiphyseal center is found at the proximal end; in irregular bones, such as the scapula or the vertebrae, one or more primary centers occur, and several secondary centers

appear. In most bones the epiphyses have fused with the diaphyses by the twentieth year. The clavicle is one important exception in that its shaft is formed by intramembranous ossification, and fusion with the epiphysis at the sternal end does not occur until the twenty-fifth year.

Skull

The development of the skull is complex, and only those aspects that are important from a medical standpoint are considered here.

The skull consists of a protective case around the brain, the *neurocranium,* and the skeleton of the jaws. Initially these parts are represented by a sheet of condensed mesenchyme that later may become converted into membrane bone or into cartilage. In some areas the cartilage undergoes enchondral ossification, while in others it persists as cartilage throughout life. The neurocranium may be divided into the cartilaginous part and the membranous part.

The *cartilaginous neurocranium* is the basal region of the developing skull and in the earliest stages extends as a plate from the anterior part of the skull to the anterior border of the foramen magnum. Later cartilaginous plates appear on either side, eventually forming the wings of the sphenoid bone. Each auditory vesicle becomes surrounded by cartilage and a cartilaginous capsule develops around each olfactory pit. By the middle of the third month, the base of the skull is a unified mass of cartilage (Fig. 23-9) known as the *chondrocranium.* Ossification of the chondrocranium begins early in the third month, and most of the bones have two or more centers of ossification.

The *membranous neurocranium* ultimately forms the large flat bones of the vault of the skull, namely the *frontals, parietals, squamous portion of the occipital,* and the *squamous temporals,* and also smaller bones, the *lacrimals* and *nasals* (Figs. 23-9 & 23-10). The bones that form the greater part of the

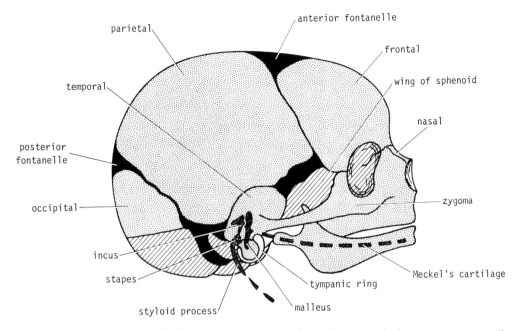

Fig. 23-9. The skull at birth. Stippled areas represent membrane bones; hatched areas represent cartilage bones; cross-hatched areas represent pharyngeal arch derivatives. The fontanelles are represented as solid.

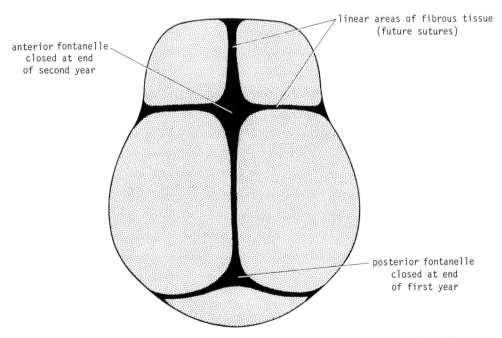

Fig. 23-10. Vault of the skull at birth. The stippled areas represent membrane bones; the solid areas represent areas of the skull that are still membranous. As the bones grow in size, they come to interdigitate with each other along the sutures.

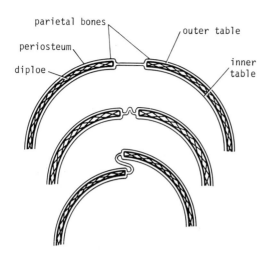

Fig. 23-11. The mobility of the bones of the vault of the skull is shown, also how the parietal bones may overlap one another during the molding process of the cranium during parturition.

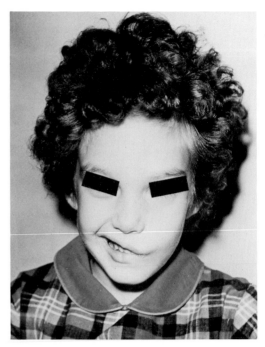

Fig. 23-12. Left-sided facial palsy following a difficult forceps delivery. (Courtesy of Dr. R. Chase.)

sides and roof of the skull are thus intra-membranous in origin. To allow for the rapid increase in size of the developing brain, these bones grow at their margins and their curvature is modified by the process of bone resorption on the inner surface and new bone deposition on the outer surface.

Most of the bones of the skull are ossified by the time of birth, but they are mobile on each other. Their mobility is most marked in the vault, and the ability to overlap provides the molding of the cranium that is so important during the process of childbirth (Fig. 23-11). In the newborn the bones of the vault are separated by fibrous tissue, the *sutures,* and at their corners by larger areas known as *fontanelles* (Fig. 23-10). From the clinical standpoint, the anterior and posterior fontanelles are the most easily examined, since they lie in the midline. Palpation of the fontanelles enables the physician to determine (1) the progress of growth in the surrounding bones, (2) the degree of hydration of the baby (e.g., if the baby is dehydrated, the fontanelles will be depressed below the sur-

face), and (3) the state of the intracranial pressure; a bulging fontanelle would indicate a raised intracranial pressure.

The *anterior fontanelle* lies between four bones: the two halves of the developing frontal bones anteriorly and the two parietal bones posteriorly (Fig. 23-10). It is usually not possible clinically to palpate the anterior fontanelle after eighteen months, since the four bones have enlarged to close the gap. The *posterior fontanelle* lies between the squamous part of the occipital bone and the posterior edges of the parietal bones. This closes by the end of the first year.

At birth the tympanic part of the temporal bone is present as a C-shaped tympanic ring (Fig. 23-9). The *tympanic membrane* is almost as large as that found in the adult, but it faces more inferiorly and less laterally; when examined with the auroscope, it therefore lies more obliquely than in the adult.

The *external auditory meatus* in the newborn is very short and wholly cartilaginous.

In the newborn the *mastoid process* is not developed, and the *facial nerve*, as it emerges from the stylomastoid foramen, is very close to the surface and thus may be damaged by forceps in a difficult delivery (Fig. 23-12). The mastoid process forms as the mastoid air cells (see Chap. 21) and the sternocleidomastoid muscle develop.

The *paranasal sinuses* are rudimentary at birth (see Chap. 9).

The development of the lower jaw or mandible is considered in Chapter 10.

Vertebral Column

In the first part of this chapter, the differentiation of each somite into a ventromedial part called the sclerotome and a dorsolateral part, the dermomyotome, was described. The sclerotome consists of rapidly dividing, loosely arranged mesenchymal cells. On each side, these cells migrate medially during the fourth week of development to surround the notochord (Fig. 23-13). In this manner the notochord becomes encased in a continuous cylinder of sclerotomic mesenchyme that still shows evidence of its segmental origin. The caudal half of each sclerotome fuses with the cephalic half of the immediately succeeding sclerotome to form the mesenchymal vertebral body (Figs. 23-13 & 23-14). Each vertebral body is therefore an intersegmental structure. The notochord degenerates completely in the region of the vertebral body, but in the intervertebral region it enlarges to form the *nucleus pulposus* of the *intervertebral discs* (Fig. 23-14). The surrounding fibrocartilage, the *annulus fibrosus,* of the intervertebral disc is derived from sclerotomic mesenchyme situated between adjacent vertebral bodies (Fig. 23-14).

Meanwhile the mesenchymal vertebral body gives rise to dorsal and lateral outgrowths on each side. The dorsal outgrowths grow around the neural tube between the segmental nerves to fuse with their fellows of the opposite side to form the mesenchymal *neural arch* (Fig. 23-13). The lateral outgrowths pass between the myotomes to form the mesenchymal *costal processes,* or primordia, of the ribs.

Two centers of chondrification appear in the middle of each mesenchymal vertebral body. These quickly fuse to form a cartilaginous *centrum* (Fig. 23-13). A chondrification center forms in each half of the mesenchymal neural arch and this spreads dorsally to fuse behind the neural tube with its fellow of the opposite side. These centers also extend anteriorly to fuse with the cartilaginous centrum and laterally into the costal processes. The condensed mesenchymal or membranous vertebra has thus been converted into a *cartilaginous vertebra.*

In the thoracic region, each costal process forms a cartilaginous rib. In the cervical region, the costal processes remain short and form the lateral and anterior boundaries of the *foramen transversarium* of each vertebra. In the lumbar region the costal process forms part of the transverse process. In the sacral region the costal processes fuse together to form the *lateral mass of the sacrum.*

At about the ninth week of development, primary ossification centers appear, two for each centrum and one for each half of the neural arch (Fig. 23-13). The two centers for the centrum usually quickly unite, but the complete union of all the primary centers does not occur until several years after birth. During adolescence, secondary centers appear in the cartilage covering the superior and inferior ends of the vertebral body and the *epiphyseal plates* are formed. A secondary center also appears at the tip of each transverse process and at the tip of the spinous process. By the twenty-fifth year, all the secondary centers have fused with the rest of the vertebra.

The *atlas* and *axis* vertebrae develop somewhat differently. The centrum of the atlas

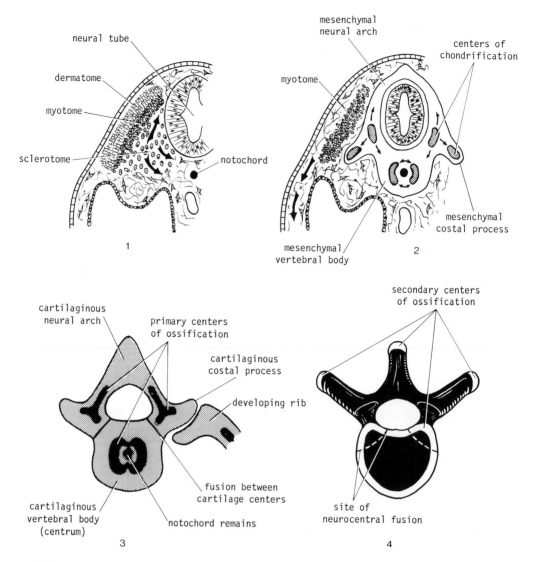

Fig. 23-13. The stages in the formation of a thoracic vertebra.

fuses with that of the axis and becomes the part of the axis vertebra known as the *odontoid process*. This leaves only the neural arch for the atlas, which grows anteriorly and finally fuses in the midline to form the characteristic ring shape of the atlas vertebra. In the *sacral* region, the bodies of the individual vertebrae are separated from each other by intervertebral discs in early life. At about the eighteenth year, the bodies start to become united by bone, and this process starts caudally; usually by the thirtieth year all the sacral vertebrae are united. In the *coccygeal* region segmental fusion also takes place, and in later life the coccyx often fuses with the sacrum.

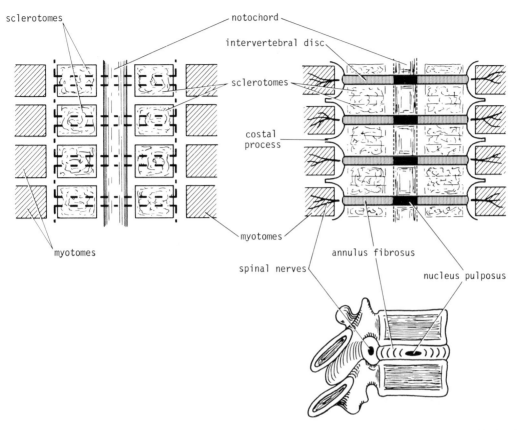

Fig. 23-14. The formation of each mesenchymal vertebral body by the fusion of the caudal half of each sclerotome with the cephalic half of the immediately succeeding sclerotome. Each vertebral body is therefore an intersegmental structure. The costal processes grow out between adjacent myotomes. Also shown is the close relationship which exists between each spinal nerve and each intervertebral disc.

RELATIONSHIP OF VERTEBRAL BODY TO THE SPINAL NERVE. Since the fully developed vertebral body is intersegmental in position, each spinal nerve leaves the vertebral canal through the intervertebral foramen and is closely related to the intervertebral disc. This fact may be of great clinical significance in cases with prolapse of an intervertebral disc (Fig. 23-14).

DEVELOPMENT OF THE CURVES OF THE VERTEBRAL COLUMN. The embryonic vertebral column shows one continuous ventral concavity. Later the sacrovertebral angle develops. At birth the cervical, thoracic, and lumbar regions show one continuous ventral concavity. When the child begins to raise its head, the cervical curve, which is convex anteriorly, develops. Toward the end of the first year, when the child stands up, the lumbar curve, which is convex anteriorly, develops.

Sternum

Bilateral plates of condensed mesenchyme appear in the ventrolateral body wall and at first have no connection with the developing ribs. Later the plates chondrify and fuse with the growing rib cartilages. As the antero-

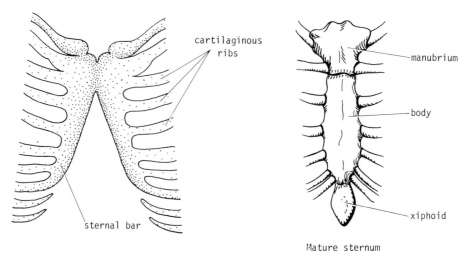

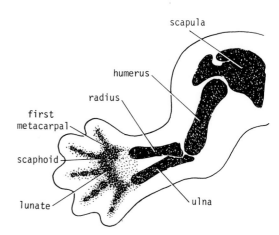

Fig. 23-15. The development of the sternum.

lateral body walls fuse with each other in the midline, the plates of cartilage come together and gradually fuse in a cephalic to caudal direction; thus the *manubrium sterni,* the *body of the sternum,* and finally the *xiphoid process* are formed (Fig. 23-15). Ossification centers develop later.

Ribs

These develop as bars of condensed mesenchyme that grow out from the primitive vertebrae (Fig. 23-13). As they extend laterally, they pass between adjacent myotomes. During the seventh week of development, they acquire a single center of chondrification. Later they sever their connection with the costal process of each vertebrae. A joint develops between the head of the rib and the vertebral body and between the tubercle of the rib and the transverse process. Later still the cartilaginous ribs become converted into bone, but the distal ends remain as the *costal cartilages.*

Appendicular Skeleton

This consists of the shoulder and pelvic girdles and the bones of the limbs. Mesen-

chymal condensations appear at the sites of the future bones during the fifth week of development (Fig. 23-16). The bones of the limbs are not derived from the sclerotomes but from the local somatic mesenchyme present within the limb bud. Differentiation of the mesenchyme occurs in the upper limb first; it occurs in a proximodistal direction in each limb. The mesenchymal models are re-

Fig. 23-16. Mesenchymal condensations at the sites of the future bones of the upper limb.

placed by cartilaginous models, the one exception being the clavicle, which is formed from membrane. Primary centers of ossification appear in the long bones during the seventh and eighth weeks of development. Secondary centers appear much later, between birth and the twentieth year.

Joints

Fibrous Joints

The sutures between the membranous bones of the vault of the skull are examples of this type of joint. The mesenchyme between the developing bones persists and becomes differentiated into dense fibrous tissue (Fig. 23-17).

Cartilaginous Joints

The joints between two vertebral bodies and the pubic symphysis are two examples of this type of joint. The mesenchyme between the bones becomes chondrified to form fibrocartilage. A layer of hyaline cartilage caps the bone on each side of the joint (Fig. 23-17).

Synovial Joints

The *knee, elbow,* and *wrist joints* are examples of this type of joint. After the cartilaginous models of the long bones have been formed, the mesenchyme between the ends of the cartilaginous bars undergoes differentiation. The peripheral mesenchyme becomes the *capsular ligament* and forms other extra-articular ligaments (Fig. 23-17). The cells in the central zone soon disappear so that a *joint cavity* is formed. The cells covering the articular surfaces and lining the capsule become flattened mesothelial cells and form the *synovial membrane.* Later, as the result of movement, the synovial membrane disappears from the surface of the articular cartilage.

In some synovial joints *fibrocartilaginous discs* project into the joint cavity from the capsule or divide the joint into two halves by forming a partition. Such discs are derived from the mesenchyme that forms the capsular ligament, and later they become chondrified (Fig. 23-17).

CONGENITAL ANOMALIES

Voluntary Muscle

MUSCLE AGENESIS. Partial or complete absence of a muscle occasionally occurs (Figs. 23-18 & 23-19). The *pectoralis major* is a muscle often involved. Defects of the *diaphragm* may cause herniation (see Chap. 14). Absence of the lower *anterior abdominal muscles* occurs in ectopia vesicae (see Chap. 15). The *palmaris longus muscle* may be absent or fail to develop completely in the forearm.

CONGENITAL TORTICOLLIS. It is now generally accepted that most cases of congenital torticollis are a result of excessive stretching of the sternocleidomastoid muscle during a difficult delivery. Hemorrhage occurs into the muscle, which may be detected as a small rounded "tumor" during the early weeks after birth. Later this becomes invaded by fibrous tissue, which contracts and shortens the muscle. The mastoid process is thus pulled down toward the sternoclavicular joint of the same side, the cervical spine is flexed, and the face looks upward to the opposite side (Fig. 23-20). Some authorities believe prenatal factors such as ischemic necrosis of the muscle may also be responsible. The condition is usually diagnosed when the child is between the ages of 5 and 7 years, when the neck elongates with growth. Mild cases can be corrected by exercises and stretching. Severe neglected cases must be treated by tenotomy of the sternocleidomastoid muscle. If they are left untreated, asymmetrical growth changes will occur in the face, and the cervical vertebrae may become wedge-shaped.

VARIATION IN MUSCLE DEVELOPMENT. Muscles show variations in size, form, and

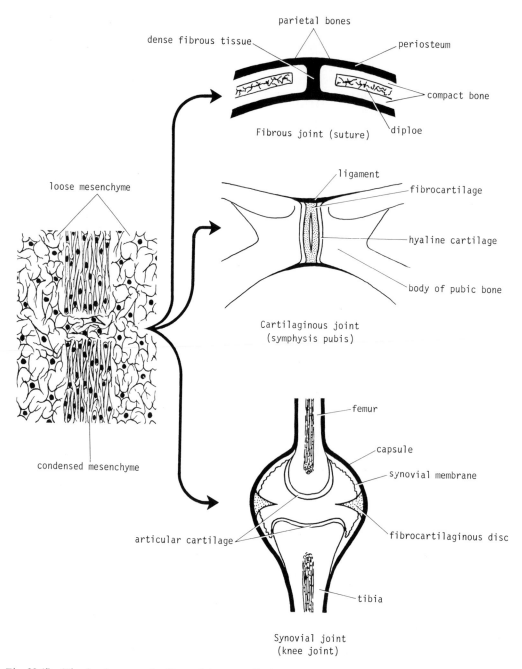

Fig. 23-17. The development of a fibrous joint, a cartilaginous joint, and a synovial joint.

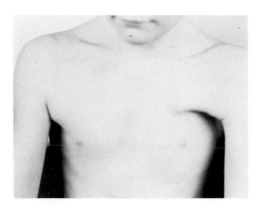

Fig. 23-18. Congenital absence of the left pectoralis major muscle. (Courtesy of Dr. M. Platt.)

attachments. Some muscles appear only occasionally in man, but they are constantly found in the primates, e.g., the *sternalis muscle*.

INFANTILE SPINAL MUSCULAR ATROPHY. This disease should be described under congenital anomalies of the spinal cord, but clinically it presents itself as a condition of hypotonia. There is progressive degeneration of the anterior horn cells of the spinal cord. The condition is inherited as an autosomal recessive trait. The hypotonia may be noticed before birth by the feeble or absent fetal movements. When the baby is held in the supine position, the head and limbs hang down. Tendon reflexes are absent. The neuronal degeneration is progressive and fatal.

BENIGN CONGENITAL HYPOTONIA. Hypotonia is present at birth or appears shortly afterward. Although the muscles are lax, paralysis is not complete. Tendon reflexes are present but weak. After a number of months, the condition improves and about 50 percent recover completely, the remainder showing some permanent muscular weakness. The cause is unknown.

SYMPTOMATIC HYPOTONIA. Lack of muscle tone is present in such conditions as mongolism and cerebral palsy, or following birth injury.

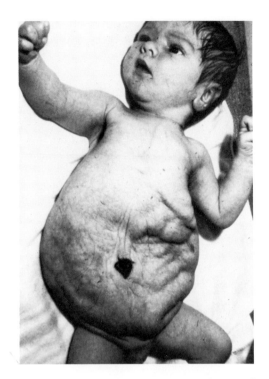

Fig. 23-19. "Prune belly." Congenital absence of abdominal muscles. (Courtesy of Dr. M. Platt.)

MYOTONIA CONGENITA. This condition is transmitted as an autosomal dominant trait but sometimes as a recessive trait (Fig. 23-21). It is present at birth or appears shortly afterward. The muscles show increased tone, and when a muscle contracts, it may remain so for half a minute. Loosening up of the muscles occurs after repeated movements, but hypertonicity is worse in cold weather.

ARTHROGRYPHOSIS MULTIPLEX. In this condition many of the limb joints are fixed as a result of the replacement of muscle by fibrous tissue (Fig. 23-22). The limbs may be in an extended or flexed position and talipes is present. It is believed that the malformation is often caused by severe loss of mobility while the fetus is in utero. Congenital muscular dystrophy and infantile muscular atrophy may also cause the condition. In cases result-

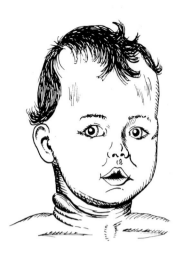
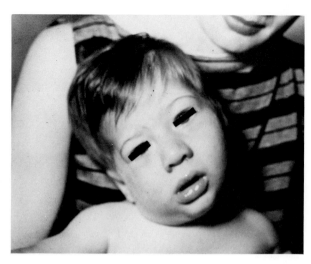

Fig. 23-20. Congenital torticollis: (1) The so-called tumor of the right sternocleidomastoid is sometimes recognized soon after birth and is caused by hemorrhage into the muscle; there is no deformity at this stage. (2) A severe case of torticollis caused by the shortening of the right sternocleidomastoid muscle. (Courtesy of Dr. J. Adams.)

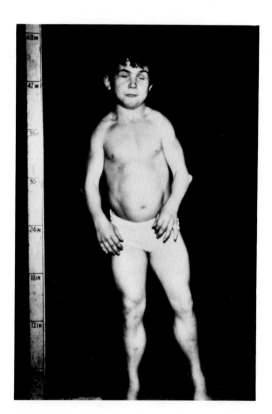
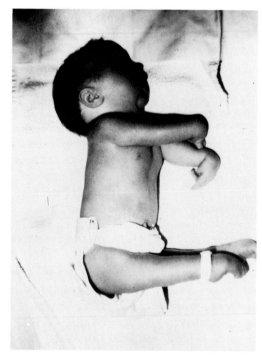

Fig. 23-22. Arthrogryphosis multiplex. (Courtesy of Dr. M. Platt.)

Fig. 23-21. Myotonia congenita. (Courtesy of Dr. M. Platt.)

376

ing from intrauterine loss of mobility, the prognosis is good; in the remainder, the prognosis is very poor.

Cartilage and Bone

ACHONDROPLASIA. This is an impairment of cartilage development in the epiphyseal plates of bones, especially long bones (Fig. 23-23). The condition is inherited as a mendelian dominant trait and is the commonest cause of dwarfism. The child has short limbs but an almost normal trunk. The skin of the thighs is thrown into folds, since the muscular development is normal and has to be confined within a reduced length. The base of the skull remains small, and premature fusion of the nasal bones leads to underdevelopment of the center of the face. Mental development is usually normal and such individuals often work in circuses.

OSTEOGENESIS IMPERFECTA. This disease is characterized by an abnormal fragility of bones and is determined by an autosomal dominant mutant gene with variable manifestation. It is a generalized mesenchymal defect. The bones are slim and delicate, and the amount of mineralized bone is greatly reduced. The basic defect is possibly the failure of the conversion of precollagen to collagen. The defect also affects connective tissue outside the skeleton, as seen by the blue sclera, which are thin and allow the choroidal pigment to show through. In the most severe form, the child is stillborn with multiple fractures. In the less severe form, the bones start to fracture with the minimum of trauma in childhood or adolescence. Union of fractures occurs easily. The fractures are treated as they occur, and the patient is protected from excessive trauma as much as possible.

OSTEOPETROSIS (ALBERS-SCHÖNBERG DISEASE). This is a rare hereditary disease in which there is defective ossification resulting from failure of normal resorption of cartilage. The bones are brittle and fracture easily. In areas where the cartilage persists, osteoid tissue accumulates, leading to the obliteration of the marrow cavity and the development of leukoerythroblastic anemia.

CRANIOCLEIDODYSOSTOSIS. This condition is caused by the inheritance of an autosomal dominant gene resulting in the incomplete formation or absence of the clavicles (Figs. 23-24 & 23-25). The membrane bones of the skull are also involved, causing the fontanelles to remain wide open. Since the clavicles are defective, the shoulders are abnormally mobile and can be brought close together.

DIAPHYSEAL ACLASIS (HEREDITARY MULTIPLE EXOSTOSIS). This is a heredofamilial condition in which multiple bony buds grow out from the diaphyses of developing bones to form large bony tumors that interfere with tendon action and cause pressure on neighboring nerves (Figs. 23-26 & 23-27).

Skull

CRANIOSCHISIS. In this condition the vault of the skull is open; it is usually associated with anencephaly (see Chap. 19). Occasionally it is combined with an open vertebral canal, *craniorachischisis* (Fig. 23-28).

PARIETAL FORAMINA. This is a localized defect of development in which symmetrical foramina occur in the parietal bones. The condition is a mendelian dominant trait.

HYPERTELORISM. The eyes are widely separated because of overgrowth of the lesser wing of the sphenoid.

CRANIOSYNOSTOSIS. In this condition, premature fusion of some of the cranial sutures occurs. If the sagittal suture is involved, the skull becomes elongated in anteroposterior diameter. If the coronal suture fuses early, the skull becomes turret-shaped because of the pushing upward of the parietal and frontal bones (Fig. 23-29). This condition may lead to a rise in the cerebrospinal fluid pressure, which in turn may lead to mental retarda-

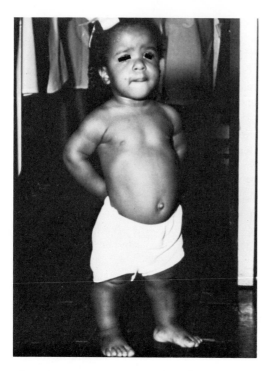

Fig. 23-23. Achondroplasia. (Courtesy of Dr. J. Adams.)

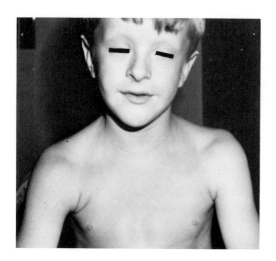

Fig. 23-24. Craniocleidodysostosis. (Courtesy of Dr. J. Adams.)

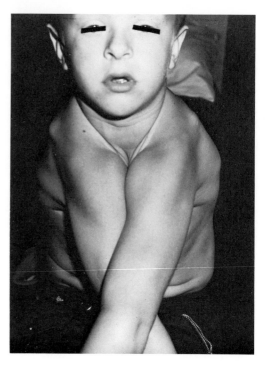

Fig. 23-25. Craniocleidodysostosis. Same patient seen in Figure 23-24.

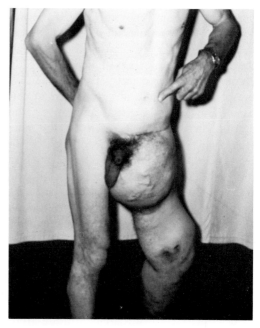

Fig. 23-26. Diaphyseal aclasis. (Courtesy of Dr. J. Adams.)

378

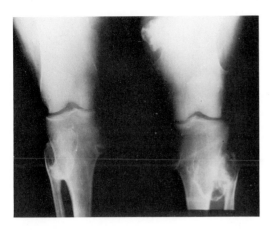

Fig. 23-27. Radiograph of region of knee of patient seen in Figure 23-26.

tion. Decompression of the skull by craniectomy, leaving the dura mater intact, may be required.

PLAGIOCEPHALY. The head is asymmetrical, possibly because of irregular fusion of the cranial bones. It may be caused by excessive pressure on one part of the developing skull in utero; however, it is not caused by the molding that normally occurs during labor. The child develops perfectly normally, but the irregular shape of the skull persists (Fig. 23-30).

Fig. 23-28. Posterior and lateral views of an anencephalic baby with an open vertebral canal, a condition known as craniorachischisis.

Vertebral Column

KLIPPEL-FEIL SYNDROME. This consists of fusion and shortening of cervical vertebrae so that the head appears to rest on the shoulders.

SCOLIOSIS. This condition is the result of a congenital *hemivertebra,* and if it occurs in the thoracic region, it is often associated with abnormalities of the ribs, such as aplasia or fusion of adjacent ribs. A hemivertebra is caused by a failure in development of one of the two ossification centers that appear in the centrum of the body of each vertebra (Figs. 23-31 & 23-32). When both centers of ossification in the centrum fail to develop adequately, *kyphosis* often occurs.

SPINA BIFIDA OCCULTA. In this condition the neural arch of one or more adjacent vertebrae fails to develop and meet in the midline (Fig. 23-33). The lumbar and sacral vertebrae are the most common sites, but the etiology is unknown. The condition is described in detail in Chapter 19.

SPONDYLOLISTHESIS. In this condition, the body of a lower lumbar vertebra, usually the fifth, moves anteriorly on the body of the vertebra below and carries with it the whole of the upper portion of the vertebral column. The essential defect is in the pedicles of the

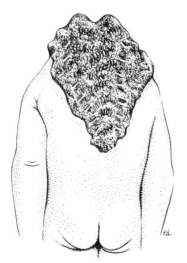

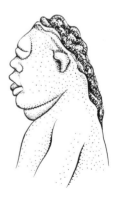

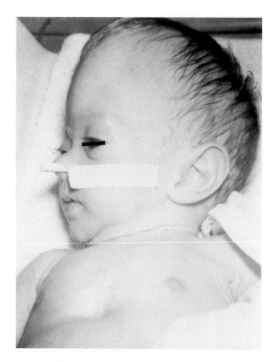

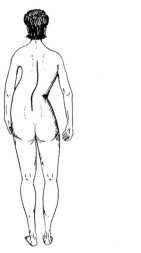

Fig. 23-31. A posterior view of a case of scoliosis resulting from a congenital hemivertebra in the lower thoracic region.

Fig. 23-29. A case of craniosynostosis caused by the premature fusion of the coronal suture of the skull. The parietal and frontal bones become pushed upward in this condition so that the skull becomes turret-shaped. (Courtesy of Dr. G. Avery.)

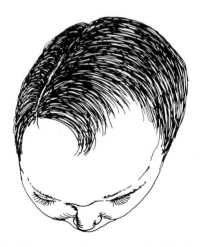

Fig. 23-30. A case of plagiocephaly. The head is asymmetrical because of irregular fusion of the cranial bones.

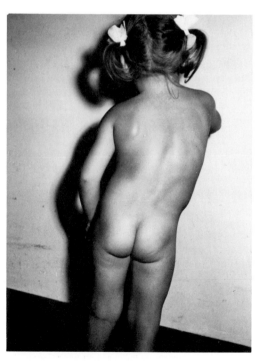

Fig. 23-32. Congenital hemivertebra in an otherwise normal child. (Courtesy of Dr. J. Adams.)

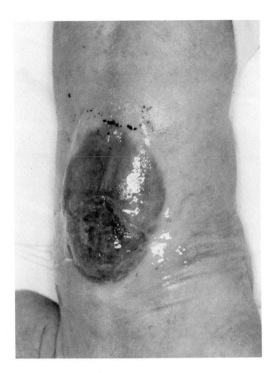

Fig. 23-33. Spina bifida. A case of thoracolumbar rachischisis. (Courtesy of Dr. L. Thompson.)

migrating vertebra (Figs. 23-34 & 23-35). It is now generally believed that the pedicles are abnormally formed in this condition and accessory centers of ossification are present that fail to unite. The spine, lamina, and inferior articular processes remain in position, while the remainder of the vertebra, having lost the restraining influence of the inferior articular processes, slips forward. Since the lamina is left behind, the vertebral canal is not narrowed, but the nerve roots may be pressed upon, causing low back ache and sciatica. In severe cases, the trunk becomes shortened and the lower ribs contact the pelvic brim. The treatment for mild cases is resting and wearing a strong lumbosacral corset. In the most severe forms, surgical lumbosacral fusion is necessary.

Thoracic Cage

Supernumerary Ribs

CERVICAL RIB. Usually an extra rib is attached to the seventh cervical vertebra (Fig.

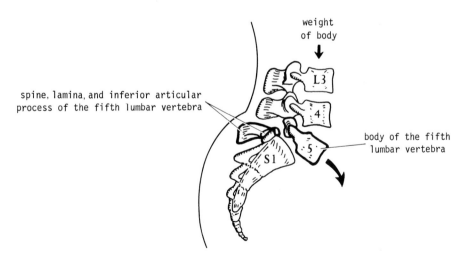

Fig. 23-34. The mechanics of spondylolisthesis involving the fifth lumbar vertebra. Shown also is a defect in the pedicles of this vertebra, allowing the vertebral body to move anteriorly and inferiorly, carrying with it the whole of the upper portion of the vertebral column.

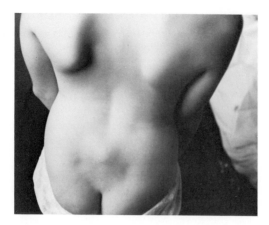

Fig. 23-35. Spondylolisthesis. Note the prominent spinous process of the fifth lumbar vertebra. (Courtesy of Dr. J. Adams.)

23-36). It may be unilateral or bilateral. Four varieties of cervical rib are recognized.

1. A *complete rib* articulating anteriorly with the manubrium or the first rib.
2. An *incomplete rib* with an expanded end.
3. An *incomplete rib* tapering off to a point that is connected by a fibrous band to the first rib.
4. A *fibrous band* extending from the seventh cervical vertebra forward to the first rib.

The majority of cervical ribs cause no symptoms. The brachial plexus and the subclavian artery have to pass over a cervical rib and in some cases pressure on these structures may give rise to pain down the arm, and there may be evidence of muscular atrophy. Removal of the rib or fibrous band is the treatment of choice.

LUMBAR RIBS. The costal processes of the first lumbar vertebra occasionally become ex-

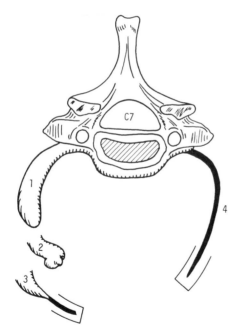

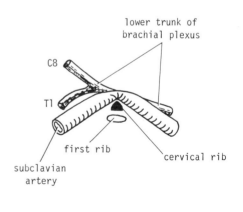

Fig. 23-36. Four types of cervical rib: (1) an almost complete rib that may articulate with the first rib or manubrium sterni, (2) an incomplete rib with an expanded end, (3) an incomplete rib connected by a fibrous band to the first rib, and (4) a fibrous band connecting the seventh cervical vertebra with the first rib. The presence of a cervical rib or fibrous band could cause kinking of the subclavian artery and pressure on the lower trunk of the brachial plexus.

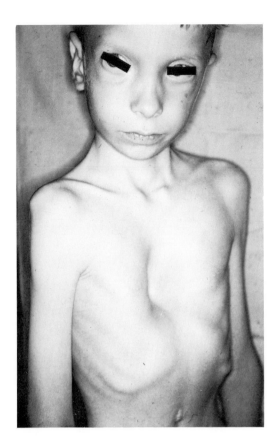

Fig. 23-37. Funnel chest. (Courtesy of Dr. J. Randolph.)

cessively large and form small additional ribs. They are symptomless and recognized by chance on a routine x-ray examination.

PIGEON CHEST. The sternum protrudes forward as a result of congenital overgrowth of the ribs or as the result of right ventricular enlargement in congenital heart disease.

FUNNEL CHEST. This is thought by some authorities to be caused by a congenital defect of the diaphragm, which has a small central tendon (Fig. 23-37). The diaphragm pulls excessively upon the lower end of the sternum, which gradually becomes depressed.

Sternum

Cleft sternum and *perforated sternum* rarely occur and are caused by incomplete fusion of the sternal plates of cartilage in the midline (Fig. 23-38). Since the process of fusion commences at the cephalic end, it is not surprising to find that *notching of the xiphoid* is the commonest anomaly.

Appendicular Skeleton

AMELIA. Absence of one or more limbs, or partial absence (*ectromelia*), may occur (Fig. 23-39). A defective limb may possess a rudimentary hand or foot at the extremity, or a well-developed hand may spring from the shoulder with absence of the intermediate portion of the limb (*phocomelia*) (Fig. 23-40). Between 1960 and 1962, as a result of the use of thalidomide during pregnancy, a large number of these deformities occurred in Western Germany and Britain (see Chap. 26).

CONGENITAL ELEVATION OF THE SCAPULA (SPRENGEL'S SHOULDER). One or both scapulae are smaller than normal and situated at a higher level (Fig. 23-41). There may be a fibrous connection with the vertebral column. The shoulder joint can be abducted to a right angle, but the arm cannot be raised further because of fixation of the scapula. Usually little disability is experienced in this condition. Occasionally the disorder is associated with the Klippel-Feil syndrome.

CONGENITAL ABSENCE OF THE RADIUS. This occasionally occurs and the growth of the ulna pushes the hand laterally (Fig. 23-42).

CONGENITAL CONTRACTURE OF THE LITTLE FINGER. There is hyperextension of the metacarpophalangeal joint and flexion at the proximal interphalangeal joint. The condition is usually bilateral and without symptoms.

TRIGGER THUMB AND FINGER. This is a localized stenosis of the tendon sheath that produces flexion deformity of the thumb or finger. The digit may be extended suddenly by passive pressure. Surgical incision of the area of stenosis corrects the deformity.

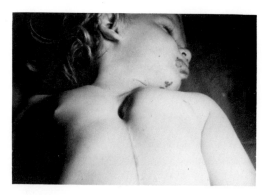

Fig. 23-38. Cleft sternum. (Courtesy of Dr. J. Randolph.)

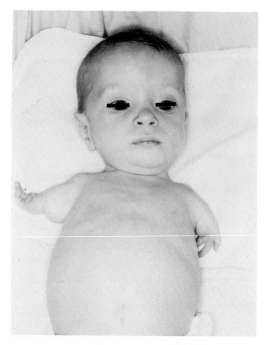

Fig. 23-40. Phocomelia. (Courtesy of Dr. G. Avery.)

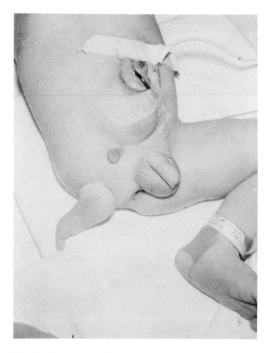

Fig. 23-39. Ectromelia. (Courtesy of Dr. G. Avery.)

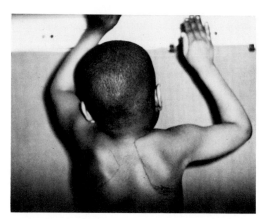

Fig. 23-41. Right-sided Sprengel's shoulder. (Courtesy of Dr. J. Adams.)

SYNDACTYLY. There is webbing of the fingers or toes. It is usually bilateral and often familial (Figs. 23-43 & 23-44). Plastic repair of the fingers is carried out at the age of 5 years. It is unnecessary to treat webbing of the toes.

LOBSTER HAND. This is a form of syndactyly that is associated with a central cleft dividing the hand into two parts (Fig. 23-45). Occasionally this condition occurs in the foot (Fig. 23-46). This is a heredofamilial disorder. Plastic surgery is indicated where possible.

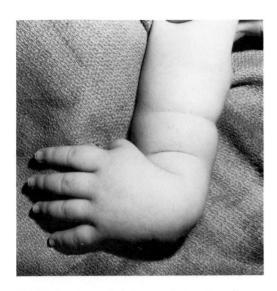

Fig. 23-42. Congenital absence of the radius. (Courtesy of Dr. J. Adams.)

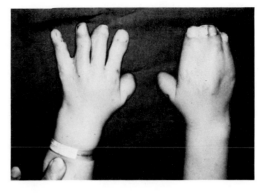

Fig. 23-44. Syndactyly of the right hand. (Courtesy of Dr. L. Thompson.)

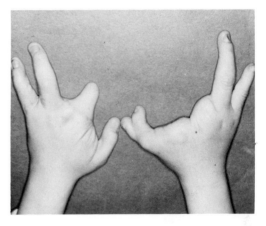

Fig. 23-45. Lobster hand. (Courtesy of Dr. L. Thompson.)

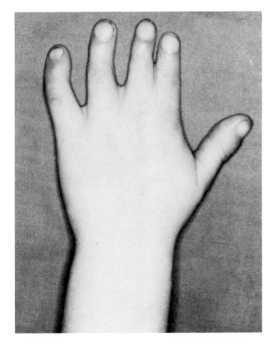

Fig. 23-43. Partial syndactyly. (Courtesy of Dr. L. Thompson.)

BRACHYDACTYLY. In this condition there is an absence of one or more phalanges in several fingers. Provided that the thumb is functioning normally, surgery is not indicated (Fig. 23-47).

FLOATING THUMB. The metacarpal bone of the thumb is absent but the phalanges are present. Plastic surgery is indicated where possible in order to improve the functional capabilities of the hand (Fig. 23-48).

POLYDACTYLY. In this condition one or more extra digits are developed (Figs. 23-49 & 23-50). It is very common in Africans and

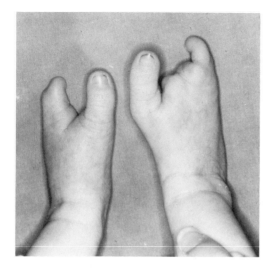

Fig. 23-46. Lobster foot. (Courtesy of Dr. L. Thompson.)

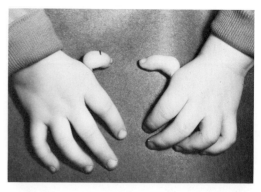

Fig. 23-48. Floating thumb. The metacarpal bone of the thumb is absent, but the phalanges are present. (Courtesy of Dr. R. Chase.)

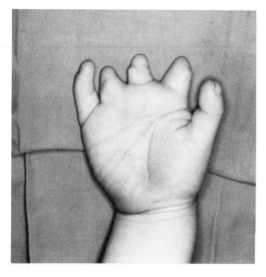

Fig. 23-47. Brachydactyly due to defects of the phalanges. (Courtesy of Dr. L. Thompson.)

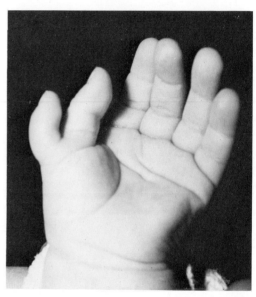

Fig. 23-49. Polydactyly of the left hand. (Courtesy of Dr. R. Chase.)

tends to run in families. The additional digits are removed surgically.

LOCAL GIGANTISM. Macrodactyly affects one or more digits; these may be of adult size at birth, but the size usually diminishes with age (Figs. 23-51 & 23-52). Surgical removal may be necessary.

CONGENITAL DISLOCATION OF THE HIP. This condition is ten times more common in female children than in male children, and it is particularly common in northern Italy (Figs. 23-53 & 23-54). Three possible causes have been suggested: (1) Generalized joint laxity; excessive laxity of the ligaments of the hip joint may predispose to this condition. (2) Breech position; the flexed hip and extended

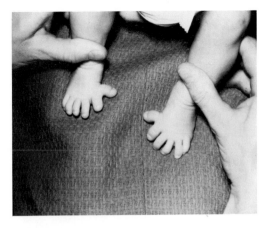

Fig. 23-50. Bilateral polydactyly of the feet. (Courtesy of Dr. L. Thompson.)

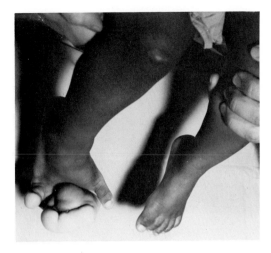

Fig. 23-52. Macrosyndactyly of the second, third, and fourth toes. (Courtesy of Dr. J. Adams.)

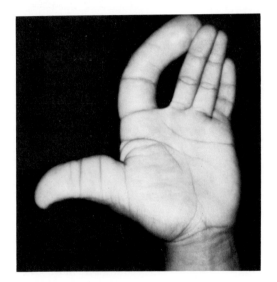

Fig. 23-51. Macrodactyly affecting the thumb and index finger. (Courtesy of Dr. R. Neviaser.)

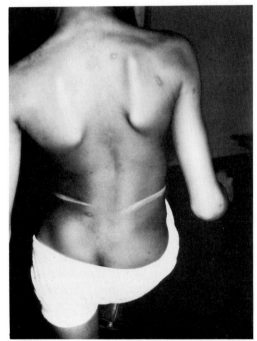

knees of the breech position may alter the normal pressure of the head of the femur on the acetabulum, and this may result in a failure of the upper part of the acetabulum to develop adequately. (3) Shallow acetabulum; the acetabulum is poorly developed, and the upper lip offers an insufficient shelf under which the head of the femur can lodge. The

Fig. 23-53. A patient with left-sided congenital dislocation of the hip. The chalk marks show that the right iliac crest did not rise when the patient stood on the left leg, indicating that the left hip joint was unstable; positive Trendelenberg's sign. (Courtesy of Dr. J. Adams.)

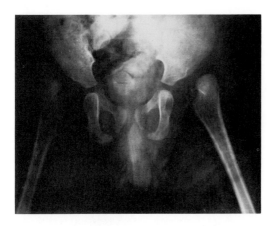

Fig. 23-54. Radiograph of bilateral congenital dislocation of the hip. The femoral heads are not within the shallow acetabular fossae. (Courtesy of Dr. J. Adams.)

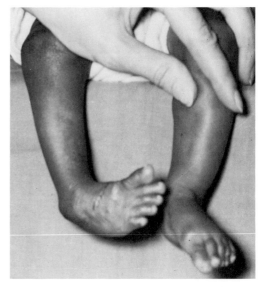

Fig. 23-55. Talipes equinovarus. (Courtesy of Dr. J. Adams.)

condition of shallow acetabulum tends to run in families. The condition should be diagnosed at birth and is treated by splinting the joint in the position of abduction.

GENU RECURVATUM. The knee joint is hyperextended. This condition is found in babies who have had a breech presentation with extended legs. No treatment is required, as the legs return to normal within a few weeks.

TALIPES. Clubfoot is often caused by abnormal position or restricted movement of the fetus in utero. A small number may be caused by muscle paralysis associated with spina bifida. The different types are named according to the position of the foot (Fig. 23-55). *Talipes calcaneovalgus* is a form of clubfoot in which the foot is dorsiflexed at the ankle joint and everted at the midtarsal joints. In *talipes equinovarus* the foot is plantar-flexed at the ankle joint and inverted at the midtarsal joints. The conditions may

be unilateral or bilateral, and they require orthopedic treatment.

METATARSUS VARUS. This is a common condition in which the forefoot is adducted on the rear part of the foot. Correction may be accomplished by manipulation and setting in plaster.

OVERRIDING TOES. This most commonly involves the fourth and fifth toes. The fourth toe is depressed and overridden by the fifth toe. This may be corrected by the application of plaster splints.

CURLY TOES. This condition most often affects the fourth and fifth toes, and commonly runs in families. The affected toe lies flexed under its medial neighbor. In mild cases there is no treatment; in severe cases the flexor digitorum longus tendon is transplanted into the extensor tendon.

Clinical Problems
Answers on page 454

1. A 6-year-old boy was taken to a pediatrician because his parents had noticed that he tended to hold his head to one side. On physical examination the child was found to hold his head so that his right ear approached the right sternoclavicular joint and the chin was rotated toward the left side. Examination of the neck revealed a shortening of the right sternocleidomastoid muscle. The face was seen to be normal. On questioning, the mother stated that she had noticed a small elongated swelling on the lower part of the neck on the right side soon after birth and that the child cried bitterly when it was touched. The swelling and tenderness disappeared after 6 months. What is the diagnosis? What is the probable cause of this condition? What was responsible for the swelling in the neck seen after birth? What happens to the face if this condition is untreated?

2. Following a normal delivery, a male child was seen to hold his arms in a position of medial rotation at the shoulder joints and his thighs in a position of lateral rotation at the hip joints. The wrists and fingers were flexed and clubfeet were present. On physical examination the joints of the limbs were noted to be rigid, but a small amount of active and passive movement was possible. The muscles around the joints appeared to be poorly developed. The child also had a cleft palate. What is your diagnosis?

3. A medical student was asked to examine a 5-year-old boy in the outpatient clinic. The first thing that he noticed was that the child's head appeared to be larger than normal. He had a prominent forehead, and yet the center of the face seemed to be relatively undeveloped, so that there was flattening of the bridge of the nose and a prominent chin. The trunk was of normal size for a 5-year-old, but the limbs were very short. The anterior abdominal wall tended to protrude and the buttocks were prominent. The skin of the thighs was thrown into folds. When asked to walk, the boy did so with a waddling gait. The child responded to questions promptly and seemed to be very intelligent. Radiological examination of the limbs revealed that the long bones were broad and short and were much broader at their ends than normal. The epiphyses showed some irregularities, but the calcification was normal. What is your diagnosis? Is this disease hereditary?

4. A 1-year-old girl was examined by a pediatrician because of multiple deformities. The mother said that at birth the baby was stunted and had a fracture of the right humerus and left femur. After the limbs had been splinted, the fractures readily united. Since that time, the left radius had been fractured when the father was holding the child in his arms while giving her a bottle of milk. On physical examination the child was observed to have blue scleras and had multiple deformities of both upper and lower limbs and chest wall, due to old fractures. Examination of the skull revealed wide membranous spaces between the bones. Radiological examination showed that the fractured bones were curved or angulated. The unbroken bones showed diffuse osteoporosis, and the long bones were unduly thin. The epiphyses and diaphyses were

normal. The skull bones were thin and osteoporotic. What is the diagnosis? What is the prognosis?

5. A routine physical examination of a 6-year-old girl showed a complete absence of both clavicles. It was possible for the child to approximate the tips of her shoulders to each other below her chin. Neither trapezius muscle had clavicular fibers. Examination of the skull showed an abnormally large transverse diameter of the cranium, so that the whole skull looked globular in shape. Examination of the mother showed that she had exactly the same condition. What is your diagnosis? Is any treatment necessary?

6. A 28-year-old man was examined by a physician because he had noticed hard swellings in the region of both knees. On questioning, the patient said that he had first noticed the swellings when he was about 10 years old and since that time they had gradually increased in size and were now interfering with the movements of his knee joints. Physical examination revealed the presence of hard swellings projecting from the posteromedial aspect of both fibulae just below their heads. The skin overlying the swellings was normal and the subcutaneous tissues moved freely over them. Each swelling measured about half an inch (1.25 cm) in diameter. The swellings were clearly pressing on the tendon of the biceps femoris muscle on each side but were not pressing on the common peronial nerves. Radiological examination showed the presence of large spurs of bone, originating from the metaphysis and growing distally away from the epiphysis, at the upper end of the shaft of the fibula on each side. What is the diagnosis? How would you treat this disease?

7. A 4-year-old boy was taken to a pediatrician because the parents were concerned about the shortness of his neck. On physical examination the child was observed to have limitation of all movements of the cervical spine. The neck looked very short and the head appeared to rest directly on the shoulders. The hairline at the back of the head extended onto the back. Radiography of the cervical spine showed gross structural irregularities of the cervical vertebrae. Only four vertebrae could be counted, and three of these appeared to be fused together. Apart from these findings the child was perfectly normal. What is your diagnosis? How would you treat this patient?

8. A 9-year-old girl was taken to a pediatrician because her mother was concerned about a lateral curvature of the child's spine, which she had noted since the child was 5 months old. The girl was otherwise perfectly healthy and active. On physical examination both legs were found to be of equal length. With the patient in the standing position, the height of the iliac crests was equal on the two sides, but the left shoulder was lower than the right. Examination of the vertebral column revealed an obvious sharp curve in the midthoracic region convex to the right with gentle compensatory curves above and below this region with convexities to the left. On flexion of the vertebral column the area of the sharp curve was noted to be rigid. Anteroposterior radiographic examination of the midthoracic region revealed a wedge-shaped vertebra at the T5 level with fusion of the left fifth and sixth ribs. What is your diagnosis? How would you explain this condition embryologically? How would you treat this case?

9. A 30-year-old man visited his physician complaining of low back pain, which he had experienced for the past year. Recently the pain had become worse. On physical examination, the patient was seen to have a severe lumbar lordosis, with

excessive prominence of the first sacral spine. A prominent fold of skin was seen on either side above the iliac crests, and the last ribs appeared to rest on the iliac crests. What is the diagnosis? What are the underlying embryological reasons for the condition?

10. A 40-year-old woman visited an orthopedic surgeon because she had experienced a dull-aching pain and a sensation of "pins and needles" down the inner side of her right forearm and hand. The symptoms had started two years previously and they were getting more severe. The condition became worse at the end of the day when she was tired. She also stated that she was having difficulty in carrying out finer movements of her fingers, such as those involved in buttoning up her coat. On physical examination of the patient it was found that the pain and paresthesia was felt in the C8 and T1 dermatomes on the medial side of the right forearm and hand. Examination of the right hand showed flattening of the thenar eminence and wasting of the interosseous muscles. The abductor pollicis, opponens pollicis, and interossei were weak. On laterally flexing the neck to the left and depressing the right shoulder, the right radial pulse could be made to disappear. What congenital anomaly in the neck could cause these symptoms and signs? What is the embryological explanation for this condition? How would you treat this patient?

11. A 7-year-old girl was examined by a pediatrician because of a deformity on the front of the chest. On physical examination the patient was found to be round-shouldered and hollow-chested. The manubrium sterni was in a normal position, but the body of the sternum and xiphoid process were depressed. The apex beat of the heart was deviated over to the left. The patient had had this condition since birth. She had no symptoms. What is the

diagnosis? What is the possible embryological cause for this deforming condition? How would you treat this patient?

12. In Britain in 1961 a pregnant woman went to her obstetrician complaining of excessive morning sickness. The patient was assured that the symptoms were limited to the early months of pregnancy and that she would soon feel much better. Two weeks later the patient returned and asked if she could take something to stop the sickness. Because she seemed to be upset and worried, the physician decided to give her thalidomide, a mild hypnotic. This drug worked satisfactorily and the patient went to term without further problems. After a normal delivery the obstetrician was horrified to find that the male child had been born without arms and legs. What is this condition called? Is there any connection between the drug administered for the control of morning sickness and the terrible congenital anomalies?

13. A 7-year-old boy was taken to a pediatrician because he was unable to raise his right arm above a right angle with the body. Although he suffered some inconvenience from this, his mother said he never complained. On physical examination it was noted that the boy held his head slightly laterally flexed to the right. The movements of his left arm and shoulder were normal. The right scapula was higher than the left, and the inferior angle pointed medially. Examination of the neck revealed a bar of bone running from the midcervical region of the vertebral column down to the superior angle of the right scapula. Examination of the right arm confirmed that he was unable to raise it above 90 degrees, and the scapula was fixed and failed to rotate in the normal manner. The boy also had a mild scoliosis. What is your diagnosis? Why

is the right scapula higher up than normal in this case?

14. A 10-year-old boy was seen by an orthopedic surgeon because he had "club hands." On examination the arms were noted to be thinner than normal and the forearms were short and stubby and had a posterior convexity. The hands were small and were deviated laterally. The ulna was present on both sides, but the radius could not be identified. The fingers were small and could grasp objects quite well. The mother said he had had this condition since birth. What is your diagnosis?

15. A mother noticed that her 6-month-old boy tended to hold his right thumb within the palm and never seemed to straighten it. On physical examination the baby could only extend the right thumb partially. By gently grasping the distal and proximal phalanges, the thumb could be passively extended, and it did so with a faint snap. On palpation a small nodule could be felt in front of the head of the first metacarpal bone in the tendon of the flexor pollicis longus muscle. What is your diagnosis? How would you treat this patient?

16. A 12-year-old boy was taken to a plastic surgeon because he had very large little and ring fingers on his right hand. On questioning, the mother said his fingers had been very large at birth, almost of adult size. The boy was otherwise perfectly normal. On examination the little and ring fingers were seen to be greatly enlarged on the right hand. The fingers were also curved laterally. The temperature of the skin and the skin sensations were normal over the affected fingers. The enlargement appeared to be confined to the distribution of the ulnar nerve. What is your diagnosis? What are the common causes of enlargement of the digits?

17. A 15-year-old girl was taken to an orthopedic surgeon because of her peculiar "duck-like" walk. When she was asked to walk away from the surgeon, it was noted that she lurched over to the right side. She had a distinct lordosis of her lumbar spine, and when asked to stand on her right leg with her left leg off the ground, the left side of her pelvis dropped. Measurement of her legs showed that her right leg was shorter than her left leg. Radiographic examination of the right hip joint showed that the right femur was displaced laterally and upward. The right femoral head was situated lateral to the dorsum of the ilium. What is your diagnosis?

18. A senior medical student was asked to examine a 1-week-old baby boy who had "something wrong with his feet." Examination revealed that both feet were plantar-flexed at the ankles and the foreparts of the feet were adducted and inverted at the talonavicular joints. The baby was otherwise perfectly normal. What is your diagnosis? How would you treat this patient?

REFERENCES

Aegerter, E., and Kirkpatrick, J. A. *Orthopedic Diseases,* 3d ed. Saunders, Philadelphia, 1968.

Arey, L. B. *Developmental Anatomy,* 7th ed. Saunders, Philadelphia, 1965.

Bardeen, C. R. The Development of the Thoracic Vertebrae in Man. *Amer. J. Anat.* 4:163, 1905.

Bardeen, C. R., and Lewis, W. H. The Development of the Limbs, Body Wall, and Back. *Amer. J. Anat.* 1:1, 1901.

Boyd, J. D. Development of Striated Muscle. In *Structure and Function of Muscle,* edited by G. H. Bourne. Academic, New York, 1960. Vol. 1.

Carlson, E. C., and Low, F. N. The Effect of Hydrocortisone on Extracellular Connective Tissue Fibrils in the Early Chick Embryo. *Amer. J. Anat.* 130:331, 1971.

Cuajunco, F. Development of the Neuro-Muscular Spindle in Human Fetuses. *Contrib. Embryol.* 28:97, 1940.

Dankmeijer, J. Congenital Absence of the Tibia. *Anat. Rec.* 62:179, 1935.

DeBeer, G. R. *The Development of the Vertebrate Skull.* Oxford University Press, London, 1937.

Devitt, R. E. F., and Kenny, S. Thalidomide and Congenital Abnormalities. *Lancet* 1:430, 1962.

Fitzgerald, J. E., and Windle, W. F. Some Observations on Early Human Fetal Movements. *J. Comp. Neurol.* 76:159, 1942.

Gardner, E. Osteogenesis in the Human Embryo and Fetus. In *The Biochemistry and Physiology of Bone,* edited by G. H. Bourne. Academic, New York, 1956.

Gardner, E. D., and Gray, D. J. Prenatal Development of the Human Hip Joint. *Amer. J. Anat.* 87:163, 1950.

Gilbert, P. W. The Origin and Development of the Human Extrinsic Ocular Muscles. *Contrib. Embryol.* 36:59, 1957.

Haines, R. W. The Development of Joints. *J. Anat.* 81:33, 1947.

Hamilton, W. J., Boyd, J. D., and Mossman, H. W. *Human Embryology,* 3d ed. Williams & Wilkins, Baltimore, 1962.

Hay, E. D. Organization and Fine Structure of Epithelium and Mesenchyme in the Developing Chick Embryo. In *Epithelial-Mesenchymal Interactions,* edited by R. Fleischmajer. Williams & Wilkins, Baltimore, 1968.

Ingalls, T. H. Epiphyseal Growth: Normal Sequence of Events at the Epiphyseal Plate. *Endocrinology* 29:710, 1941.

Jolly, H. *Diseases of Children,* 2d ed. Davis, Philadelphia, 1968.

Leblond, C. P., and Greulich, R. C. Autoradiographic Studies of Bone Formation and Growth. In *The Biochemistry and Physiology of Bone,* edited by G. H. Bourne. Academic, New York, 1956.

Lenz, W. Thalidomide and Congenital Abnormalities. *Lancet* 1:1219, 1962.

Lewis, W. H. The Development of the Arm in Man. *Amer. J. Anat.* 1:145, 1902.

Lewis, W. H. The Cartilaginous Skull of a Human Embryo 21 mm in Length. *Contrib. Embryol.* 9:299, 1920.

Noback, C. R. The Developmental Anatomy of the Human Osseous Skeleton During the Embryonic, Fetal and Circumnatal Periods. *Anat. Rec.* 88:91, 1944.

Patten, B. *Human Embryology,* 3d ed. McGraw-Hill, New York, 1968.

Peacock, A. Observations on the Prenatal Development of the Intervertebral Disc in Man. *J. Anat.* 85:260, 1951.

Ruth, E. B. A Study of the Development of the Mammalian Pelvis. *Anat. Rec.* 53:207, 1932.

Sensenig, E. C. The Early Development of the Human Vertebral Column. *Contrib. Embryol.* 33:21, 1949.

Sissons, H. A. The Growth of Bone. In *Biochemistry and Physiology of Bone,* edited by G. H. Bourne. Academic, New York, 1956.

Vickers, T. H. Congenital Abnormalities and Thalidomide. *Med. J. Aust.* 1:649, 1962.

Well, L. J. Development of the Human Diaphragm and Pleural Sacs. *Contrib. Embryol.* 35:107, 1954.

The series of processes by which the baby, the fetal membranes, and the placenta are expelled from the genital tract of the mother is known as *labor,* or *parturition.* Normally labor takes place at the end of the tenth lunar month, at which time the pregnancy is said to be at *term.*

ATTITUDE, LIE, AND PRESENTING PART OF THE FETUS AT TERM

Toward the end of pregnancy the fetus is curved and folded upon itself and occupies the smallest possible space within the uterine cavity. The usual *attitude* is one of flexion, with the back flexed, the head bent forward, the arms crossed on the chest, the thighs flexed on the abdomen, and the knees bent. The umbilical cord lies between the upper and lower limbs. The fetus commonly changes its position during the early months of pregnancy, but during the tenth month it becomes more or less stationary. The *lie* of the fetus is then usually such that its long axis is parallel with the long axis of the uterus. Occasionally the body of the fetus lies transversely, a position referred to as *transverse lie.*

The part of the body which lies lowest in the uterus is called the *presenting part,* and this is most commonly the head. Sometimes the buttocks present first, and this is known as a *breech presentation.* The most common attitude, lie, and presentation of the fetus are shown in Figure 24-1.

POSITION OF THE UTERUS AT TERM

As the fetus enlarges and the uterus increases in size, the fundus gradually rises out of the pelvic cavity (Fig. 24-2). The ascent of the fundus is fairly uniform. At the fourth month, it lies just above the symphysis pubis; at the fifth month about halfway between the symphysis and the umbilicus; at the sixth month it is on a level with the umbilicus; at the eighth month it lies halfway between the umbilicus and the xiphoid process; at nine months it has reached the xiphoid process; and at ten months, in the first pregnancy, the fetus sinks downward as the presenting part enters the pelvic cavity and the fundus again takes up the position halfway between the xiphoid and the umbilicus (Fig. 24-3). In mothers who have had multiple pregnancies, the presenting part of the fetus descends at a later date. At term, the uterus is a large, thin-walled, muscular sac. The fetus

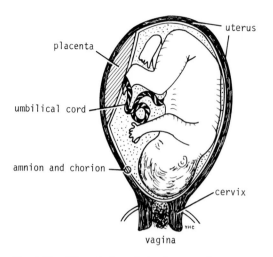

Fig. 24-1. The relation of the fetus to the uterus, placenta, and fetal membranes at the tenth month of pregnancy.

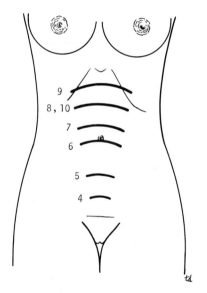

Fig. 24-2. The height of the fundus of the uterus at each month of pregnancy.

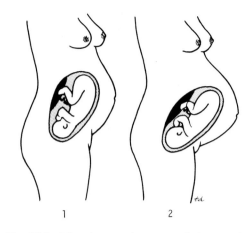

Fig. 24-3. The change of contour of the anterior abdominal wall that takes place after the fetal head has descended into the pelvis at the tenth month of pregnancy.

DATE OF DELIVERY

The actual birth of the child is called *delivery*. The approximate date of delivery may be estimated by counting forward 280 days from the first day of the last menstrual period. Practically, a simpler method is used: 7 days are added to the date of onset of the last period and 3 months are then subtracted. For example, if the last period began on July 10th, the addition of seven days gives July 17th; counting back 3 months indicates April 17th as the approximate date on which delivery may be expected. This method is accurate to within 10 days before or after the estimated date in the majority of deliveries. It is assumed of course that the mother has a normal, regular menstrual history.

ONSET OF LABOR

The cause of the onset of labor is not definitely known. Why the uterine contractions, which have occurred painlessly, arrhythmically, and weakly throughout pregnancy should suddenly become painful, rhythmic,

and amniotic fluid are contained within the amniotic and chorionic membranes. The average fetus at term is about 20 inches long (50.8 cm) and weighs about 7½ lb. (3,500 gm).

and forceful at the onset of labor is still a matter for conjecture. The pain is almost certainly caused by the anoxia of the uterine muscle resulting from the stronger and more prolonged contractions that reduce the blood flow through the muscle. The uterine musculature in the region of the placenta remains largely inactive up to the time of birth to allow the placental circulation to function satisfactorily. It is known that in animals the local injection of progesterone into the uterine muscle decreases its spontaneous activity. It has also been established that in the human subject there is a rising production of progesterone from the placenta after the fourth month of pregnancy, and it is probable that progesterone exerts a local inhibitory action on the uterine muscle cells near the placenta. Accompanying this local action of progesterone, the uterine muscle away from the placental site gradually hypertrophies, probably in response to a rise in estrogen influence. It has been shown in the rabbit, for example, that estrogen is capable of causing hypertrophy of the uterine muscle in preparation for parturition. By the end of pregnancy the contractility of the uterus has been fully developed in response to estrogen, and at this time it is particularly sensitive to the actions of *oxytocin*. In women the onset of labor does not appear to be caused by a great change in the blood levels of either estrogen or progesterone. In some laboratory animals the onset of parturition can be delayed by giving large injections of progesterone. It is possible that the onset of labor in the human subject can be attributed to a sudden withdrawal of progesterone or one of its metabolites, too small in amount to be detected by present biochemical techniques.

It is interesting to note that uterine muscular activity is largely independent of the extrinsic innervation. In animals, normal parturition may take place following sympathectomy or section of the spinal cord. In women in labor, spinal anesthesia does not interfere with the normal uterine contractions. However, it is known that severe emotional disturbances may cause premature parturition.

LABOR

Forceful uterine contractions occurring at regular intervals indicate the onset of labor. The process of labor is divided into three stages: The *first stage*, or *stage of dilatation*, begins with the onset of regular, forceful uterine contractions and ends with complete dilatation of the cervix. The *second stage*, or *stage of expulsion*, begins with the complete dilatation of the cervix and ends with complete delivery of the baby. The *third stage*, or *placental stage*, begins immediately following the delivery of the baby and ends with the expulsion of the placenta and fetal membranes.

Duration of Labor

This depends on (1) the strength and frequency of the uterine contractions and (2) the resistance offered to the passage of the baby by the bony pelvis and the soft tissues of the lower part of the genital tract, namely the cervix, the vagina, the pelvic floor, and the perineum. The approximate length of each stage in the primigravida is as follows: first stage 9½ hours, second stage 50 minutes, and third stage 10 minutes. In the multigravida the duration of the first and second stages is shorter because of the reduced resistance offered by the maternal soft tissues.

The Processes of Labor

During the first stage of labor, the liquor amnii and the fetal membranes are forced down into the cervical canal as a hydrostatic wedge, and the cervix slowly dilates (Fig. 24-4). The pulling away of the membranes from

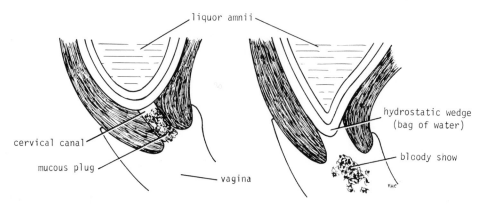

Fig. 24-4. The cervix dilating during the first stage of labor as the result of the fetal membranes being forced down into the cervical canal as a hydrostatic wedge.

the uterine wall in the region of the internal os of the cervix causes a little bleeding, and this, together with the cervical plug of mucus, forms the so-called *bloody show*. The rupture of the membranes and the escape of the liquor amnii usually occur when the first stage of labor is well advanced. The escape of the liquor amnii allows the uterus to exert pressure directly on the baby and force it down. During the second stage of labor, the combined actions of the now very strong uterine contractions and the reflex and voluntary contractions of the abdominal muscles force the baby through the maternal passages (Fig. 24-5).

After birth of the child, the pulsations in the exposed umbilical cord cease within a few minutes. The cord is tied with a ligature and divided, and thus the baby is separated from the mother.

The third stage of labor now commences, and the uterus contracts downward so that the fundus lies at the level of the umbilicus. Rhythmic uterine contractions continue, as in the second stage, but they are painless. Separation of the placenta from the uterine wall now takes place. As the uterus diminishes in size, there is a decrease in the surface area at the site of placental attachment. The placenta, being unable to accommodate itself to the decreased area, begins to fold up and is

squeezed off the uterine wall (Fig. 24-6). Separation takes place at the spongy layer of the decidua basalis, and some bleeding occurs. In a similar manner the fetal membranes and the remains of the decidua parietalis are squeezed from the remainder of the uterine wall. As the placenta is finally expelled from the uterus by the uterine contractions, the membranes that are attached to it are dragged after it and peeled off from the inner surface of the uterus. The expelled placenta and fetal membranes are often referred to as the *afterbirth*. The uterine muscle now becomes firmly contracted and little bleeding occurs.

THE PUERPERIUM

This is the period from the end of labor until the mother returns to her prepregnant physiological state, and it usually lasts from 6 to 8 weeks. For about 3 weeks after birth, a discharge occurs from the genital tract of the mother. This is known as the *lochia,* and at first it is bright red and consists of blood and decidual remains; later this becomes brown, and then yellow, and finally it stops. Meanwhile the denuded walls of the uterine cavity become lined with endometrium within 2 to 3 weeks after delivery. This occurs as a result

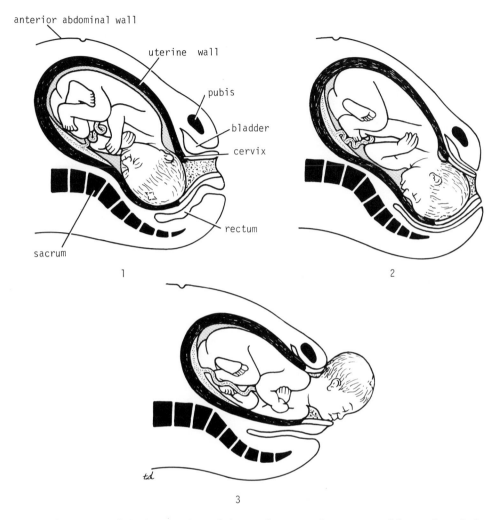

Fig. 24-5. The position of the fetal head in relation to the maternal passages at different times during the second stage of labor.

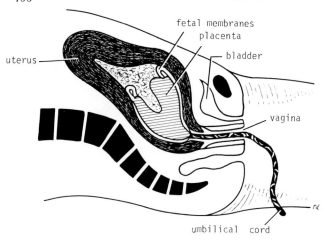

Fig. 24-6. The third stage of labor showing the separated placenta with the attached fetal membranes about to be expelled through the vagina.

of the proliferation of the cells of the glands and stroma of the remains of the decidua basalis. The placental site requires a longer time for repair, which should be complete in from 6 to 8 weeks. The uterine muscle undergoes rapid involution, but it never completely regains its pregravid state. The shrinkage of the uterine muscle is caused chiefly by autolysis of the muscle fibers, and the end products are removed by the bloodstream. Menstruation will generally occur 6 to 8 weeks after parturition, but it may be delayed several months in mothers who breast-feed their babies.

Clinical Problems
Answers on page 457

1. A fourth-year medical student was asked to define the following terms: (a) labor, (b) attitude of the fetus, (c) transverse lie, (d) presenting part. How would you define them?
2. A 30-year-old pregnant woman expecting her first child attended a prenatal clinic for a routine checkup. On physical examination the fundus of the uterus was found to lie at the level of the xiphoid process. Can you use this information to determine approximately the period of gestation?
3. After completing his physical examination, the obstetrician told the patient she was pregnant. The patient then asked him the date of the expected time of delivery. Given that the day of onset of her last period was November 10 and that prior to that time she had had a history of normal regular menstrual periods, how would you answer that question?
4. A nurse specializing in midwifery was asked to discuss the possible causes of the onset of labor in a normal patient. How would you reply?
5. Define each of the three stages of labor.
6. A pregnant woman telephones you and says that she thinks her labor has started. What are the signs and symptoms of the onset of labor?
7. An obstetrician, when asked how long Mrs. N ---- had been in the second stage of labor, replied, "Three hours." Is this

normal for (a) a primigravida? (b) a multigravida?

8. What is the so-called bloody show?

9. During the third stage of labor, when the placenta is separating from the uterine wall, at which layer of the decidua basalis does separation actually take place?

10. What is the so-called afterbirth?

11. What is the lochia? Does this change in color during the puerperium?

12. A medical student was asked at an examination how long the walls of the uterine cavity remain denuded after delivery is completed? How would you answer that question?

REFERENCES

Baird, D. *Obstetrics and Gynaecology,* 8th ed. Livingstone, Edinburgh, 1969.

Huffman, J. W. *Gynecology and Obstetrics.* Saunders, Philadelphia, 1962.

GENERAL APPEARANCE OF THE NEWBORN

The newborn baby is a wonder to behold but he is not a thing of beauty. The head is large but the face and jaws are relatively small. The neck is short, the thorax is narrow, and the abdomen is prominent, mainly because of the relatively large size of the liver. The arms and legs are short and are in a position of flexion. If the presentation was a breech, the legs are flexed on the abdomen and the knees are extended. The skin is tight and rounded because of the thick layer of subcutaneous fat, and it is partly covered by a coat of cheesy *vernix caseosa*. *Lanugo hair* may still be present over the shoulders, back, and forehead. The baby is pinkish-red in color, but there may be slight cyanosis of the skin of the hands and feet. The cry of the newborn should be lusty from birth and is usually accompanied by a flexing of the arms and legs and clenching of the fists. The thumb or clenched fist quickly finds its way to the mouth, and sucking begins almost immediately following birth.

THE NEONATAL PERIOD

At the moment of birth, the baby suddenly has to make drastic physiological adjustments necessary for the change from intra-uterine to extra-uterine life. Prior to birth he was given a continuous supply of nourishment and oxygen, and waste materials were removed through the placental circulation. The liquor amnii provided a constant warm fluid environment and was a medium that allowed easy movement and protection from external injury. The extra-uterine life is dry and cold; in fact the temperature of the new environment may fluctuate considerably during each 24-hour period. The lungs suddenly have to be inflated for the purpose of obtaining oxygen and the excretion of carbon dioxide. Nourishment now comes intermittently by a new route and has to be worked for by sucking. No longer is the baby protected from pathogenic organisms and physical trauma. The first 4-week period after birth is referred to as the *neonatal period;* during this critical time of adjustment, the greatest mortality rate in childhood occurs. The first day of life is the most dangerous, more deaths occurring on that day than during the whole period from the age of 12 months to 25 years. While there has been a considerable improvement in the mortality rates for infants from 1 to 12 months of age as a result of better feeding methods and the use of antibiotics in the treatment of infection, the neonatal mortality rates still remain high. Premature births, postmature births, birth injuries, physiological failures of adjustment, and congenital anomalies are some of the problems responsible and are now the subject of intensive research.

The sudden emergence of the baby from a protective environment in which he has existed as a parasite for 10 months into a relatively hostile world where he must begin a separate existence is the subject of this chapter. The care of the child during this critical period and the understanding of the fundamental changes which are taking place within its body at this time are essential for a student of medicine.

CHANGES THAT TAKE PLACE AT BIRTH

Respiratory System

In 1964 McLain injected a radiopaque contrast medium into the amniotic fluid of 75 pregnant women and was unable to detect it within the lungs of a single fetus in utero. It is now generally accepted that rhythmic respiratory movements do not take place in the mature fetus in utero unless it is subjected to partial asphyxia or is stimulated physically.

During labor, as soon as the placental circulation ceases, the respiratory system must function to take over from the placenta the activity of gaseous exchange with the uptake of oxygen and the excretion of carbon dioxide. There would appear to be two phases in the respiratory efforts. The first phase requires considerable exertion to achieve expansion of the lungs with air. The cohesive state of the alveoli, the elastic resistance of the lungs, the movement of the thoracic cage, the descent of the diaphragm against the resistance of the abdominal viscera all have to be overcome. During this phase, the baby exhibits strong gasping efforts. The second phase is the establishment of rhythmic breathing movements.

The exact mechanism by which respiration is initiated is not precisely known. It is probable that the respiratory center in the medulla responds to the summation of a number of subliminal stimuli. During labor, the oxygen tension of the fetal blood is lowered, the carbon dioxide tension rises, and the blood becomes increasingly acidotic. The tying of the umbilical cord further accentuates this condition, and the respiratory center is stimulated through chemoreceptor reflexes from the aortic and carotid bodies. Cutaneous stimulation by the birth process and exposure to the cold air provides additional stimulation of the respiratory center. The first breath is taken normally within seconds after delivery and is brought about by a strong contraction of the diaphragm, causing an increase in volume of the thoracic cavity, resulting in air being forced into the respiratory tract. This is usually quickly followed by a lusty cry. A normal baby establishes rhythmic breathing movements within 1 minute after delivery. If the onset of breathing is delayed, the asphyxia increases, and this will ultimately depress the respiratory center. Under these circumstances, resuscitation procedures should be started immediately.

The average *respiratory rate* in the newborn is approximately forty times per minute and is regular. In the earliest stages, the ribs are nearly horizontal in position and very little movement of the thoracic cage takes place. Respiration is mainly brought about by the diaphragm, and this is accompanied by reciprocal movement of the muscles of the anterior abdominal wall. At birth the baby's skin is usually slightly cyanotic, but within a few minutes it becomes pink. However, slight circumoral cyanosis and cyanosis of the hands and feet may persist for a few hours until the peripheral circulation opens up.

It is important to realize that the lungs are not fully expanded with the first breath. Some degree of *atelectasis* may indeed be present for several days after birth. The presence of adequate amounts of *surfactant* to overcome the surface-tension forces within the alveoli, together with the presence of residual air left within the alveoli between each breath, makes each subsequent inspiration easier. The amniotic fluid present within the respiratory tree before birth is largely expelled through the mouth in vertex deliveries by compression of the thorax by the birth canal. Any residual fluid is probably removed by way of the pulmonary lymphatics. As soon as respiration has been established, the pulmonary arterioles and capillaries dilate so that there is a great fall in the pulmonary vascular resistance, and this allows blood in the pulmonary artery to be diverted from the ductus arteriosus into the lungs.

Circulatory System

Immediately after birth the *umbilical cord* is tied, thus severing the placental extension of the fetal circulation. In cases in which the umbilical cord is not tied, the blood flow may continue for several minutes after delivery, although at a rapidly decreasing rate. A number of factors may contribute to this diminishing flow: (1) the contraction of the uterus and the effect of this on the placental attachment and (2) constriction of the umbilical vessels as the result of mechanical stimulation or the presence in the fetal circulation of catecholamines. The fetal blood volume may be increased by as much as 100 ml if the tying of the cord is delayed. However, it is generally agreed that there is no advantage in delaying the tying beyond a minute after delivery.

The interruption of umbilical flow when the cord is tied results in an immediate fall in blood pressure in the inferior vena cava. This fact, coupled with the increased left atrial pressure from the increased pulmonary blood flow, causes the *foramen ovale* to close. From that moment onward the valve of the foramen ovale is kept closed by the hemodynamic changes, and within a few days of birth the valve becomes attached to the edge of the foramen ovale.

The diminished pulmonary vascular resistance associated with inflation of the lungs results in the direction of flow through the ductus arteriosus from right to left to be changed to the neonatal route of left to right. The *ductus arteriosus* constricts as a reaction of its muscle to the raised oxygen tension. It later closes and becomes the *ligamentum arteriosum*. One week after birth its lumen is 2 mm or less in diameter, and by the end of the first month the majority have closed.

The heart in the newborn is relatively large and is higher in the thorax and in a more horizontal position than it is in later life. The *pulse rate* is rapid with an average of 130 beats per minute. The rate may rise considerably with crying and fall to around 80 during sleep. The peripheral circulation is initially slow in the newborn. The hands and feet may be cold and slightly cyanotic for the first few hours after birth.

Blood Changes

At birth the infant has a large number of *erythrocytes,* 5 to 6 million per cu mm, and a high *hemoglobin* level, 15 to 20 gm per 100 ml of blood. The time of tying the umbilical cord after delivery will influence these values. The erythrocytes of the newborn are larger than those of the older child, and the hemoglobin content is correspondingly high. The high values found at birth are a result of the necessity of providing adequate amounts of oxygen in the fetus in utero. At the end of the first week of life, the high values begin to fall, until by the end of the first month all infants develop *physiological anemia.* The decrease in hemoglobin and in the volume of packed erythrocytes is much more rapid than the fall in erythrocyte count. This is because of the replacement of the fetal macrocytes by postnatal normocytes. At the end of 3 months, the *erythrocyte count* may be as low as 4 million cells per cu mm and the hemoglobin level may be down to 12 gm per 100 ml of blood. Physiological anemia of the newborn is symptomless and recovery is spontaneous.

There is a wide variation in the normal *leukocyte count* in the newborn; values of 10,000 to 35,000 per cu mm are considered within normal limits. The majority of the cells are polymorphonuclear *neutrophils*. On the third or fourth day, the count drops rapidly. After the third week, the relative proportion of neutrophils and lymphocytes is reversed, and this predominance of *lymphocytes* persists until the fourth year.

Icterus Neonatorum (Physiological Jaundice)

In nearly half of all healthy babies, the bilirubin content of the blood is raised sufficiently to cause a slight degree of jaundice. This occurs during the first week of life, usually during the second or third day, and is greater and occurs more often in infants born before term. The condition is mainly a result of temporary impairment of the excretion of bilirubin by the liver and also of increased destruction of erythrocytes at this time. It is symptomless and disappears after 2 weeks. Infants who are severely jaundiced within the first 24 hours should be suspected of having hemolytic disease.

Body Temperature

In the newborn the heat-regulating mechanism is in an immature state. The small body has a large surface area from which to lose heat. Almost immediately after birth the temperature falls by as much as 3 degrees, even though the baby is covered with blankets in a warm room. However, increased muscular activity, increased general metabolic activity, and improved vasomotor control of the peripheral blood vessels results in the temperature rising and becoming stabilized within 8 hours. Recently attention has been drawn to the fact that *brown adipose tissue* may play an important role in heat production in the newborn infant. Brown adipose tissue is found in the root of the neck, in the axillae, between the scapulae, and around the vessels and organs in the thorax and posterior abdominal wall.

Gastrointestinal System

In utero the fetus, as early as the fourth month, swallows large quantities of amniotic fluid, and a fecal material called *meconium* begins to form. After birth a baby shows signs of hunger by becoming restless, crying fretfully, and sucking on his fingers or anything he finds close to his mouth. The sense of smell is acute and the mouth is turned toward the source of milk, which the baby can smell. The baby may be hungry at birth or show no desire for food for 24 or 36 hours.

Sucking is assisted by the presence of transverse corrugations of the mucous membrane of the palate, and the *buccal pad* of fat prevents the cheeks being indrawn. The mechanism of sucking is accomplished by the combined action of the tongue, cheeks, and palate. The lips play only a small part in the process, which explains how babies with cleft lip suck quite well whereas babies with cleft palate find it impossible to suck.

The various digestive juices appear to be present in the newborn, except for pancreatic amylase. Digestion of proteins and carbohydrates can take place after birth, but starch is poorly tolerated.

The first stools to be passed are *meconium*.

This is a sticky, dark green, odorless material consisting of a mixture of digestive secretions, bile pigments, desquamated cells, and lanugo and vernix caseosa swallowed with the amniotic fluid. After 3 or 4 days the meconium ceases, and loose, greenish-yellow stools are passed, consisting of a mixture of meconium and milk stools. After the fifth day, the yellow milk stools appear.

Renal System

Although in utero the placenta is responsible for the excretion of all waste substances, nevertheless the kidneys are developed early in fetal life and excretion begins about the ninth week. The urine secreted by the kidneys before birth is acid, is hypotonic to plasma, and contains very little sodium or chloride and no phosphate. The presence of urates in the amniotic fluid confirms that urine is voided by the fetus. Normally the fetus swallows the amniotic fluid and absorbs it from the gastrointestinal tract, so maintaining a fluid balance and completing the cycle.

At birth the child continues to produce urine in much the same manner as in utero. The biochemical characteristics of the urine are the same. There is evidence of functional immaturity in that the infant's kidney cannot concentrate urine as well as that of the adult. However, under normal conditions, the renal function is quite adequate for the needs of the newborn. Large amounts of uric acid are excreted in the newborn. The glomerular filtration rate is low and the kidney may have difficulty in excreting excessive amounts of water and electrolytes, and this fact should be remembered when instituting intravenous therapy.

The baby often empties his bladder immediately after birth, but emptying of the bladder may be delayed for as long as 24 hours. The total amount of urine passed per day varies from 30 to 60 ml, and at the end of the first week this rises to about 200 ml per day.

Umbilical Cord

The umbilical cord stump shrivels, dries, and sloughs off by the sixth to the tenth day. Just prior to separation it is nothing more than a black string. At the site of separation, a small granulating surface persists for several days until healing occurs. Later the thrombosed umbilical vessels become fibrosed and contract and invaginate the skin at the root of the cord, producing the typical umbilicus.

Weight Loss

A normal full-term baby weighs between 6 and 10 lb., with an average of approximately 7½ lb. (3,500 gm). During the first 3 to 5 days, the child loses up to 10 percent of his birth weight by loss of fluid from the body and a relatively low fluid intake. By the eighth to fourteenth day, this weight has been regained, and during the next 3 months the baby will gain 1.0 oz. (30 gm) per day, approximately.

Posture, Behavior, and Reflex Movements

Posture

A newborn baby delivered with a cephalic presentation is most comfortable in the general position of flexion, i.e., the position he was confined in in utero. A baby born with a brow or face presentation tends to lie with the head extended. In breech deliveries, the legs are extended at the knees.

If the baby who has had a normal cephalic presentation is placed on his back, the arms and legs are semiflexed and the head is turned to one or the other side (Fig. 25-1). He is unable to raise his head. The hip joints are partly abducted, externally rotated, and semi-

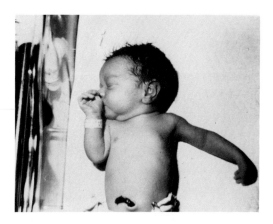

Fig. 25-1. Erb's palsy. During a difficult delivery the upper trunk of the left brachial plexus was damaged. Note that the elbow joint of the left upper extremity is held in the position of extension, and the forearm is pronated. Active abduction of the left shoulder joint was not possible. (Courtesy of Dr. M. Platt.)

flexed. When the baby moves his arms, they remain flexed at the elbows and move at the shoulder joint. At the end of the first month, the position of flexion becomes less. The fists remain clenched for about 2 months. When the baby is placed in the prone position, the legs become even more flexed, and he can raise his head momentarily and rotate it from side to side.

Behavior

When the baby is awake, alternating movements of flexion and extension take place. He often yawns and stretches. He may sneeze, and he often hiccoughs after feeding. If the upper respiratory tract is irritated, he may respond by coughing or spluttering. The baby startles easily, and his chin, arms, and legs may tremor for a short time after a fright.

A newborn baby cries vigorously without tears. The first cry is usually heard immediately following delivery; thereafter crying generally occurs when he is hungry or uncomfortable. Mild stimulation, such as contact with a cold hand, change in position, or distension of the gut with air, may initiate it. A newborn infant usually sleeps most of the time, waking because of discomfort from hunger or a wet diaper.

Reflex Movements

Motor activity in the newborn is largely a continuation of the movements exhibited by the fetus. A study of aborted fetuses has shown that simple reflex movements can be elicited as early as 3 to 4 months, and the movements may be sufficiently vigorous to be felt by the mother during the fifth month. Reflex movements of the lips and tongue are the first to appear, and a little later movements of the arms can be induced by passive displacement of the head. The movements involved in sucking and swallowing begin before birth.

At birth, therefore, certain reflex activities have reached a surprising degree of maturity, and for the most part they are carried out without the assistance of higher centers. Later, as anatomical and physiological development of the nervous system progresses, intricate connecting nerve pathways start to function so that the simple spinal reflexes become influenced by higher centers and the movements become more complex.

A baby should have good *neuromuscular tone* and should not be completely limp. His posture and the way in which he performs voluntary and involuntary movements depend on muscle tone. When a newborn infant is lifted, the head and neck require support, but there should be a feeling of resistance when, for example, an attempt is made to extend the limbs passively.

Behavioral responses during the neonatal period reflect the progressive development of the nervous system. As noted previously, certain reflexes are well developed at birth and a patient observer can elicit these, provided the baby is fully awake and is in a quiet room.

The *sucking reflex* present at birth is easily demonstrated by touching the lips. The *rooting reflex* occurs before feeding time and is a side-to-side movement of the head with the mouth open in response to perioral touch. It is a search for the nipple. The *grasp reflex* is easily demonstrated by placing an object in the palm near the base of the fingers, whereupon the fingers will close around it with a firm grasp. Pressure applied to the sole of the foot causes the toes to flex in a grasping movement. The *plantar reflex* (Babinski's reflex) may be elicited by stroking the lateral plantar surface, which will cause extension of the toes.

The *knee jerk* may be elicited if the child is quiet and relaxed. However, it usually spreads and involves other reflexes on the same side and even on the opposite side of the body. This lack of selectivity is indicative of the state of immaturity of the nervous system in the newborn. The *superficial abdominal reflexes,* which consist of contraction of the abdominal muscles when the skin is stroked, are seldom elicited in the newborn. The *tonic neck reflex* is elicited when the baby lies on his back and turns his head to one side. The arm and leg on the side to which the head faces are extended and the opposite arm and leg are flexed. This is essentially a reflex that is subcortically mediated and is further evidence of immaturity of the nervous system. The *startle reflex* is a response of the infant to a sudden, threatening change of posture. It is best elicited by having the child lying quietly, unclothed, on a table in the supine position. When the table is suddenly jarred the baby throws out both arms laterally, opens his hands and abducts his fingers, and then brings both arms forward in an embrace position; the legs are fully flexed and he usually gives a sharp cry. This reflex requires certain nerve tracts connecting the higher centers of the brain with the spinal cord and, of course, intact peripheral nerves. A failure to obtain a satisfactory reflex response may be an indication of cerebral injury.

In a normal child the grasp reflex, the tonic neck reflex, and the startle reflex have disappeared by the fourth month.

Eyes and Ears

A newborn baby perceives light and closes his eyes whenever he is in a bright light. Eye movements are at first uncoordinated, and the eyes may squint. This condition may last several months until the ability of the eyes to focus develops. Toward the end of the neonatal period, the eyes will follow a bright object. By the age of 3 months, focusing and following an object are well coordinated. At birth the iris is light in color and the permanent darker color does not appear until between 3 months and 1 year. The lacrimal glands do not function at birth and tears do not appear with crying until the end of the third or fourth week.

A newborn baby can hear at birth and responds to loud noises. However, the sensitivity of hearing improves after a few days as a result of aeration of the middle ear and the draining away of amniotic fluid.

Skeleton

The head of the newborn is large and accounts for one-fourth of the body length. The vault of the skull has areas of residual membranes, called *fontanelles,* which allow considerable molding of the head during labor and delivery. When molded, the parietal bones commonly override each other and the occipital bone, and this gives the head an elongated shape at birth. The head assumes its normal shape by the end of a week. The face may be asymmetrical at birth, caused by fetal posture and pressure in utero. This usually disappears within a few days after birth.

A diffuse swelling may be present in the scalp at birth, called the *caput succedaneum*. This is caused by edema that has formed as a result of pressure of the scalp against the dilated cervix during the early stages of labor. The swelling diminishes rapidly in size after delivery and usually disappears in 2 days.

Changes After Withdrawal of Maternal Hormones

During fetal life, maternal and placental hormones enter the fetal circulation and activate the tissues of the mammary gland, uterus, and vagina.

The mammary glands of both sexes may become enlarged and tense during the first week of life, and a milky fluid called *witch's milk* may be expressed from the nipples. The condition resolves spontaneously as the estrogen level in the blood falls.

The female external genitalia show congestion and moisture, and the vaginal epithelium is hypertrophied. As the hormonal levels in the blood become reduced, there may be uterine bleeding, vaginal desquamation, and a mucoid vaginal discharge. By the end of the second week after birth, the congestion of the genitalia disappears and the vaginal discharge ceases.

DEFENSE AGAINST INFECTION

One of the great dangers to the newborn is infection. Immediately after delivery, an infant has numerous sites where organisms can enter the body: for example, the stump of the umbilical cord; the skin of the body, which is delicate and easily damaged; the mucous membranes of the mouth and respiratory tract, which may be damaged by suction tubes used in resuscitation; at the time of birth the lungs may aspirate contaminating material; or infected milk may gain entrance to the gastrointestinal tract. Moreover, the newborn lacks specific antibodies, and his ability to form new antibodies is slow during the first few months of life. This is compensated for in part by the acquisition of passive immunity by the passage of maternal antibodies across the placenta before birth. These antibodies are for the most part antitoxic and not bactericidal, and their concentration falls rapidly after birth. Antibodies to diphtheria and tetanus and antiviral immune bodies against measles, smallpox, mumps, and poliomyelitis pass to the fetus from the mother in this manner. The newborn is also susceptible to certain organisms which are nonpathogenic to adults; the *Escherichia coli* is an example.

Clinical Problems
Answers on page 458

1. Having assisted at the delivery in his first obstetric case, a medical student was astonished to see that the baby was covered by a coat of white, cheese-like material. The baby also had long fine hair on his shoulders and back. What is this cheese-like material? Where does it originate from? Will the baby always have hair on his shoulders and back?

2. A pediatrician commonly uses the term *neonatal period*. What is this period?

3. During a ward round an obstetrician asked a medical student if a mature fetus in utero ever performs the movements of inspiration or expiration. How would you answer that question?

4. A pediatrician examined a newborn baby and found that the respiratory rate was

40 times per minute. Observation of the child showed that there was considerable movement of the anterior abdominal wall as breathing took place, but there was little movement of the thoracic cage. Would you comment on these observations?

5. When a child takes his first breath, are the lungs fully expanded? What part does the substance surfactant play in the process of expansion of the lungs?

6. A senior medical student was concerned at finding some degree of circumoral cyanosis and cyanosis of the hands and feet in a child born a few hours previously. Would you be concerned? What would you do?

7. An obstetrician asked a student if he thought it was necessary to tie the umbilical cord in a newborn infant. He also asked if there is any advantage to delaying the tying of the cord? How would you answer these questions?

8. What is the pulse rate of a newborn infant?

9. A 2-week-old baby was suspected of suffering from right-sided lobar pneumonia. The resident asked for a total leukocyte count and a differential leukocyte count. What is the normal leukocyte count in a newborn? Does the relative proportion of neutrophils and lymphocytes remain constant in the normal child

in the early weeks or months following birth?

10. A premature baby weighing 5 lbs. (2,272 gm) was observed to be jaundiced during the first week after birth. Is this a common finding in premature infants? If so, why?

11. Does the body temperature of a newborn baby fall even though it is covered with blankets in a warm room?

12. What is the normal appearance of the first stools passed by a newborn baby?

13. A mother was surprised to find that her newborn son had not wet his diaper for 24 hours. Is this a common occurrence?

14. During the first week of life a child may lose up to 10 percent of his birth weight. Is this a true statement?

15. A father was worried because his 1-month-old baby daughter kept her hands clenched. He thought she might have a congenital anomaly. What would you tell this father?

16. In a newborn baby are the toes flexed or extended when the lateral plantar surface is stroked?

17. Can a baby hear well and cry tears at birth?

18. What is the caput succedaneum?

19. What is witch's milk?

20. The newborn's ability to form new antibodies is slow during the first few months of life. Is this statement true?

REFERENCES

Avery, M. E. *The Lung and Its Disorders in the Newborn Infant.* Saunders, Philadelphia, 1964.

Beintema, D. J. *A Neurological Study of Newborn Infants.* Spastic International Medical Publications, in Association with William Heinemann. Medical Books, Ltd., London, 1968.

Dawes, G. S. *Foetal and Neonatal Physiology.* Year Book, Chicago, 1968.

Hubble, D. *Paediatric Endocrinology.* Davis, Philadelphia, 1969.

Jonxis, J. H. P., Visser, H. K. A., and Troelstra, J. A., eds. *The Adaptation of the Newborn Infant to Extra-Uterine Life.* Thomas, Springfield, Ill., 1964.

Parmelee, A. H. *Management of the Newborn,* 2d ed. Year Book, Chicago, 1959.

Wolstenholme, G. E. W., and O'Connor, C. M., eds. *Somatic Stability in the Newly Born.* Ciba Foundation Symposium. Little, Brown, Boston, 1961.

Ziegel, E., and Van Blarcom, C. C. *Obstetric Nursing,* 5th ed. Macmillan, New York, 1964.

A *congenital malformation* may be defined as any anatomical defect present at birth. The term therefore excludes inborn errors of metabolism but includes gross and microscopic structural defects. Most embryos with severe structural defects die early and thus represent an important cause of miscarriage and stillbirth. If they do survive until late pregnancy, they may be born prematurely. These anomalies may be compatible with intra-uterine existence, but at birth the newborn infants are unable to adjust themselves to the profound physiological changes associated with extra-uterine life and die soon after delivery. Such anomalies are responsible for about 15 percent of deaths in the neonatal period. It has been estimated that about 2 percent of all newborn infants have defects that are either lethal or will cause death or disability if left untreated. This figure is remarkably constant throughout the world. For this reason it is important that correctable congenital malformations be recognized as soon as possible after birth. Prompt operative treatment may save an infant's life, and in the less urgent cases the anxious parents may be quickly advised about the most suitable form of treatment.

EARLY RECOGNITION OF CONGENITAL MALFORMATIONS

It is important that medical personnel caring for a woman during the antenatal period should obtain a thorough medical history from her. Delicate but firm inquiries into the possibility of a family history of congenital abnormalities should be made. The general health of the woman, especially during the early weeks of pregnancy, should be ascertained, and the possibility that she might have been exposed to rubella should be considered. Has she received medication while pregnant? Has she been exposed to irradiations? Has she felt fetal movements? Answers to these questions may have an important bearing on the early recognition and subsequent treatment of a malformed child.

Repeated careful physical examinations of the mother during the antenatal period may reveal a congenital defect before birth. *Hydramnios* is frequently associated with fetal *anencephaly* and *esophageal atresia*. *Oligohydramnios*, although rare, is usually associated with a fetus with multiple deformities. The condition is recognized by the fact that the fundus of the uterus is lower than

413

normal for the date of pregnancy and the fetus can only be moved with difficulty. *Hydrocephalus* may be recognized before birth by the presenting part, the head, remaining above the pelvic brim, and on abdominal palpation the enlarged head is felt to be softer than normal and more globular. In the more severe cases, the head fails to descend even after labor has been in progress for several hours. *Breech* presentation and other malpresentations commonly occur in this condition. Hydrocephaly and anencephaly may also be recognized on radiological examination. Congenital malformations are about twice as common in *twins* as in single births.

At the time of the delivery, the physician should be especially alert to the possibility of finding a malformation. A *single umbilical artery* is always an ominous sign. Once the newborn infant has been successfully separated from its mother in the delivery room, he should be carefully examined. Malformations are often multiple (Fig. 26-1), and if one is present others should be looked for; for example, *hydrocephalus* is associated with *spina bifida, talipes,* and *cleft palate; mongolism* with *congenital heart disease* and *duodenal atresia; agenesis of the kidneys* with *lung abnormalities.*

Particular attention should be paid to the following signs during the first few days after birth:

1. *Cyanosis.* Severe degrees of cyanosis may occur following cerebral hemorrhage caused by intracranial injury or respiratory difficulty. However, *congenital malformations of the heart, tracheo-esophageal fistula,* and *diaphragmatic hernia* must be excluded.

2. *Feeding difficulties.* Having excluded the possibility of weakness of sucking resulting from general body weakness in the immature infant, brought on by the effect of maternal anesthesia during labor, or by shock as the result of a difficult delivery, a careful exami-

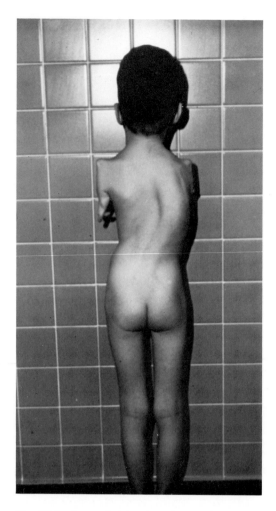

Fig. 26-1. Congenital hemivertebra in the thoracic region associated with phocomelia. (Courtesy of Dr. J. Adams.)

nation of the mouth may reveal a *cleft palate,* a poorly developed mandible, nasal obstruction, or mental deficiency associated with mongolism.

3. *Failure to defecate and vomiting.* Distension of the gut producing enlargement of the abdomen, vomiting, and failure to pass meconium should suggest some form of intestinal obstruction. *Congenital atresia* or *stenosis of the gut, imperforate anus,* or *Hirshsprung's disease* may be responsible.

Persistent vomiting alone after the first few days of life, provided the infant has not had cerebral injury, should suggest some form of obstruction to the intestinal tract. *Congenital pyloric stenosis* seldom produces projectile vomiting before the second week. *Congenital inguinal hernia, meconium ileus,* or *atresia of the ileum* may be present.

4. *Retention of urine.* Most normal infants pass urine at the time of delivery or during the first 24 hours of life. Continued failure to void urine should suggest in the male the possibility of *congenital urethral obstruction.*

5. *Genital organs.* Abnormalities of the external genitalia should be carefully looked for. The presence or absence of the testes in the scrotum should be confirmed. Signs of the *adrenogenital syndrome* should be excluded.

6. *Hip joints.* The hip joints should always be carefully examined, especially in the female, for signs of instability associated with *congenital dislocation of the hip.* Cases of breech delivery are very prone to this condition, and there is often a strong family history of it.

INCIDENCE

An accurate overall figure of the number of infants delivered that have a congenital malformation, however minor in nature, is impossible to obtain at the present time. Errors in diagnosis, different methods of recording observations, variations in the interpretation of terms, failure to record minor defects—all these facts make it difficult to compare the reported incidence of congenital defects from one center to another and even more difficult from one country to another. A further problem that may be misleading is the fact that the incidence of malformed children born in a hospital is always higher than that of children born at home. In Great Britain mothers admitted for hospital delivery are a specially selected group and usually consist of those with a poor obstetric history, elderly mothers, those with multiple pregnancies, those with complications such as hydramnios and toxemia. Conclusions should also be drawn only from long-term surveys, for it is known that certain defects exhibit seasonal variation, and in some areas of the world there are years of peak incidence. It should also be remembered that in some defects, as for example congenital heart disease, the incidence cannot be ascertained at birth and requires a follow-up study of some years. The above problems underline the desirability of establishing an international agreement for standardization of diagnosis so that statistically accurate incidence rates can be recorded.

In a 1966 worldwide survey reported by the World Health Organization, some interesting observations were made on the incidence of congenital malformations. This survey covered almost half a million hospital births and was collected from 24 centers in 16 different countries. Confining our attention to *neural tube defects, tracheo-esophageal fistulas* and *stenoses,* and *cleft lip* and *cleft palate,* the following facts emerge: The overall incidence of neural tube defects was 2.6 per 1,000 total single births. The variation between one country and another was very wide, from 0.6 per 1,000 in Calcutta to 10.2 per 1,000 in Belfast. In the case of *spina bifida,* the incidence in Manila was 0.03 per 1,000 single births and in Belfast 2.59 per 1,000 single births. The incidence of *tracheo-esophageal fistulas* and *stenoses* was 0.11 per 1,000 total single births; the incidence in Manila was 0.03 per 1,000 births, and in São Paulo 0.49 per 1,000 births. The figures for *cleft lip* and *cleft palate* were 0.64 per 1,000 total single births; the incidence for Mexico City was 0.28 per 1,000 births, and for Kuala Lumpur, 1.25 per 1,000 births.

In another worldwide survey (1967) based on birth certificates and hospital and clinic records, the incidence of congenital malformations ranged from 0.15 percent when the sources of the records were birth certificates and official records, through a mean of 1.26 percent when the data were derived from hospital records, and 4.5 percent when the information was obtained by special examinations. In the latter group, the incidence was highest in the United States at 8.76 percent and lowest in Germany at 2.2 percent.

Because of the wide variations that exist in the incidence of different defects in different parts of the world, and the wide diversity of criteria of diagnosis and in methods of recording, it is difficult to arrive at even an approximate figure for the incidence of congenital malformations. However, if for practical purposes one remembers that about 2 percent of all newborn infants have defects which are either lethal or will cause death or disability if left untreated, the magnitude of the problem will be realized. Furthermore, this figure can be nearly doubled if we include those defects that are discovered by the end of the first year.

ETIOLOGY

It must be emphasized that a congenital malformation is not necessarily caused by any single etiological factor. Some congenital defects are purely genetically determined; others are caused by environmental factors such as maternal medication, infection, or irradiation. A single factor probably accounts for no more than 25 percent of all congenital malformations. The majority appear to be a result of a complex interaction of genetic and environmental factors (Fig. 26-2).

Chromosome Abnormalities

Relatively simple techniques have now been established for the examination of human chromosome structure. The normal human somatic cell contains 46 chromosomes consisting of 1 pair of sex chromosomes and 22 pairs of autosomes. In the male cell, the sex chromosomes are represented by an X chromosome and a much shorter Y chromo-

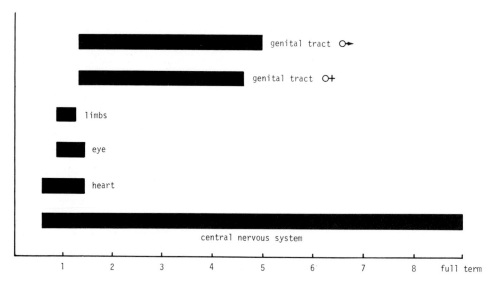

Fig. 26-2. Timetable of critical stages of human development during which mutant genes, drugs, or environmental factors may alter normal development of specific structures. (After Tuchmann-Duplessis, 1969.)

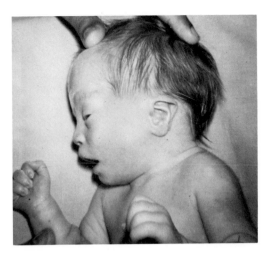

Fig. 26-3. Translocation of chromosome 18. Shows deformed ear and fish-like mouth. (Courtesy of Dr. G. Avery.)

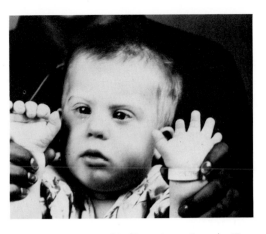

Fig. 26-4. Trisomy 21 (Down's syndrome). Note the characteristic facies and the short, broad hands. (Courtesy of Dr. M. Platt.)

some. In the female cell, the sex chromosomes are represented by two X chromosomes. It soon became apparent that there exists a relationship between specific congenital malformations or syndromes with certain abnormalities of chromosome number and structure. The presence of an additional chromosome to a pair is a condition referred to as *trisomy,* and the person is said to be *trisomic* for that particular chromosome. If the additional chromosome is not free but is attached to another chromosome, the condition is known as *translocation* (Fig. 26-3). The absence of one chromosome of a pair is rare and is known as *monosomy.* It is important that chromosome examinations be carried out not only on the affected infants but also on their parents, so that accurate information may be obtained about recurrence risks.

Trisomy 21 (Down's Syndrome, Mongolism)

This is the most common form of trisomy, occurring in Western countries about 1 in 600 births (Fig. 26-4). The incidence in infants varies with maternal age, rising steeply after the mother has reached the age of 35 years. In young mothers, the incidence is no more than 1 in 1,000 births.

Because the incidence rises with advancing maternal age, it is believed that the chromosomal abnormality occurs during oogenesis rather than spermatogenesis. There are four types: (1) In about 90 percent of cases, 47 chromosomes are present instead of the normal 46. (2) In about 6 percent, the chromosomes are double trisomic, making 48 chromosomes in each cell (XXY plus trisomy 21). (3) In about 3 percent of cases, the chromosomal number is apparently 46, the additional chromosome 21 having become translocated and joined to one of the others, e.g., 13, 14, or 15, or 21–22. An examination of the parents may show that one parent also has translocation of chromosome 21 although clinically normal. A person who shows translocation of a chromosome but is clinically normal is referred to as a *carrier.* (4) About 1 percent of cases of Down's syndrome are *chromosome mosaics* having some normal cells with 46 chromosomes and other cells with 47 chromosomes. This latter group is more difficult to recognize clinically, since the individuals are often intelligent and possess only a few of the signs of the condition.

In parents with normal chromosomes and with a mongoloid child, the chance of having a second mongoloid child is not more than 2 percent. If one of the parents is a carrier of a translocated chromosome 21, the chance of having a second mongoloid child rises to 33 percent. Fortunately cases of trisomy 21 are rarely fertile so that direct inheritance only rarely occurs. In monozygotic twins, both infants will be affected.

In complete mongolism the eyes are small and the palpebral fissures slant downward at the medial ends. The epicanthal folds are prominent on either side, and the iris may have a white spotted appearance. The skull is small and brachycephalic, with a flattened occipital region. The mouth is small and the tongue protrudes and is fissured. The hands are short and broad, with a deep transverse crease across the palms. Mongoloids are mentally defective and exhibit generalized hypotonia and retardation of physical development. The incidence of *congenital heart disease, umbilical hernia,* and *duodenal atresia* is very high. The majority die young but some live to an old age.

The discovery of abnormal chromosomes in Down's syndrome stimulated laboratories throughout the world to initiate the study of human chromosomes in other cases of congenital abnormalities. The following conditions have been described.

Trisomy 17–18

This condition is less common than Down's syndrome. The infant has a receding chin and a prominent occiput. The fingers are rigidly flexed across the hand and *syndactyly* may be present. There is also *mental retardation.* The child usually dies soon after birth.

Trisomy 13–15

This is very rare. The head is small, the nose deformed, and the jaw underdeveloped. *Con-*

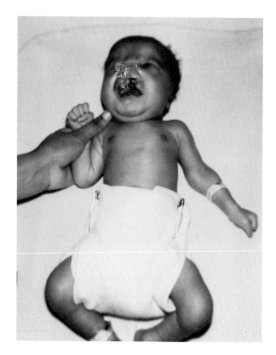

Fig. 26-5. Trisomy 13–15 with cleft lip and cleft palate. (Courtesy of Dr. G. Avery.)

genital heart disease, cleft lip, and *cleft palate* are common in this condition (Fig. 26-5). Deafness and eye defects may also be present. Most infants die soon after birth.

Cri du Chat Syndrome

This is caused by a partial deletion of the short arm of one of the chromosome 5 pair (Fig. 26-6). The condition is characterized by the infant's having a weak high-pitched cry, like that of an animal in distress. There may be *congenital heart defects* present and some infants are *microcephalic.*

Klinefelter's Syndrome

This condition occurs only in the male. The cells have 47 chromosomes with a sex chromosomal constitution of XXY. Up until the age of puberty, the boy appears normal. At puberty the secondary sexual characteristics develop, but the testicles remain small.

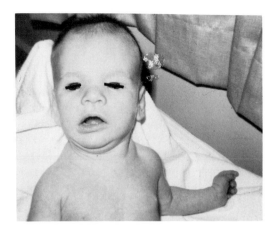

Fig. 26-6. Cri du chat syndrome. (Courtesy of Dr. G. Avery.)

The seminiferous tubules show degeneration, but the interstitial cells are normal. Gynecomastia is usually present, and the patients grow very tall. Some are mentally retarded. Patients with Klinefelter's syndrome are sterile. Some patients have 48 chromosomes, that is, 44 autosomes and 4 sex chromosomes, XXXY. A number of cases exhibit mosaicism.

Turner's Syndrome

This condition occurs in females (Fig. 26-7). The cells have 45 chromosomes with a sex chromosomal constitution of X0, i.e., only a single X chromosome. The external genitalia and mammary glands remain infantile after puberty because of a lack of estrogen. The ovaries are hypoplastic or absent. Other associated abnormalities include *webbing of the neck,* skeletal deformities, *congenital heart defects, lymphedema of the extremities, mental retardation,* and stunting of growth. A few cases exhibit chromosomal mosaicism.

Abnormalities of the Genes

It is now known that some congenital malformations are caused by defects in the genes. It is important to realize that a single defec-

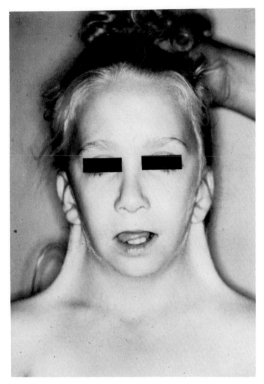

Fig. 26-7. Turner's syndrome. (Courtesy of Dr. L. Thompson.)

tive dominant gene can produce a multiplicity of effects and may involve tissues derived from more than one germ layer. Equally important is the knowledge that the same effect can be produced by many different defective genes. In *retinitis pigmentosa,* for example, a dominant gene may be responsible or a sex-linked gene may be defective, or one of several recessive genes may be to blame. Congenital malformations that occur with a frequency in excess of one in a thousand births are not simply inherited, for a seriously harmful gene cannot attain frequencies of this order. In these cases, environmental factors must be involved in addition to the genetic element.

Autosomal dominant inheritance accounts for such conditions as *lobster claw hand, achondroplasia, osteogenesis imperfecto, craniocleidodysostosis, congenital cataract,* a rare form of *cleft lip,* and *cleft palate.* Autosomal recessive inheritance is responsible for cases of *albinism* and *deaf-mutism. Fibrocystic disease of the pancreas* is one of the commonest disorders resulting from a recessive gene. The *testicular feminization syndrome* and the *adrenogenital syndrome* are also caused by recessive genes. Sex-linked genes are the underlying cause in certain cases of *hydrocephalus, hemophilia,* and *ichthyosis.* Hydrocephalus is not usually a genetically determined disorder; sex-linked hydrocephalus is caused by aqueduct stenosis and is rare. The family history will reveal that it occurs in males and is transmitted to them by unaffected carrier females. For further information on genetics in the etiology of congenital malformations, the reader is referred to *An Introduction to Medical Genetics* by Fraser Roberts.

Infection

It has definitely been established that if a pregnant woman has an attack of rubella (German measles) during the first 3 months of pregnancy, there is a 10 to 20 percent chance that her child will be born with a congenital malformation. The rubella virus causes defects of organs only if the fetus is infected during the period of organogenesis. It has been shown that the virus persists in an individual for as long as 12 months after the patient has clinically recovered from the infection, and this may account for the congenital defects that occur in infants born to mothers who had an attack of German measles some time before the pregnancy started. The virus has been shown to cause defects in the following organs: the eye (*cataract* and *glaucoma*); the ear (*destruction of the organ of Corti,* resulting in deafness); the heart (*septal defects,* and persistent

patent ductus arteriosus); and the brain (*microcephaly* and *mental deficiency*). The infection of the organ appears to occur at a time when there is marked cellular proliferation; for example, cataracts result from infection during the sixth week, a time when the lens is being actively formed. A suitable vaccine is now available to protect pregnant women.

Other viruses may be implicated in the causation of defects. There is suggestive evidence in respect to *influenza, infective hepatitis, mumps, coxsackie B,* and *smallpox vaccination.* There is definite evidence that the *cytomegalic virus* can cause congenital malformations. Cytomegalic virus infection is caused by a group of viruses rather than a single one. It is thought that the mother is asymptomatically infected and the viruses cross the placental barrier. The developing brain and liver are the chief organs affected. *Microcephaly* with *mental retardation, choroidoretinitis,* and *hepatosplenomegaly* occur with this condition.

Maternal infection with the protozoan *Toxoplasma gondii* has been shown to cause congenital *hydrocephalus, microcephaly,* and abnormalities of the eye. It would appear that the mother must have been recently infected and infection must have occurred during the second half of pregnancy when the parasite can cross the placental barrier. The diagnosis is established by performing serological tests on the mother and infant.

The fetus can become infected with *Treponema pallidum,* which crosses the placental barrier and causes *congenital syphilis.* If infected early in pregnancy, abortion or stillbirth may occur. The signs of congenital syphilis usually make their appearance at the end of the first 2 weeks after birth. These signs may include a purulent nasal discharge, a hoarse cry, and a maculopapular rash. Congenital syphilis is prevented by effective antenatal treatment of the mother.

Drugs

The widespread use of *thalidomide* as an antinauseant drug for pregnant women in Britain and Western Germany between 1960 and 1962 led to a great increase in the incidence of congenital malformations. This tragedy resulted in the withdrawal of this drug from the market and initiated a complete reappraisal of all drugs prescribed during pregnancy. Teratogenic drugs, like viruses, affect the fetus during the first 3 months of pregnancy, a period during which organs are undergoing active development. It is impossible to estimate the dose or duration of treatment necessary to produce congenital defects. It would appear that some fetuses are particularly sensitive to this drug, and a single small dose given at the right time may produce widespread gross deformities. These deformities include malformation of the limbs (*micromelia, ectomelia, phocomelia*), *congenital heart disease, intestinal atresia,* and *atresia of the external auditory meatus.*

There is suggestive evidence that other drugs such as *quinine, aminopterin, mercaptopurine,* and *cyclophosphamide* are also teratogenic. Antithyroid drugs, including *thiouracil, carbimazole, iodides,* and *radioactive iodine* may affect the fetus. The infant may develop *hypothyroidism* and may also develop a *goiter* that is sufficiently large to cause respiratory obstruction.

Hormones

Endocrine preparations such as *ethisterone* and *norethisterone,* which are strong progesterone-like substances given in the treatment of threatened abortion, also have a virilizing effect on female fetuses. The degree of masculinization varies from slight enlargement of the clitoris with or without fusion of the labia minora to hypoplasia of the uterus and vagina in the severe cases. The condition may be differentiated from congenital adrenal hyperplasia by finding that the urinary excretion of 17-ketosteroids in the newborn infant is within normal limits.

Although with modern treatment pregnancy involves little risk for the mother suffering from *diabetes mellitus,* nevertheless the risk for the fetus remains high. *Abortions, stillbirths,* and *neonatal death rates* are high in diabetic patients, and meticulous care in the control of the maternal diabetes is necessary for a successful conclusion. Infants born of diabetic mothers are larger than normal and often show hyperplasia of their islets of Langerhans in the pancreas. At the present time, there is no evidence that diabetic mothers are more likely to bear infants with congenital malformations than nondiabetic mothers.

In experimental animals, the administration of *cortisone* has been shown to cause *cleft palate* in the offspring. It is presumed that the hormones suppress the growth of the palatal processes of the maxilla and they fail to fuse with each other in the midline. There is no definite evidence to show that this can occur in man.

Irradiation

Exposure of the fetus to *x-irradiation* or *radium* during the early weeks of development may lead to malformation. Although there is no evidence that diagnostic x-irradiation of the pregnant mother is hazardous, it is wise to leave such examination until after the first 3 months of pregnancy. Radiotherapy, on the other hand, where large doses of ionizing radiations are used, can cause widespread congenital defects including *microcephaly, skull defects, spina bifida,* and *cleft palate.* Infants born to pregnant women who were exposed to the atomic bomb explosions of 1945 within 1,500 meters of the hypocenter had an increased incidence of abnormalities of the central nervous system such as *microcephaly* and *mental retardation*. A long-term risk to the community is the possibility that irradiation of the gonads of either parent may result in *gene mutation,* so that congenital malformations may appear in future generations.

Mechanical Pressure

There can be little doubt that intra-uterine pressure on the fetus, especially in association with *oligohydramnios,* will produce congenital malformations. The development of *talipes equinovarus* and *talipes calcaneovalgus* appears to be caused by intra-uterine molding forces. It would seem probable that a malplaced limb can cause pressure on the head or trunk leading to distortion of growth. The common association of breech deliveries with *congenital subluxation of the hip joint* would suggest that a flexed hip joint in association with extended knees alters the normal pressure forces that are necessary for the development of an adequate acetabulum. It has also been suggested that *retrognathia* may be caused by hyperflexion of the fetal neck. *Dimples,* or thinning of the skin over bony points, may occur at sites where persistent pressure has occurred.

Antenatal Vascular Accidents

Animal experimentation provides evidence that interference with the blood supply of a developing organ could produce the congenital malformations found after birth. Many authorities now believe that fetal vascular accidents explain the genesis of bile duct and bowel atresias. The presence of bile below the site of complete obstruction of the gut would add support to the idea that at one time the lumen of the gut was patent and that obstruction occurred later. The physiological herniation of the midgut loop into the umbilical cord, and its eventual return to the abdominal cavity, provide a situation in which the vascular supply to a segment of the gut could become twisted and result in a partial or complete necrosis of a portion of the gut wall.

Immunity Reactions

It has been suggested that maternal autoimmunization to the thyroid may be responsible for *athyrotic cretinism*. It has been shown that the serum of a number of women who have given birth to athyrotic cretins contained antithyroid antibodies. More recently Brent has shown in experiments using pregnant rats that it was possible to immunize the mother against kidney and placenta extracts. The offspring of such a mother were found to possess many congenital malformations. This is a new field in experimental embryology and one which may ultimately help to explain the causes of many human malformations.

Nutrition, Age, and Parity of the Mother

There is little evidence that nutrition is an important factor in human congenital malformations. In animal experiments, however, defects can be produced with deficiencies of certain vitamins, namely, A, D, or E, and some of the B group.

Mongolism is definitely more common in infants born to mothers of more advanced age. Although different authors suggest that all congenital malformations are more common in children of older mothers, a statistical analysis does not support this.

Parity does appear to influence the incidence of certain defects. Neural tube defects, including spina bifida, anencephaly, and hydrocephalus, and congenital dislocation of the hip are more common in the first-born infants.

Other Factors

There are a number of known etiological factors the effects of which are not understood. Some congenital malformations which do not involve sex-linked genes nevertheless occur more often in one sex than the other. *Hirschsprung's disease, pyloric stenosis,* and *cleft lip* occur more often in the male, while *anencephaly, spina bifida, patent ductus arteriosus, congenital dislocation of the hip,* and *cleft palate* occur more often in females.

Racial and geographical influences are also important. For example, *anencephaly* and *spina bifida* appear to be much less common among African Negroes than among Caucasians. *Preauricular skin tags* and *polydactyly* are more common in Negroes. In Western countries, *cleft lip* and *cleft palate* are less common than in Japan. In Britain there is a higher incidence of anencephaly in the western half of England and Wales than in the eastern half.

Years of peak incidence have been reported for certain congenital abnormalities, and this may be related to the weather. An excessively severe and long winter has been found to favor *anencephaly, spina bifida,* and *congenital dislocation of the hip.* A good summer has been associated with *pulmonary stenosis* and abnormalities of the *lower alimentary tract.* It is most unlikely that factors such as these per se are directly responsible for causing congenital defects. Rather, it is more probable that weather influences the chances of infection of the mother by known and unknown teratogenic organisms.

Clinical Problems
Answers on page 459

---

1. Approximately what percentage of newborn infants have defects that are either lethal or will cause death or disability if left untreated?
2. List three congenital anomalies which you might suspect or be able to detect in the fetus before birth.
3. If, following delivery, you find that a child has a congenital anomaly, you should immediately look for the possible existence of other anomalies. Give examples of congenital anomalies which tend to occur together in the same child.
4. Name two congenital anomalies that may be responsible for each of the following clinical signs: (a) cyanosis, (b) difficulty in sucking at the breast, (c) failure to defecate, (d) persistent vomiting, (e) failure to urinate.
5. Does the incidence of congenital anomalies differ in different parts of the world? If so, can you give some examples?
6. List six etiological factors which are known to be responsible for congenital anomalies.
7. Having fully examined a 6-month-old child, a pediatrician made the diagnosis of Down's syndrome. What is the incidence of this condition? What signs and symptoms would you look for to make a diagnosis of this condition?
8. Name three congenital syndromes in which an examination of the chromosome structure would enable you to make an accurate diagnosis.
9. Do you think it is important to give an expectant mother advice about (a) the danger of taking drugs and (b) the risk of contact with a person suffering from German measles?
10. The parents of a child with a severe con-

genital deformity come to you as a physician for advice and guidance. They are greatly distressed and want to know whether either of them is to blame, whether they could have done something to prevent the anomaly. "What are the chances that it may recur in the next child that we may have?" they ask. How would you handle this situation?

REFERENCES

Anderson, W. J. R., Baird, D., and Thomson, A. M. Epidemiology of Stillbirths and Infant Deaths due to Congenital Malformation. *Lancet* 1:1304, 1958.

Apgar, V. Drugs in Pregnancy. *J.A.M.A.* 190:840, 1964.

Barnes, A. C., ed. *The Fetal Environment: Drugs and Chemicals in Intrauterine Development.* Lea & Febiger, Philadelphia, 1968. P. 362.

Barr, M. L., and Carr, D. H. Correlations Between Sex Chromatin and Sex Chromosomes. *Acta Cytol.* (Balt.) 6:34, 1962.

Blizzard, R. M., Chandler, R. W., Landing, B. H., Pettit, H. D., and West, C. D. Maternal Auto-Immunization to Thyroid as a Probable Cause of Athyrotic Cretinism. *New Eng. J. Med.* 263:327, 1960.

Brent, R. L. Production of Congenital Malformations Using Tissue Antisera. *Proc. Soc. Exp. Biol. Med.* 125:1024, 1967.

Carr, D. Chromosome Studies in Spontaneous Abortion. *Lancet* 2:603, 1963.

Carr, D. M. The Chromosome Abnormality in Mongolism. *Canad. Med. Ass. J.* 87:490, 1962.

Carter, M. P. A Probable Epidemic of Congenital Hydrocephalus 1940–41. *Develop. Med. Child. Neurol.* 7:61, 1965.

Coffey, V. P., and Jessop, W. J. E. Maternal Influenza and Congenital Deformities. *Lancet* 2:935, 1959.

Cohlan, S. Q. Fetal and Neonatal Hazards from Drugs Administered During Pregnancy. *New York J. Med.* 64:493, 1964.

Collman, R. D., and Stoller, A. A Survey of Mongoloid Births in Victoria, Australia, 1942–1957. *Amer. J. Public Health* 52:813, 1962.

Cusher, I. M. Irradiation of the Fetus. In *Intrauterine Development,* edited by A. C. Barnes. Lea & Febiger, Philadelphia, 1968. P. 378.

Doll, R. Hill, A. B., and Sakula, J. Asian Influenza in Pregnancy and Congenital Defects. *Brit. J. Prev. Soc. Med.* 14:167, 1960.

Dudgeon, J. A. Maternal Rubella and Its Effect on the Foetus. *Arch. Dis. Child.* 42:110, 1967.

Edwards, J. H., Harnden, D. G., Cameron, A. H., Crosse, J. M., and Wolff, O. W. A New Trisomic Syndrome. *Lancet* 1:787, 1960.

Edwards, J. H., Norman, R. M., and Roberts, J. M. Sex-Linked Hydrocephalus. *Arch. Dis. Child.* 36:481, 1961.

Fraser, F. C. Genetics and Congenital Malformations. In *Progress in Medical Genetics,* edited by A. G. Steinberg. Grune & Stratton, New York, 1961. P. 38.

Fraser, F. C. The Use of Teratogens in the Analysis of Abnormal Developmental Mechanisms. In *Proceedings of the First International Conference on Congenital Malformations.* Lippincott, Philadelphia, 1961. P. 179.

Gal, I., Kirman, B., and Stern, J. Hormonal Pregnancy Tests and Congenital Malformations. *Nature* (London) 216:83, 1967.

Hadorn, E. *Developmental Genetics and Lethal Factors.* Methuen, London, 1961.

Hay, J. D. Population and Clinic Studies of Congenital Heart Disease in Liverpool. *Brit. Med. J.* 2:661, 1966.

Hibbard, E. D., and Smithells, R. W. Folic Acid Metabolism and Human Embryopathy. *Lancet* 1:1254, 1965.

Hoet, J. P., Gommers, A., and Hoet, J. J. Causes of Congenital Malformations: Role of Prediabetes and Hyperthyroidism. In *Congenital Malformations.* Ciba Foundation Symposium, edited by G. E. W. Wolstenholme and C. M. O'Connor. Little, Brown, Boston, 1960.

Ingalls, T. H. Environmental Factors in Causation of Congenital Anomalies. In *Congenital Malformations.* Ciba Foundation Symposium, edited by G. E. W. Wolstenholme and C. M. O'Connor. Little, Brown, Boston, 1960.

Jolly, H. *Diseases of Children,* 2d ed. Davis, Philadelphia, 1968.

Kennedy, W. P. Epidemiologic Aspects of the Problem of Congenital Malformations. In *Birth Defects,* edited by D. Bergsma. New York, National Foundation of the March of Dimes, 1967. Vol. 3, p. 1.

Klinefelter, H. F., Reifenstein, F. C., and Albright, F. Syndrome Characterized by Gynecomastia, Aspermatogenesis Without aLeydigism and Increased Excretion of F.S.H. *J. Clin. Endocr.* 2: 615, 1942.

Koenig, E., Lubs, M., and Brandt, T. Congenital Malformations and Autosomal Abnormalities. *Yale J. Biol. Med.* 35:189, 1962.

Korones, S. B., Ainger, L. E., Monif, G. R., Roane, J., Sever, J. L., and Fuste, F. Congenital Rubella Syndrome: New Clinical Aspects with Recovery of Virus from Affected Infants. *J. Pediat.* 67:166, 1965.

Langman, J., and Welch, G. W. Excess Vitamin A and the Development of the Cerebral Cortex. *J. Comp. Neurol.* 131:15, 1967.

Leck, I., and Record, R. G. Seasonal Incidence of Anencephalus. *Brit. J. Prev. Soc. Med.* 20:67, 1966.

Leck, I., and Smithells, R. W. The Ascertainment of Malformations. *Lancet* 1:101, 1963.

Leibow, S. G., and Gardner, L. I. Genital Abnormalities in Infants Associated with Administration of Progesteroids to Their Mothers. *Pediatrics* 26:151, 1960.

Lenz, W. Thalidomide and Congenital Abnormalities. *Lancet* 1:1219, 1962.

Long, N. L., and Holtzman, G. B. Hazards to the Fetus from Maternal Diabetes. In *Intrauterine Development,* edited by A. C. Barnes. Lea & Febiger, Philadelphia, 1968. P. 427.

Manson, M. M., Logan, W. P. D., and Loy, R. M. *Rubella and Other Virus Infections During Pregnancy.* Her Majesty's Stationery Office, London, 1960.

Medearis, D. N. Observations Concerning Human Cytomegalovirus Infection and Disease. *Bull. Johns Hopkins Hosp.* 114:181, 1964.

Moore, K. L. *The Sex Chromatin,* edited by K. L. Moore. Saunders, Philadelphia, 1966.

Neel, J. V. Study on Major Congenital Defects in Japanese Infants. *Amer. J. Hum. Genet.* 10:398, 1958.

Neel, J. V. *Genetic Effects of Radiation.* Thomas, Springfield, Ill., 1963.

Preisler, O. Is Prolonged Cortisone Treatment in Pregnancy Damaging to the Infant? *Zbl. Gynaek.* 18:675, 1960.

Rasmussen, D. M. Syphilis and the Fetus. In *Intrauterine Development,* edited by A. C. Barnes. Lea & Febiger, Philadelphia, 1968. P. 419.

Roberts, J. A. F. *An Introduction to Medical Ge-netics,* 5th ed. Oxford University Press, London, 1970.

Rubin, A., and Murphy, D. P. Studies in Human Reproduction. III. Frequency of Congenital Malformations in Offspring of Non-Diabetic and Diabetic Individuals. *J. Pediat.* 53:579, 1958.

Rugh, R., and Grupp, E. Congenital Defects Following Low Level X-Irradiation. *Anat. Rec.* 138:380, 1960.

Sever, J. L., Nelson, K. B., and Gilkeson, M.R. Rubella Epidemic, 1964: Effect on 6,000 Pregnancies. *Amer. J. Dis. Child.* 110:395, 1965.

Smithells, R. W. Incidence of Congenital Abnormalities in Liverpool, 1960–1964. *Brit. J. Prev. Soc. Med.* 22:36, 1968.

Smithells, R. W. The Incidence and Causation of Congenital Defects. In *Neonatal Surgery,* edited by P. P. Rickham and J. H. Johnston. Butterworth, London, 1969.

Somers, G. F. Thalidomide and Congenital Abnormalities. *Lancet* 1:912, 1962.

Stevenson, A. C., Johnston, H. A., Stewart, P., and Golding, D. R. Congenital Malformations: A Report of a Study of Series of Consecutive Births in 24 Centres. *Bull. WHO* 34 (Suppl.), 1966.

Tondury, G., and Smith, D. W. Fetal Rubella Pathology. *J. Pediat.* 68:867, 1966.

Tuchmann-Duplessis, H. The Effects of Teratogenic Drugs. In *Scientific Foundations of Obstetrics and Gynecology,* edited by E. E. Philipp, J. Barnes, and M. Newton. Heinemann, London, 1970. Pp. 636–648.

Vallance-Owen, J., Braithwaite, F., Wilson, J. S. P., Edwards, J. R. G., and Maurice, D. G. Cleft Lip and Palate Deformities and Insulin Antagonism. *Lancet* 2:912, 1967.

Warkany, J., Beaudry, P. H., and Hornstein, S. Attempted Abortion with Aminopterin: Malformations of the Child. *A.M.A. J. Dis. Child.* 97:274, 1959.

Warkany, J., and Kalter, H. Congenital Malformations. *New Eng. J. Med.* 265:993, 1961.

Wilson, J. S. P., and Vallance-Owen, J. Congenital Deformities and Insulin Antagonism. *Lancet* 2:940, 1966.

Wolstenholme, G. E. W., and O'Connor, C. M., eds. *Congenital Malformations.* Ciba Foundation Symposium. Little Brown, Boston, 1960.

Wood, J. W., Johnson, K. G., and Omori, V. In Utero Exposure to the Hiroshima Atomic Bomb. *Pediatrics* 39:385, 1967.

Answers to Clinical Problems

1. Many men in their 80s and 90s are capable of engaging in satisfactory sexual intercourse. Provided that they are physically fit, there should be no reason why normal intercourse should not take place. Those who experience pain due to arthritis or some other disability are usually able, with the cooperation of a loving and understanding partner, to adopt a position which causes the minimum of discomfort.

   About one-quarter of the male population becomes impotent by age 70 (McCary, 1967—see Chap. 1 references). Some men at this age believe, or are made to believe, that they are sexually impotent. Aging of the testis is a gradual process and, after the age of 45 years, spermatogenesis decreases regularly. The number of Sertoli cells remains unchanged, but fewer spermatogonia are noted. The percentage of nonviable and abnormal spermatozoa increases with age. Nevertheless, abundant spermatozoa have been found in the testes of extremely old men, and many such men have successfully fathered children. With our present knowledge, the examination of a masturbation specimen of human semen cannot prove or disprove the fertilizing ability of the spermatozoa.

2. Erection of the penis may occur in normal boys soon after birth. Orgasm has been noted as early as 5 months. The first ejaculation usually occurs between 11 and 15 years of age. Active spermatogenesis starts at about the age of 13 and a few dozen fathers under the age of 15 are recorded annually (Parkes, 1970—see Chap. 1 references). Reassure the mother that her son has and is displaying a perfectly normal behavioral pattern. Describe to her the bodily changes which are taking place in her son. It is hoped that the life-style of the parents will provide the growing boy with a model upon which he can develop his own moral responsibilities.

3. Mumps is a virus infection of the salivary glands, most commonly the parotid, and other tissues, notably the testis, pancreas, and central nervous system. The orchitis usually develops 1 or 2 weeks after the salivary gland enlargement and is most common in postpuberal males.

   The inflammatory process within the testis results in pressure on the seminiferous tubules from the inflammatory edema. The tough, fibrous tunica albuginea seriously restricts the swelling of the organ, so that the condition is extremely painful and is usually followed by some atrophy of the seminiferous tubules. Fortunately, the condition is commonly unilateral; even if it is bilateral, it is rarely followed by sterility.

4. It is now generally agreed that if a child's testes remain within the abdominal cavity or in the inguinal canal beyond the age of 5 years, irreversible degenerative changes take place within the seminiferous tubules. If a testicle is not in the scrotum by the time of puberty, it will be incapable of producing spermatozoa thereafter. It should be emphasized that an intra-abdominal testis is perfectly capable of producing testosterone from its interstitial cells. The temperature within the scrotum (2 to 3° C lower than the intra-abdominal temperature) is sufficiently low to allow normal spermatogenesis to take place. If the testis should remain within the abdomen beyond the age of 30, testicular fibrosis may result in diminished hormone secretion. Moreover, the undescended testis is very likely to undergo neoplastic change. For these reasons, both testes should be surgically placed in the scrotum in this patient.

5. Puberty in the female may be defined as the series of bodily and behavioral changes which take place in response to the interactions between the hypothalamus, pituitary, and gonads. Normally puberty begins with the appearance of pubic hair and budding of the breasts at the age of 10 or 11. At the same age the external genitalia and the uterus undergo a rapid increase in size. The axillary hair makes its appearance and cyclic menstruation begins by age 13 to 14.

Menarche is the time of onset of cyclic menstrual bleeding. It is a dramatic event, occurring at an average age of 13 years. The appearance of the menarche before the age of 9 or after the age of 17 is considered to be abnormal.

Adolescence becomes evident by the appearance of a growth spurt in body height, development of secondary sexual characteristics, and gradual attainment of psychosexual maturity. The child undergoes emotional changes such as bursts of great energy, inconsistency, and unpredictability.

Menopause is the time when the menstrual periods cease. This may occur abruptly, but more commonly the menstrual bleeding gradually becomes scanty, and the periods become irregular and more widely spaced. The average age at which menopause occurs is between 49 and 50 years; the normal range is from the midforties through the mid-fifties. It signifies the decline in ovarian function.

Most girls are anovulatory for the first 12 to 18 months after menarche; the uterine bleeding during this phase results from estrogen stimulation and withdrawal. The uterus is incompletely matured at this time. A girl at this stage is thus usually infertile.

6. The use of a progesterone-containing pill as an ovulation-inhibiting agent has become an increasingly popular method of controlling conception. The progestogens completely suppress ovulation by inhibiting the output of pituitary gonadotropins. The combination of both progesterone and estrogen in a single pill that is taken orally each day for 21 days, or the sequential use of estrogen pills for 15 days followed by progesterone pills for 6 days, allows the endometrium to be built up. The short periodic interruption of the drug therapy for 7 days results in vasoconstriction of the endometrial blood vessels; an interval of withdrawal bleeding occurs, which may be likened to the normal menstrual flow. The interruption of the hormone therapy thus prevents the excessive buildup of the endometrium and excessive breast stimulation. On the fifth day after the onset of the withdrawal bleeding, the patient begins another 21-day treatment with the pill program.

7. The administration of pregnant-mare serum gonadotropins, which have large

amounts of follicle-stimulating activity (FSH), followed by the administration of human chorionic gonadotropin isolated from pregnant women's urine and containing large amounts of luteinizing hormone, has been successful in some cases. A greater number of successes have occurred with the use of human pituitary gonadotropin extracts followed by human chorionic gonadotropin.

Clomiphene citrate, a nonsteroid substance, has also been used with success. This substance is believed to act on the pituitary or hypothalamus, causing the release of the luteinizing hormone (LH), which in turn stimulates ovulation and corpus luteum development.

The two complications which may follow these two types of therapy are cystic enlargement of the ovary and a greatly increased frequency of multiple births.

CHAPTER 2

1. According to Green (1971) (see Chap. 2 references), the reported percentage of couples with absolute infertility ranges from 10 to 20 percent. The following factors may be responsible for the infertile condition: (a) male seminal factor: 25 to 35 percent; (b) ovarian factor: 15 to 25 percent; (c) uterine tubal factor: 25 to 35 percent; (d) uterine cervical factor: 15 to 20 percent.
2. Endocrine disorders (hypothyroidism, diabetes, adrenal and pituitary disorders); acute infections (mumps); chronic infections (tuberculosis); nutritional factors (vitamin A, B, and C deficiency); chronic renal failure; toxic exposures to heavy metals or radioactive substances; drugs affecting spermatogenesis (Myleran [busulfan] used in the treatment of leukemia and methotrexate used in the treatment of psoriasis).
3. Numerous cases of varicocele associated with infertility have been reported. In many of these cases, ligation of the testicular veins has restored normal spermatogenesis. The reason why a varicocele should inhibit spermatogenesis is not fully understood. One theory is that the static blood raises the temperature of the scrotal contents and thus inhibits spermatogenesis. Another theory is that there is often free communication between the veins draining both testes. If the valves of one or both veins are incompetent, toxic metabolites can flow down to both testes and affect sperm production. Assuming the surgeon performed a careful operation and did not damage the vas deferens, this patient should have normal spermatogenesis.

4. *Males.* Congenital diseases (hypospadias, epispadias, undescended testes [see Chap. 16]); trauma (injuries to the groin, including operations for hernia with damage to the vas deferens); acute infections (mumps, venereal disease); chronic infections (tuberculosis of vas deferens, chronic prostatitis).

Females. Congenital diseases (anomalies of the uterus and vagina [see Chap. 16]); trauma (previous abortions or miscarriages); acute infections (previous venereal diseases principally involving the uterine tubes); previous acute pelvic inflammatory disease (e.g., pelvic abscess following appendicitis); chronic infections (tuberculosis, particularly involving the uterine tubes); neoplastic disease (uterine fibroids causing tubal obstruction).

5. While it is not possible in the human subject to detect the precise time of ovulation, the following two tests will indicate whether ovulation is or is not taking place.

Basal body temperature test. The patient is asked to take her oral temperature each morning before rising. This is recorded on a chart for four cycles. During the secretory phase of the menstrual cycle the temperature rises by approximately 1° F. The biphasic temperature curve for each cycle will indicate normal regular ovulation.

Endometrial biopsy. A histological examination of the endometrium during the secretory phase of the menstrual cycle and within a few days of the calculated onset of the period will determine whether or not estrogen and progesterone have developed a normal endometrium suitable for implantation.

Patency of the uterine tubes. This may be tested by insufflation of carbon dioxide under pressure or by hysterosalpingography. In the first test, carbon dioxide is introduced into the cervix under pressure. A sudden fall in pressure, followed later by pain over the shoulder when the patient sits up, indicates that one or both uterine tubes are patent. The pain over the shoulder occurs because the escaping gas passes into the peritoneal cavity, and when the patient sits upright, it passes up under the diaphragm and stimulates the phrenic nerve. Pain is referred along the supraclavicular nerves to the point of the shoulder. In hysterosalpingography, a harmless radiopaque fluid is introduced into the cervical canal. If the canal, uterine cavity, and uterine tubes are patent, the fluid will clearly outline these structures and will eventually enter the peritoneal cavity. A series of radiographs are taken during the filling process. Blockage, abnormal dilatation, or congenital anomalies such as bicornuate uterus may be diagnosed by this method.

Culdoscopy. In this procedure, a lighted instrument, fitted with lenses similar to those of a telescope, is introduced into the pelvic peritoneal cavity through a small incision in the posterior fornix of the vagina. This direct observation of the uterus, uterine tubes, ovaries, and pelvic peritoneum enables one to make an accurate diagnosis of pelvic pathology. The passage of solutions of dyes into the peritoneal cavity through the uterine tubes and the presence of fibrous adhesions can easily be detected.

Cervical mucus. A sample of cervical mucus is removed by aspiration through a glass cannula soon after coitus. The physical and chemical properties of the mucus can then be ascertained, and the presence or absence of normal numbers of sperm can be determined.

6. After a careful examination of the external genitalia, testes, and vasa deferentia and prostate (rectal examination), a seminal analysis should be made. A masturbation specimen of semen should be examined for volume, viscosity, sperm count, sperm motility, and sperm morphology.

7. The operation of bilateral vasectomy is a simple procedure performed under local anesthesia. There is minimal postoperative pain, and there are no immediate after-effects. Spermatozoa may be present in the first few postoperative ejaculations, but that is simply an emptying process. There is no effect on testosterone production by the testis, and no adverse effect on the prostate or seminal vesicles. There is some evidence to show that back pressure of accumulated spermatozoa in the testes and epididymides may result in spermatozoa extravasating into the interstitial tissue and entering the lymphatic and blood vessels. This condition could produce an induction of an immune response with the development of serum antibodies against the sperm. Further research into the possibility of the development of an auto-immune response in cases of vasectomy is clearly indicated.

Vasovastostomies have been performed which were followed by the return of spermatozoa to the ejaculate; in many cases, successful fertilization resulted.

8. Tubal ligation is a method of producing permanent sterility. Restoration of the continuity of the uterine tubes has been attempted, and in about 20 percent of such cases the women have become fertile again (Green, 1971—see Chap. 2 references).

9. Large doses of estrogen administered postcoitally, during the immediate postovulatory portion of the cycle, will prevent pregnancy. Estrogen's action in this respect is not fully understood. It is believed to accelerate the transport of the fertilized ovum along the uterine tube; it also leads to an abnormal buildup of the endometrium and so interferes in some way with implantation. It may have a direct effect on the blastocyst. It should not be used as a regular form of contraception since estrogen in large doses causes nausea, breast soreness, and irregular, prolonged menstrual flow. Further, if implantation should occur before the hormone is administered, it fails to prevent pregnancy.

10. Normal implantation takes place in the endometrium of the body of the uterus, most frequently on the upper part of the posterior wall. Implantation of the blastocyst outside the uterine cavity is called an *ectopic pregnancy*. Implantation in the wall of the uterine tube is a serious condition. Because there is no decidua formation in the tube, the eroding action of the trophoblast quickly destroys the wall of the tube. Tubal abortion or rupture of the tube, with the effusion of a large quantity of blood into the peritoneal cavity, is the common result.

11. This patient has a hydatidiform mole. The ovum has died, but the chorionic villi have continued to grow. The grapelike swelling of the villi in such cases is due to the fact that they continue to absorb fluid from the maternal decidua, and the fluid remains within the villi, since the fetal circulation is absent. Moreover, the trophoblastic villi continue to grow and invade the decidua and frequently involve the myometrium. This condition is thus a neoplasm of the trophoblast. In view of this woman's age, hysterectomy would be the treatment of choice. In younger women desirous of childbearing, curettage of the uterine cavity is the best treatment.

12. This woman has a chorioepithelioma with metastases in the lower lobe of the left lung. This is a malignant neoplasm of the trophoblast and fortunately is rare. About half the cases follow a hydatidiform mole; the remainder occur following an abortion or normal pregnancy. The treatment of choice in this case is hysterectomy, followed by the administration of an antimetabolite drug such as methotrexate.

CHAPTER 3

1. *Abortion* is the term used to denote the termination of pregnancy before the fetus is viable. The blastocyst normally becomes implanted in the endometrium of the body of the uterus, most frequently on the upper part of the posterior wall near the midline. On implantation the blastocyst remains confined to the compact layer of the endometrium and never lies deeper than a few millimeters from the surface. The pregnant uterine wall is very vascular and soft and could easily be perforated by the uterine probe or curettage. However, an experienced obstetrician, having first carefully determined with the uterine probe the depth of the uterine cavity and its direction, dilates the cervix and is then able with a sharp curet to remove the entire

stratum compactum without damage to the uterine muscle. Unless the operation is performed under sterile conditions, infection of the uterus is a common complication.

2. Teratomas vary in structure from simple cysts to a mass of material composed of numerous well-differentiated tissues. The tumors usually arise in or near the midline and just anterior to the vertebral column. The common sites are within the pelvis, retroperitoneal and mediastinal. They are thought to arise from undifferentiated embryonic cells which retain some or all of their totipotentiality. Their common midline position has lead pathologists to suggest that they arise from the primitive streak.

CHAPTER 4

1. Before starting any operation which involves the introduction of a surgical instrument into the uterine cavity, great care must be taken to ascertain that the patient is not pregnant. The *decidua* is the name given to the endometrium of the pregnant uterus. As the result of the continued production of progesterone from the enlarging corpus luteum, the endometrial stromal cells lying close to the trophoblast enlarge, become polyhedral in shape, and are filled with glycogen and lipid material. The capillaries of the endometrium become congested and dilated to form intercommunicating sinusoids. The enlarged stroma cells or decidual cells are first seen in the immediate area of implantation, but they are soon found throughout the lining of the uterus.

The decidua may be divided into three different regions or areas: (a) the decidua basalis, (b) the decidua capsularis, and (c) the decidua parietalis (see p. 41). The placenta may be divided into (a) the fetal part formed by the chorion frondosum and (b) the maternal part formed by the stratum compactum of the decidua basalis.

2. This patient has hydramnios. The very large volume of amniotic fluid excessively distends the uterus and impairs the movements of the diaphragm—hence the breathlessness. The distended uterus is tender because of the excessive stretching of its wall. The pressure of the uterus on the inferior vena cava impairs the venous return from the legs, causing edema of the feet and ankles. The large volume of amniotic fluid enables the fetus to be moved about easily but at the same time makes palpation of its parts difficult. The large volume of fluid also serves as a barrier to the fetal heart sounds. The normal volume of liquor amnii at term averages 1 liter. The liquor is thought to be produced early in development by the cells forming the wall of the amnion. Later, when the kidneys of the embryo start to function, urine is added to the fluid, and the kidneys become the major source of the fluid. Anencephaly and esophageal atresia are two common congenital anomalies associated with hydramnios. In these conditions the fetus is unable to swallow the amniotic fluid; in the case of anencephaly the cerebrospinal fluid is added to the amniotic fluid, thus increasing its volume.

3. A protuberance of fused amnion and chorion is pushed down into the canal of the cervix at the onset of labor. This occurs as the result of a rise in pressure in the liquor amnii caused by contractions of the uterus. As the membranes stretch and descend, they tear away from the uterine wall and push out the plug of mucus which closes the cervical canal. The tearing process is accompanied by slight bleeding.

4. With the onset of uterine contractions the

amnion and chorion are pushed down into the canal of the cervix as described in answer 3. With each uterine contraction the two membranes with the contained liquor amnii serve as a fluid wedge (hydrostatic wedge) and assist in the dilation of the canal of the cervix. The rupture of the membranes and the escape of the liquor amnii usually occur when the first stage of labor is well advanced. By this time the advancing head of the fetus has entered the cervix and plugs the canal. It is not until the end of labor that the remaining liquor amnii escapes, coming out with a gush after delivery of the child's body.

5. The possible explanations are: (a) The woman is mistaken in the date of her last menstrual period, and thus the uterus is smaller than the estimated period of gestation warrants. (b) Fetal death. This can be verified by listening for the fetal heart. (c) The fetus may be excessively small due to fetal or maternal disease. (d) Oligohydramnios.

6. Oligohydramnios is a gross deficiency in the amount of liquor amnii (less than 300 ml). It is a rare condition. It is usually due to congenital absence of the fetal kidneys. The excessive pressure of the uterus on the fetus may cause deformities of the skull, limbs (talipes), and trunk. Amniotic adhesions could produce amputations of the limbs. The baby's skin is dry and leathery.

7. Liquor amnii is normally clear, pale, and straw-colored. The green color is due to the presence of meconium (see p. 164) and, except in cases of breech delivery, would indicate that the fetus is in distress. You should listen to the fetal heart sounds. If they are normal there is nothing to worry about. If they are very rapid, very slow, or weak and irregular, the fetus is in distress and you should look for the cause.

8. Amniocentesis is a common method used for the evaluation and management of many disorders in the fetus. It is used for the following: (a) spectrophotometric study of the amniotic fluid in cases of Rh sensitization (by this method the amount of bilirubin excreted by the fetus into the amniotic fluid may be determined); (b) detecting genetic disorders in the fetus (superficial fetal skin cells are present in the fluid); (c) assessment of fetal maturity (the more mature the fetus the greater the number of fat droplets present in the fetal skin cells in the fluid). The determination of the concentrations of creatinine, lecithin, and sphingomyelin is also helpful in establishing the degree of maturity.

In this procedure, the amniotic fluid is aspirated through a needle passed through the anterior abdominal wall, peritoneal cavity, uterine wall, chorion, and amnion. Needless to say, it is important to avoid the mother's bladder, the placenta, and the fetus.

9. The umbilical cord contains two umbilical arteries which carry deoxygenated blood from the child to the placenta, and one umbilical vein which carries oxygenated blood from the placenta to the child. At birth the vein can easily be seen. Drugs can be injected into it and milked toward the child and so enter the general circulation.

10. A small part of the extra-embryonic coelom occasionally remains within the root of the umbilical cord. A piece of intestine could then herniate into the cord and become included in a ligature placed close to the umbilicus. A fine ligature could sever the cord; Wharton's jelly, with its covering of amnion, could be easily cut. A second ligature is necessary only when the placenta in utero is shared by a second fetus, a uniovular twin (see p. 63). The stump of the cord

may become infected, the common organism being *Staphylococcus aureus*. In cases of umbilical sepsis, hemorrhage may occur from the stump. The umbilical scar may stretch during the postnatal period, producing an acquired infantile umbilical hernia. The majority become smaller and disappear without treatment as the abdominal cavity enlarges.

11. A normal umbilical cord measures about 20 to 24 in. (50 to 60 cm) long. An excessively long cord may become wound once, twice, or three times around the neck of the fetus. This occurs most commonly during the middle months of pregnancy, when the relative amount of liquor in relation to the fetus is greatest. It also occurs in cases of hydramnios. The mobility of the fetus is responsible for the long cord becoming wrapped around the neck. An excessively short cord may prevent the descent of the fetus during labor and lead to premature separation of the placenta, fetal distress, and uterine hemorrhage. An excessively long cord may form loops through which the fetus passes, thus producing knots. These knots should be distinguished from irregularities of the cord which are due to a heaping up of Wharton's jelly. An excessively long cord may prolapse through the cervix and vagina at the onset of labor when the membranes rupture.

12. The normal placenta is flattened and circular in shape, with a diameter of about 8 in. (20 cm) and a thickness of about 1 in. (2.5 cm). The maternal surface is dark red in color and oozes blood from the torn maternal vessels. It has a sponge-like consistency. The outer surface is rough, and the margins of the lobules or cotyledons may be recognized. The fetal surface is smooth and shining and is covered by amnion, which is fused with the underlying chorion. The umbilical cord is attached near its center,

and the umbilical vessels radiate out under the amnion from the point of attachment. The amnion may be peeled from the chorion up to the umbilical cord. This procedure should always be carried out following delivery to determine if the chorion is complete and to make sure that some part has not been retained in the uterus adherent to the decidua.

13. From a practical point of view the obstetrician must determine whether or not any part of the placenta or the fetal membranes has been retained within the uterus. Retention of these structures interferes with the contraction of the uterine wall and may result in puerperal hemorrhage or infection. The presence of accessory lobes (placenta succenturiata) or holes in the placenta (placenta fenestrata) may lead to confusion if they are not recognized.

14. Chorionic gonadotropin is produced by the placenta and maintains the corpus luteum during early pregnancy. It is excreted in the urine. It reaches its peak between the sixteenth and seventeenth days of gestation and then gradually falls to a low level. Excessively high levels are found in multiple pregnancies, hydatidiform mole, and chorion epithelioma. Estrogens are produced by the placenta in large quantities, and they are excreted in the urine. Estrogens are concerned with the growth of the uterus and the mammary gland. They serve to increase the contractility of the uterine muscle and sensitize it to oxytocin at the time of parturition. Progesterone is produced in massive amounts by the placenta. It is excreted in the urine and feces. Its production is essential for normal pregnancy. It inhibits the contractility of the uterine muscle and stimulates the growth of the uterus.

15. The functions of the placenta in terms of respiration, nutrition, excretion, protec-

tion and as an endocrine organ are fully described on page 55. The permeability of the placental membrane reaches its maximum during the thirty-sixth week and then rapidly declines during the last few weeks of pregnancy. This normal physiological change is accompanied by the deposit of fibroid material on the maternal surface of the chorionic villi, which tends to thicken the placental membrane. As the placenta undergoes these senile changes, it is still able to meet the fetal requirements during labor. Pre-eclampsia, hypertension, and diabetes may accelerate these senile changes. Placental infarction involving large areas of the placenta can seriously interfere with its function, and the death of the fetus may follow.

16. The placenta serves as a protective barrier against many infecting organisms and drugs. Bacteria are unable to cross the barrier unless the placenta itself becomes involved in the inflammatory process. *Treponema pallidum,* tubercle bacilli, protozoa of malaria, and toxoplasmosis can reach the fetal circulation. Rubella virus can easily pass through the barrier and may cause many congenital anomalies if the mother is infected during the eighth to twelfth week. The Rh antigen can cross the placenta. Morphine, barbiturate drugs, and general anesthetics easily cross into the fetal circulation and depress the respiratory center of the fetus. Teratogenic drugs, such as thalidomide, can cross the placental membrane and produce numerous congenital defects.

17. Normally the placenta is situated in the upper half of the uterus. Should implantation occur in the lower half of the body of the uterus, the condition is called *placenta praevia.* As the lower half of the body of the uterus dilates towards the end of pregnancy, the placenta is separated from the uterine wall and hemorrhage occurs. The bleeding is painless since the blood escapes through the cervix, and the uterus does not contract and is not distended.

CHAPTER 5

1. According to Oettle (1953) (see Chap. 5 references), there is no doubt that heredity influences the tendency to polyzygotic births, but it is uncertain whether or not heredity affects the frequency of monozygotic twins. In polyzygotic births the children have different physical and mental characteristics; in monozygotic births the children have identical physical and mental characteristics. White and Wyshak (1964) (see Chap. 5 references), after studying 4,000 records, found that the genotype of the father does not affect the frequency of twinning.

2. The results of many studies have shown that increasing maternal age increases the possibility of multiple pregnancies.

3. There is a marked variation in the incidence of multiple births among different races. In the United States twinning is more common in whites than in Negroes, and in Japanese women the incidence of twinning is about half as common as in the United States. Multiparous women are more likely to have twins than nulliparous women.

4. Identical twins occur when a single fertilized ovum splits, eventually to form two babies. Rarely, the process of splitting occurs late in the blastocyst stage, and the inner cell mass may be incompletely split so that the primitive streak and the embryonic disc are incompletely divided, and conjoined twins result. The union may vary from slight skin fusion to a double monster, in which heads, trunks, organs, and limbs are shared.

5. In the United States the incidence of twins is about 1 in 95 births; of triplets, about

1 in 10,750 births. The use of drugs to stimulate the ovaries artificially in the treatment of amenorrhea or anovular menstruation may result in multiple pregnancies. Follicle-stimulating hormone, chorionic gonadotropic hormone, and clomiphene are good examples of agents that may cause the maturation and liberation of several ova that may become fertilized.

6. Congenital malformations are about twice as common in twins as in single births. Premature delivery is common, and the birth weight of twins is less than that of a nontwin. Perinatal mortality is about 10 percent, in comparison to less than 3 percent in single births. The mortality of the second twin is twice that of the first. This may be explained on the basis of (a) placental separation after delivery of the first twin and (b) the greater frequency of abnormal positions of the second twin. The mother is more susceptible to pre-eclampsia and premature labor. Pressure side-effects due to the greatly distended uterus may cause edema of the ankles, varicose veins, and breathlessness.

7. The dead fetus is usually retained within the uterus until the end of pregnancy. It becomes partially mummified and compressed by the enlarging normal fetus. Provided that the remaining fetus is normal and is receiving an adequate placental circulation, the pregnancy should continue until term.

8. The presence of two fetal heads, or two backs, or both, is diagnostic. The finding of an unduly large uterus for the period of gestation and the presence of what appears to be an excessive number of limbs make the diagnosis almost certain. The hearing of two fetal hearts is not reliable since a loud, vigorous heart beat may be heard over a large area of the abdominal wall. The diagnosis can be confirmed by radiology after the thirtieth week. In an obese woman with strong abdominal muscles, especially in a primigravida, it is sometimes extremely difficult to palpate the different parts of the fetus.

9. (a) monozygotic or dizygotic. (b) monozygotic or dizygotic. (c) monozygotic. (d) monozygotic or dizygotic. (e) monozygotic. (f) dizygotic. (g) monozygotic or dizygotic. (h) monozygotic.

CHAPTER 6

1. A premature baby is defined as one with a birth weight of 5½ lbs (2,500 gm) or less, regardless of the estimated period of gestation. The cheesy material is vernix caseosa. The period of gestation is approximately 32 weeks. Provided that the baby is kept warm, carefully fed, and expertly nursed, he has a good chance of survival.

2. The embryonic period extends from week 4 to week 8 inclusive. It is the time of rapid growth and differentiation. All the major organs of the body are formed during this time. The fetal period extends from week 9 to the tenth month inclusive. It is the time of further growth and development of all the previously established organs in the body.

3. This condition is called *dysmaturity* and is due to intra-uterine malnutrition. The commonest cause is placental insufficiency. It is found in cases of twins when both fetuses have a single placenta, but one fetus develops at the expense of the other.

CHAPTER 7

1. This child has a large sternal defect through which the pulsations of the heart can be seen and felt. This condition is known as *incomplete ectopia cordis.*

2. The condition is known as *situs inversus;* if it is complete, it involves the heart and other thoracic organs. The condition in

which the heart and its apex are directed toward the right is called *dextrocardia*. Dextrocardia alone is much less common than dextrocardia associated with complete situs inversus.

3. Atrial septal defects allow the oxygenated blood in the left atrium to be shunted across into the right atrium, the blood pressure in the left atrium being higher than that in the right atrium. The increased blood flow through the pulmonary valve is responsible for the systolic murmur and the enlargement of the pulmonary artery as seen on x-ray examination. The increased amount of blood on the right side of the heart is responsible for the right-sided cardiac enlargement seen on x-ray examination. The increased blood flow through the lungs is the cause of the increased pulmonary vasculature seen on x-ray examination.

Atrial septal defects may be due to a failure of the foramen ovale to close or to a persistence of the ostium primum; defects of the ostium primum are less common (for details, see p. 92). Small septal defects produce no symptoms and are of no clinical significance. Large atrial septal defects overload the right ventricle and the pulmonary circulation and should be closed by operation.

4. Normally, the ventricular septum is formed from two sources: the inferior muscular part grows up from the floor of the primitive ventricle; the membranous part is formed from the fusion of the lower ends of the bulbar ridges and the septum intermedium (endocardial cushions). The complete septum is formed when the membranous part fuses with the muscular part. Defects are almost invariably found in the membranous part of the septum.

The complications which follow a ventricular septal defect are due to the overloading of the right side of the heart. Blood under high pressure is shunted from the left ventricle through the septal defect into the low-pressure system in the right ventricle. Enlargement of the right ventricle follows, and if the defect is large right-sided heart failure will eventually occur. Small ventricular septal defects are more common than large defects; small defects are asymptomatic and cyanosis is absent.

5. The tetralogy of Fallot consists of (a) a large ventricular septal defect; (b) stenosis of the pulmonary trunk that may occur at the infundibulum of the right ventricle, or at the pulmonary valve; (c) the exit of the aorta immediately above the ventricular septal defect; (d) right ventricular hypertrophy secondary to the ventricular septal defect and the pulmonary stenosis.

The delay in the appearance of the cyanosis is usually due to the delay in the closure of the ductus arteriosus.

The pulmonary stenosis results in an impaired pulmonary circulation, with consequent poor oxygenation of the blood. Even at rest there is insufficient oxygenation of the blood, as revealed by cyanosis and clubbing of the fingers and toes. Lack of oxygen also results in impaired growth and development. It is not surprising, therefore, that the increased oxygen need that occurs on exertion would produce excessive breathlessness. Breathing is easier in the squatting position.

6. Transposition of the great vessels occurs more commonly in males than females. It arises as the result of the aorticopulmonary septum's being formed in the wrong direction so that the aorta exits from the right ventricle and the pulmonary trunk exits from the left ventricle. This condition is incompatible with life since the deoxygenated blood returning to the right atrium of the heart from the tissues is immediately pumped out to the tissues again via the right ventricle and aorta. The child usually dies soon after birth. The presence of a

large atrial septal defect in this patient allowed some mixing of the blood on the two sides of the heart. The prognosis is poor in untreated cases, and the great majority of patients die in early infancy from congestive heart failure.

7. This rare condition is due to a failure of the development of the spiral aorticopulmonary septum in the upper part of the bulbus cordis (the truncus arteriosus). The breathlessness, cyanosis, and clubbing of the fingers were due to the mixing of the bloods from the two sides of the heart. The right ventricle was enlarged due to the higher pressure on the right side of the heart as the result of the large ventricular septal defect; the ventricular septal defect was responsible for the loud systolic murmur. The prognosis of this condition depends on the status of the pulmonary arteries. If the pulmonary arteries arise from the truncus arteriosus, then a large volume of blood will pass through the lungs and cyanosis may be minimal. If the pulmonary arteries are absent, then only the bronchial arteries supply the lungs and there is deep cyanosis. The majority of children die within 6 months of birth.

8. Congenital aortic stenosis is caused by a failure of the mesenchyme to break down and form separate cusps of the aortic valve. The result is that the edges of the valve cusps are often fused together, forming a diaphragm with an eccentric orifice. This condition should be distinguished from subaortic stenosis.

    The systolic murmur was caused by the blood being forced through the narrowed aortic valve during the ejection phase of the heart. The left ventricular hypertrophy was produced by the increased effort required to force the blood through the narrowed aortic valve.

9. There are two types of pulmonary stenosis: (a) pulmonary valve stenosis, which is caused by a failure of the mesenchyme to break down and form separate cusps of the valve, and (b) infundibular stenosis, which is due to a failure of the lower end of the bulbus cordis to expand to form a normal-sized infundibulum. This defect usually occurs in association with tetralogy of Fallot.

    In this case there was pulmonary valve stenosis. The systolic murmur was caused by the blood being forced through the narrowed pulmonary valve during the ejection phase of the heart. The right ventricular hypertrophy was produced by the increased effort required to force the blood through the narrowed pulmonary valve.

CHAPTER 8

1. The ductus arteriosus represents the distal portion of the sixth left aortic arch artery and connects the left pulmonary artery to the descending aorta. In fetal life it is the normal bypass of blood to the aorta from the pulmonary trunk. At birth, the ductus arteriosus normally constricts in response to a rise in arterial oxygen tension (see p. 108). Later it closes and becomes the ligamentum arteriosum. A failure of the ductus arteriosus to close results in aortic blood passing into the pulmonary artery, producing the machinery-like murmur. The shunting occurs during both systole and diastole because of the higher blood pressure in the aorta and the lower blood pressure in the pulmonary artery. Because of this leak from the aorta the left ventricle initially shows hypertrophy. Later, due to the raised pressure in the pulmonary circulation, enlargement of the pulmonary trunk occurs and hypertrophy of the right ventricle takes place.

    Because of the risk of bacterial infection of the wall of the pulmonary artery and cardiac failure, a patent ductus arteriosus should be ligated and divided surgically.

2. This boy has coarctation of the aorta, which

is a narrowing of the aorta just proximal to, opposite, or distal to the site of attachment of the ligamentum arteriosum. The possible explanation for this condition is given on page 108. The absent femoral pulse is due to the failure of the small aortic pulse wave to reach the femoral arteries. The high blood pressure in the arteries of the upper limbs (and cerebral circulation) is due to an attempt by the heart to force blood through the narrowed aorta and maintain a reasonable blood flow through the trunk and lower limbs. In order to compensate for the diminished volume of blood reaching the lower part of the body, an enormous collateral circulation opens, involving the internal thoracic, subclavian, and posterior intercostal arteries.

The raised arterial blood pressure proximal to the aortic narrowing may later result in cerebral hemorrhage and heart failure. The continued passage of high-pressure blood through the narrowed aorta may lead to bacterial invasion of the tunica intima at the site of the narrowing (bacterial endocarditis—the word *endocarditis* is a misnomer here).

3. Normally the right and the left coronary arteries are branches of the ascending aorta. They develop as solid endothelial buds from the undivided truncus arteriosus. One must assume that in this case the endothelial bud of the right coronary artery arose abnormally from that part of the truncus arteriosus which later became the pulmonary trunk. In this case, after birth, the blood pressure in the pulmonary trunk was much less than that in the aorta; thus, the right coronary artery received deoxygenated blood under low pressure. Within months of birth, degenerative changes occurred in the myocardium and the child died of heart failure.

4. The superior vena cava is formed from the terminal portion of the right anterior cardinal vein and the right common cardinal vein. Normally the right and the left anterior cardinal veins become connected in the lower part of the neck by a transverse anastomosis, and a portion of the left common cardinal vein disappears. By this means, blood from the left side of the head and neck becomes shunted over to the right side to drain into a single right-sided superior vena cava. A persistence of the left common cardinal vein in its entirety results in the presence of a left-sided as well as a normal right-sided superior vena cava as seen in this case. The left-sided superior vena cava drains into the coronary sinus, which is enlarged. There are no functional disturbances and no treatment is required.

5. The foramen ovale is closed after birth by the valve-like flap formed by the lower part of the septum primum pressing against the septum secundum and fusing with it. This takes place as the result of the rise in blood pressure in the left atrium which occurs once the child takes a deep breath and the pulmonary circulation is established. During fetal life, oxygenated blood passes through the foramen ovale from the right atrium to the left atrium.

CHAPTER 9

1. Unilateral cleft lip is caused by a failure of the maxillary process on one side to fuse with the globular process. The palate should always be examined in these cases since cleft palate is commonly associated with cleft upper lip. The child should have a complete physical examination since congenital malformations are often multiple. The cleft lip and cleft palate complex occurs more frequently in boys than in girls (Warkany, 1971—see Chap. 9 references). According to Fraser Roberts (1962) (see Chap. 9 references), the genetic prognosis is worse for affected females, for they have

a higher incidence of malformed offspring with this complex than do affected males. Provided that the infant is thriving, surgical repair of the cleft lip should be performed during the first two months of life. In the majority of children the cosmetic results are excellent.

2. The diagnosis is microstomia associated with micrognathia. This condition frequently occurs with trisomy 18 and trisomy 13–15. Microstomia occurs as the result of excessive fusion of the maxillary processes with the mandibular processes of the first pharyngeal arch. Micrognathia is due to the poor development of the mandibular process of the first pharyngeal arch.

3. On examination this baby was found to have a median cleft palate which involved the uvula, the soft palate, and the greater part of the hard palate; there was no evidence of a cleft lip. The difficulty with the feeding was that the cleft in the palate prevented the child from actively sucking milk from the breast. With this condition the child should be fed by manual expression of the milk from the breasts or carefully fed with a spoon or dropping pipette. Because of the risk of aspiration pneumonia, great care must be taken to prevent the milk from pouring down the throat into the larynx. Surgical repair of the palate should be undertaken at 18 months, i.e., before the child starts to speak.

4. This baby has a congenital obstruction of the right nasolacrimal duct. During development the duct is formed from a solid cord of ectodermal cells which sink beneath the surface of the face. Later the cord becomes canalized, but in this case, the duct on the right side remained blocked by epithelial cells. The stagnated tears in the lacrimal sac became infected soon after birth—hence the presence of pus in the lacrimal sac. First the infection should be treated with antibiotics and then the duct should be probed under a general anesthetic to remove the obstruction. Tears do not begin to form until the third or fourth week of life; thus, the condition is not recognized during the first week of life.

CHAPTER 10

1. This patient has a branchial cyst. Normally the cervical sinus becomes obliterated by apposition and fusion of its walls. Should this fail to occur, a branchial cyst forms. Such cysts are lined with stratified squamous epithelium and are filled with a creamy fluid containing cholesterol crystals. Because they tend to increase gradually in size and may become infected, they should be removed surgically.

2. This patient has a branchial sinus. In this condition the second pharyngeal arch has failed to bury the pharyngeal clefts completely, and the cervical sinus remains in communication with the surface of the neck. The sinus is present at birth, but the external opening is often very small and inconspicuous. Infection of the tract causes pain and abscess formation. The tract is lined with stratified squamous epithelium in its lower part and sometimes with columnar epithelium in its upper part. Occasionally, the sinus extends up the neck between the internal and external carotid arteries and opens into the pharynx. It is then more correctly referred to as a branchial fistula. A branchial sinus or fistula should be removed in its entirety by careful surgical dissection.

3. This child had an auricular appendage. Normally the pinna or auricle of the ear is formed from the fusion of a number of small swellings around the external auditory meatus. Three of the swellings are derived from mesenchymal proliferations from the first pharyngeal arch, and three similar swellings are derived from mesenchyme of the second pharyngeal arch (see

p. 127). Occasionally, additional swellings are formed from these pharyngeal arches and produce the auricular appendages, which are made up of skin but may also contain a small piece of cartilage. They usually are found just anterior to the normal auricle. Surgical removal is the treatment of choice.

4. This child has a preauricular sinus. It is thought to result from incomplete fusion of the small swellings derived from the first and second pharyngeal arches, which normally form the auricle of the ear. Most sinuses are harmless. However, should they become infected, the track may become blocked, with the resulting formation of a cyst or an abscess. Preauricular sinuses may become the site of a chronic discharge. In the event of complications, they must be completely removed surgically to obtain a lasting cure.

5. This patient has a cystic hygroma of the neck. It occurred as the result of a failure of a portion of the jugular lymph sacs to join up with the remainder of the lymphatic system. On section the swelling is found to consist of a large number of small cysts filled with clear lymph. As the cysts enlarge, they extend out widely into the surrounding connective tissue. Complete surgical removal is the treatment.

6. Uniform enlargement of the tongue in infancy should make one think of Down's syndrome (see p. 417) and cretinism (see p. 272). Congenital muscular hypertrophy of the tongue may occur in an otherwise perfectly normal child; the cause is unknown. Cystic hygroma and neurofibromatosis should also be considered.

7. This patient has a ranula of the tongue. It should be regarded as a retention cyst of part of the sublingual salivary gland. If present from birth, it is due to a failure of one of the ducts of the sublingual gland to become canalized during development. In this case the cyst had gradually enlarged

since birth and was first noticed when the child was 3 years of age. The ranula should be removed surgically. Larger cysts that sometimes extend down into the neck are thought to be branchial cysts.

8. This patient has a dentigerous cyst involving the right lower third molar tooth. The cyst is formed after the enamel has been laid down. Degeneration and accumulation of fluid occur in the remains of the stellate reticulum, and a cyst is formed, the walls of which are derived from the outer epithelial layer of the dental bud. The crown of the tooth lies within the cavity of the cyst and the root is outside the cyst. The treatment is to open the cyst, curet out the lining, and remove the unerupted tooth.

9. This child has micrognathia associated with a cleft palate, and a small tongue. The condition is referred to as the *Pierre Robin syndrome*. Basically, in this condition the mandibular processes of the first pharyngeal arches fail to grow, and the tongue remains between the palatal processes. The presence of the tongue prevents the palatal processes from fusing in the midline—hence the cleft palate. Provided that the child can be carefully fed without causing aspiration pneumonia, the lower jaw will continue to grow and assume a nearly normal appearance. The cleft palate can be dealt with surgically at the appropriate time (see p. 118).

CHAPTER 11

1. A history of normal feeding for the first 15 days of life followed by a history of projectile vomiting, the presence of a palpable swelling below the right costal margin, and visible gastric peristalsis make the diagnosis of congenital hypertrophic pyloric stenosis certain. If untreated, the child becomes dehydrated (as seen by dry skin and depression of the anterior fon-

tanelle) and rapidly loses weight. The stools are small in quantity and infrequent, and the child becomes very restless. In this case, in which there was a history of vomiting for 5 days and the child shows obvious evidence of dehydration, surgical treatment is necessary. After the fluid and electrolyte imbalance has been corrected, a longitudinal incision is made through the hypertrophied circular fibers of the pyloric sphincter. Very careful postoperative feeding is required. The prognosis is excellent.

The exact cause of this condition is unknown. Recent research has shown that the autonomic ganglion cells in this region are fewer in number than normal. Prenatal neuromuscular incoordination may be responsible for the hypertrophy of the circular muscle of the pylorus.

2. This child has complete obstruction of the duodenum at a level below the entrance of the common bile duct. The presence of bile in the vomitus and the absence of bile in the meconium (pale in color) enables a determination of the approximate site. The visible gastric peristalsis would indicate that the obstruction is at a high level in the gastrointestinal tract, but the absence of a firm swelling below the right costal margin rules out congenital hypertrophic pyloric stenosis; the latter condition usually presents itself between the second and fourth weeks after birth. The projectile type of vomiting is characteristic of a high level of obstruction. The failure of x-ray examination to reveal air in the gut indicates a high level of obstruction.

When the fluid and electrolyte imbalance is corrected, the baby should be operated upon and the obstruction removed or bypassed (duodenojejunostomy). Failure to make an early diagnosis inevitably results in death. During the early development of the duodenum, the lining cells proliferate so that the lumen becomes

obliterated. Normally the duodenum becomes recanalized at a later date. Failure of recanalization leads to duodenal atresia or stenosis. In some cases the duodenum is obstructed by the presence of an annular pancreas (see p. 151).

3. This patient has an annular pancreas. In this condition the ventral pancreatic bud becomes fixed, so that when the stomach and duodenum rotate, the ventral bud is pulled around the right side of the duodenum to fuse with the dorsal bud of the pancreas, thus encircling the duodenum (see p. 151). This is a common congenital defect associated with Down's syndrome. The condition is treated surgically by bypassing the obstruction by performing a duodenojejunostomy.

4. This child has congenital atresia of the common bile duct. This condition is due to a failure of the bile ducts to canalize during development. There are many different forms of the condition (see p. 152). In this case no bile pigments are entering the duodenum through the common bile duct. However, as the clay-colored stools pass through the intestine, a small amount of bile is secreted along with the mucus from the mucous glands—hence the stools are pale yellow in color. The urine in such cases is deep yellow in color. Some degree of fibrosis invariably occurs in the portal canals and in some instances is very extensive, causing obstruction of the portal vein and enlargement of the liver and spleen, as in this case. A child with this condition should be operated on as soon as the diagnosis is made. In this case the hepatic ducts and the gallbladder were normal, and the gallbladder was anastomosed to the duodenum.

CHAPTER 12

1. This child has atresia of the middle part of the ileum. The lower the level of ob-

struction, the less forceful the vomiting and the greater the degree of abdominal distension, as in this case. The exact embryological explanation for this condition is unknown. It may be due to failure of the lumen to become recanalized after epithelial proliferation of the cells of the mucous membrane but is more likely to be due to peritonitis followed by adhesions or vascular damage to the intestine. Once the water and ionic imbalance has been corrected, such a patient should be operated on. Wide resection of the area of intestinal atresia should be performed, followed by ileal anastomosis.

2. Duplication of the digestive system may occur anywhere from the mouth to the anus. For the embryological explanation, see page 165.

3. Incomplete rotation and malrotation of the midgut loop are fully explained on page 165. To begin with, the child had obstruction of the third part of the duodenum, which would explain the projectile vomiting of bile-stained fluid. However, the obstruction was partial since normal meconium was passed per rectum during the first 3 days. The sudden appearance of blood-stained meconium on the third day accompanied by generalized abdominal distension was due to the rotation of the terminal ileum and ascending colon, producing the condition of volvulus. Twisting of the intestine, or volvulus, is very likely to occur in cases of incomplete rotation or malrotation of the midgut loop where the mesenteric attachment to the posterior abdominal wall is narrow.

4. This patient has a gastric ulcer in a Meckel's diverticulum. In many cases of Meckel's diverticulum a small area of ectopic gastric mucosa is present which is capable of producing hydrochloric acid and pepsin. This child has a chronic ulcer in the adjoining mucous membrane that is responsible for the umbilical pain.

The sudden severe hemorrhage from an artery in the floor of the ulcer is responsible for the rectal bleeding and fainting attack.

After restoration of the blood volume and hemoglobin to a normal level a child with this condition should be operated on and the diverticulum widely excised. The cut ends of the ileum are then joined by an end-to-end anastomosis.

5. This child has a vitello-intestinal fistula. This condition is due to a persistence of the vitello-intestinal duct. Feces pass from the terminal part of the ileum to the umbilicus, where they are discharged onto the skin. In such a case, the child should be operated on and the entire remains of the vitello-intestinal duct removed.

6. This patient has a patent urachus. The allantois in the early fetus connects the primitive bladder to the umbilical cord. Normally this channel becomes a fibrous cord, the urachus. In male children with urethral obstruction (posterior urethral valves—see p. 236) the channel may persist, allowing the urine to escape from the bladder through the umbilicus. Rarely, the channel may persist without congenital urethral obstruction and is recognized in the male only in old age when prostatic enlargement hinders the passage of urine. In this case the urine passed along the patent urachus and discharged through the umbilicus as a watery fluid.

7. This child has meconium ileus, which is part of a more general disease known as *fibrocystic disease of the pancreas*. The ileum is filled with viscid mucus mixed with meconium which has caused intestinal obstruction. Where possible the ileal loop is opened surgically and the contents removed. In this case the intestine was greatly distended, and a segment of the ilium had to be resected.

8. On return of the midgut loop to the abdominal cavity, the cecum and appendix

lie at first in close contact with the right lobe of the liver. Later the cecum and appendix normally descend into the right iliac fossa, so that the ascending colon and hepatic flexure of the colon are formed. In this case the final descent of these structures into the right iliac fossa did not occur, and chronic appendicitis gave rise to the mistaken diagnosis of chronic cholecystitis.

9. This is a case of primary megacolon (Hirschsprung's disease). The condition is due to the failure of development of the parasympathetic ganglion cells in the constricted part of the bowel. In this case the constriction occurred in the sigmoid colon. Immediately above this section of the bowel, the colon was hypertrophied as the result of attempting to force the meconium and feces onward. The greater part of the descending colon and transverse colon were greatly distended by the accumulation of flatus and feces.

   The treatment in such a case is transverse colostomy, in which a part of the transverse colon is temporarily made to open onto the anterior abdominal wall, followed by resection of the aganglionic constricted part of the colon at the age of about 1 year.

10. This child has an ectopic anus. The anus was minute in size and opened into the posterior part of the vagina. This anomaly is probably caused by a failure in the complete development of the urorectal septum.

CHAPTER 13

1. Tracheo-esophageal fistula may be explained by failure of the margins of the laryngotracheal groove to fuse adequately, leaving an abnormal opening between the laryngotracheal tube and the esophagus. In this case the esophagus was completely obstructed, because the tracheo-esophageal septum formed by the fusion of the margins of the laryngotracheal groove was deviated posteriorly and fused with the posterior wall of the esophagus.

   The accumulation of saliva in the mouth was due to the complete obstruction of the esophagus. The abdominal distension was due to air being forced from the trachea through the fistula and down the distal end of the esophagus into the stomach, which expanded like a balloon.

   Following careful preoperative nursing in the head-down position, the child should be operated on, the esophageal ends anastomosed to one another, and the fistula to the trachea closed. The operative mortality is high.

2. Neonatal lobar emphysema is believed to be due to a failure of development of a bronchial cartilage. As a result, the bronchus collapses. Air is inspired through the collapsed bronchus but is trapped during expiration, and the lobe of the lung becomes distended.

3. This boy has congenital cysts of the lung. They are believed to be caused by sequestration of the lung tissue during development. They seldom give rise to symptoms unless they become infected or distended with air; in the latter case they may produce pressure symptoms.

4. This child died of the respiratory distress syndrome (hyaline membrane disease). It has been shown that the lungs of infants dying from this condition do not contain surfactant. This substance is necessary to overcome the surface tension forces in the alveoli when the lungs are inflated. The eosinophilic membrane is due to effusion of fluids containing fibrinogen from the pulmonary circulation. The fibrinogen is converted into fibrin, which forms the membrane.

   The condition is common in premature infants, infants of diabetic mothers, and infants born by cesarean section. The child should be treated in an intensive care unit, where every effort is made to improve the uptake of oxygen and the giving up of carbon dioxide from the blood. Mechanical assistance for breathing may be necessary.

CHAPTER 14

1. This child has an exomphalos, or omphalocele. The anterior abdominal wall is closed by a process of folding of the embryonic disc (see Chap. 3). Failure of the formation of adequate lateral folds causes a defect in the umbilical region, which is filled by amnion only. The wall of the sac is thus composed of amnion only. Once the baby starts to swallow air, the loops of small intestine become distended and the sac increases in size. During the first 24 hours after birth the wall of the sac becomes dry and opaque and may rupture, causing evisceration. Bacteria at once gain entrance to the peritoneal cavity, producing peritonitis.

   The sac of amnion should be surgically excised as soon after birth as possible, and the contained viscera returned to the abdominal cavity. The defect in the anterior abdominal wall must then be closed. When the defect cannot be closed easily, some form of plastic surgical procedure must be undertaken, using skin flaps. This condition is very commonly associated with other congenital anomalies.

2. This is a case of gastroschisis. The small intestine herniated through a defect in the anterior abdominal wall adjacent to the umbilicus. Gastroschisis is caused by a defect in the development of one of the lateral folds of the embryo, resulting in a full-thickness defect of the abdominal wall. The umbilical cord is attached to the anterior abdominal wall in a normal manner.

   The intestine should be covered with a warm, moist dressing and should be gently returned to the abdominal cavity. Surgical closure of the defect in the abdominal wall should then be attempted. The mortality is high. This is largely due to the difficulty experienced in closing the defect in the anterior abdominal wall.

3. This child has a diaphragmatic hernia through the left pleuroperitoneal canal. It was caused by a failure of fusion of the left pleuroperitoneal membrane with the septum transversum (see p. 196). The treatment is surgical reduction of the hernia and repair of the defect. It should be noted that in some cases the lung on the affected side is hypoplastic and may take a long time to expand to fill the pleural cavity.

4. This child has an esophageal hiatal hernia. This is due to an excessively large esophageal hiatus and a weakness of the muscle of the right crus of the diaphragm. The cardiac end of the stomach herniates upward into the thorax. The associated incompetence of the cardio-esophageal junction allows the stomach contents to flow up into the esophagus, which was responsible for the projectile vomiting that occured when the child was laid on its back. Repeated esophageal reflux will result in esophagitis, which may lead to stricture formation. Such a child always should be nursed and made to sleep in an upright position.

CHAPTER 15

1. This child has agenesis of the right kidney which is asymptomatic. It has an incidence of 1 per 1,400 autopsies. The ureter as well as the kidney is usually absent. The left kidney is hypertrophied in this case. The condition is caused by a failure of the mesonephric duct to give rise to a ureteric bud. The presence of the ureteric bud induces the mesenchyme in the intermediate

cell mass to form the metanephrogenic cap. Unilateral renal agenesis is compatible with a normal life expectancy.

2. This child has infantile polycystic disease of the kidneys with accompanying biliary cysts of the liver. The possible causes for this condition are discussed on page 209.

3. This man has the adult form of polycystic disease of the kidneys. Although the renal function tests showed diminished function, nevertheless the results indicated that there still existed a reasonable amount of normal kidney tissue. Because of this it was decided to incise the cysts and aspirate as many as possible to relieve pressure on the remaining renal tissue. Such patients will ultimately die in uremia as the result of the destruction of the renal tissue by the enlarging cysts.

4. This woman has a horseshoe kidney. This is caused by a fusion of the most medial subdivisions of the ureteric bud, resulting in union of the caudal ends of both kidneys. The low medial position of both kidneys can be explained on the basis that, as both kidneys began to ascend from the pelvis, they became trapped behind the inferior mesenteric artery. The symptoms in this patient were almost certainly due to urinary stasis in the ureters, which were kinked as they passed down anterior to the connecting bridge of renal tissue. Surgical division of the renal bridge corrects the condition.

5. An aberrant renal artery represents a persistent lateral splanchnic artery, a branch of the aorta. Normally the lower lateral splanchnic arteries to the kidney disappear (see p. 214). If they persist, the majority cause no ill effects; in some cases they cause obstruction of the ureter, with resulting hydronephrosis.

6. This boy has a left-sided hydronephrosis with some degree of hydroureter. The cause of the obstruction is the presence of a bifid ureter on the left side. At opera-tion it was found that the ureter draining the lower part of the kidney crossed and partially obstructed the ureter draining the upper part of the kidney. It was decided to separate the two ureters and re-implant the obstructed ureter into the bladder. The cause of bifid ureter is a premature division of the ureteric bud during the early stages of development. In this case, the ureters opened independently into the bladder; the ureter draining the upper pelvis and calyces opened into the bladder below the orifice of the other ureter (see p. 214). In cases in which there are marked hydronephrosis and renal infection which are confined to one part of the kidney, heminephrectomy is the treatment of choice.

7. Megalo-ureter is a congenital condition in which the ureter is dilated, but there is no evidence of obstruction within the bladder or urethra and no neurogenic disturbance involving the urinary tract. Defects in the ureterovesical junction, allowing regurgitation of urine from the bladder, may be the cause in some cases. A maldevelopment of the muscular coats of the ureter may explain hydroureter in other cases. Valves in the lower end of the ureter are rarely responsible.

8. This child has extrophy of the bladder. It is believed that the condition is caused by a failure of the embryonic mesenchyme to invade the embryonic disc caudal to the cloacal membrane. (For a full description see p. 215). Because of the urinary incontinence and the almost certain occurrence of ascending infection, surgical treatment is necessary. Moreover, it has been reported that patients who are not treated and live until middle age develop carcinoma of the bladder mucous membrane.

Surgical reconstruction of the bladder may be attempted. Excision of the bladder and transplantation of the ureters into the colon or an ileal loop diversion is now a more common form of treatment. The defects in the anterior abdominal wall and the genitalia are corrected at a later date.

9. This boy has a urachal cyst. Both ends of the urachus (allantois) had closed during development in this case. The cells of the lining mucous membrane had produced secretion in the unobliterated midportion, and so a cyst had gradually formed.

CHAPTER 16

1. This patient has an anterior inversion of the testis. The epididymis is situated anteriorly, and the testis and the tunica vaginalis posteriorly. The condition is relatively common but is of little clinical significance. It may cause confusion in the diagnosis of testicular diseases.

2. This boy has a right-sided incomplete descent of the testis. Examination revealed the presence of the testis within the inguinal canal. In fat children it is sometimes very difficult to palpate the undescended testis in the inguinal canal. The exact cause of incomplete descent of the testis is not known. The mechanism of normal testicular descent is discussed on page 233. It is possible that there has been some mechanical interference with the descent, due to failure of normal development of the inguinal canal. Bilateral failure of descent may be due to deficiency in the secretion of pituitary gonadotropins.

This child should be examined every 6 months. In the majority of cases in which the testis remains in the inguinal canal close to the superficial inguinal ring, it will descend by itself within a few months after birth. If the testis has not descended into the scrotum by the fifth year it should be treated surgically and placed in the scrotum. Only rarely is hormone treatment used. The higher temperature in the inguinal canal or within the abdominal cavity causes irreversible destructive changes in the seminiferous tubules of the testis, and for this reason surgical treatment is necessary.

3. This child has a maldescent of the right testis. Instead of descending by its normal path into the scrotum, the right testis was shunted off into the perineum. While the mechanism is not fully understood, it is possible that in this case the gubernaculum was malformed, or split, or fixed by fibrous tissue. Under these circumstances the testis never reached the scrotum.

The presence of the testis in the perineum makes it very liable to injury and torsion. Moreover, it is now recognized that patients with a maldescended testis commonly suffer from neoplastic changes in the testis in later life. For these reasons, a maldescended testis should be placed in the scrotum by surgical means.

4. This child has a congenital hydrocele. The processus vaginalis has remained in direct communication with the peritoneal cavity by a narrow channel, and peritoneal fluid is forced down into the processus when the child cries. Toward the end of an active day the peritoneal fluid tends to accumulate in the processus; thus, the swelling is larger at night and smaller in the morning. The neck of the processus vaginalis in this case is not wide enough to permit the passage of some of the abdominal contents, and, therefore, there is no inguinal hernia present. Because the condition persists and may later be complicated by the development of an inguinal hernia, the processus vaginalis should be removed surgically in its entirety.

5. This patient has a right encysted hydrocele of the spermatic cord. This is a cyst in the remnant of the upper part of the processus vaginalis and is connected to the tunica vaginalis by a fibrous strand (a further remnant of the processus). The

cyst is formed by the accumulation of fluid in the isolated segment of the processus vaginalis. The size of the cyst may remain stationary or gradually increase over a period of years. On pulling down the testis and the tunica vaginalis, the cyst in this case was pulled medially by the fibrous strand.

Because the cyst is causing symptoms and because it may increase in size, it should be removed surgically.

6. The child has a right indirect inguinal hernia with a preformed sac, due to the failure of the upper part of the processus vaginalis to become obliterated prior to birth. The contents of such a hernia usually consist of omentum and coils of small intestine; with gentle pressure it is possible to push the contents back into the abdominal cavity. The movement of gas in the bowel is responsible for the gurgling sounds. When the child cries, additional contents are forced down into the hernial sac. When a loop of intestine becomes incarcerated in the sac, all the signs and symptoms of intestinal obstruction may develop and may lead to strangulation of the intestine and death. It is very possible that in this case a loop of small intestine did become temporarily fixed within the sac during the previous week, causing the screaming attack, fretfulness, and loss of appetite. In such a case the child should be operated on, the contents of the hernial sac should be returned to the abdominal cavity, and the hernial sac (i.e., the remains of the processus vaginalis) should be completely removed.

7. This child has congenital posterior urethral valves situated just below the summit of the urethral crest in the prostatic urethra. The chronic urinary obstruction since before birth has produced severe back pressure effects on the bladder, ureters, and kidneys. The condition is believed to be caused by a failure of the mesonephric ducts to integrate normally with the developing urethral wall. The treatment in this case was directed first to relieving the upper urinary tract damage by improving the drainage with an indwelling catheter. Later the valves were removed surgically.

8. This child has hypospadias associated with chordee. The proximal portion of the penile urethra is normally formed by the fusing together of the two genital folds on the ventral surface of the penis. By this means the urethral groove, whose floor is formed by the entodermal urethral plate, is converted into the tubular penile urethra. The fusion of the genital folds extends progressively along the shaft of the phallus to the root of the glans penis. A bud of ectodermal cells on the tip of the glans grows into the substance of the glans and joins the entodermal cells lining the penile urethra. This cord of cells later becomes canalized so that the penile urethra opens at the tip of the glans. In this case, the urethral folds failed to unite on the ventral surface of the developing penis, so that the urethra opened on the ventral surface of the penis. This deformity is invariably associated with some degree of chordee.

The condition should be treated surgically. The first step is to correct the ventral curvature of the penis (chordee). This unfortunately makes the hypospadias worse, since the external urethral meatus comes to be situated further posteriorly. Following the initial operation, the second step is to undertake plastic construction of the penile urethra. Treatment should start at about the age of 2 years and be complete before the child goes to school. Little boys like to look the same as other little boys.

9. This case is a typical example of Turner's syndrome, in which there is complete failure of both ovaries to develop. In

Turner's syndrome the cells have only 45 chromosomes because one X chromosome is missing (XO) (see p. 419). In this case the clinical signs and symptoms make the diagnosis obvious. A simple buccal smear and the finding of absent nuclear sex chromatin make the diagnosis absolute. In difficult cases, where the diagnosis is in doubt, culdoscopy shows the absence of ovaries in the pelvis. Since these individuals are females in appearance and psychological outlook, they should be brought up as females. The cyclic administration of estrogen and progesterone in this case will bring about the development of normal female secondary sexual characteristics and cyclic menstrual function.

10. This girl has the condition known as uterus bicornis unicollis. The left uterine tube, the left part of the uterine body, and the cervix are normal and in free communication with one another. The right uterine tube and the right part of the uterine body are distended with blood and old menstrual secretions, with only a very small communication with the canal of the cervix. This condition has resulted in a backup of the menstrual flow on the right side with each period—hence the soft right-sided pelvic mass attached to the uterus and the severe abdominal pain with each period. The exact diagnosis was made at exploratory laparotomy. The abnormal right uterine tube and right half of the body of the uterus were excised in this case. The left hemiuterus was perfectly capable of supporting a normal pregnancy. This condition is due to a failure in the normal development of the right paramesonephric duct, together with a failure of the right and left ducts to fuse completely.

11. This girl has an imperforate hymen. The pelvic discomfort and the absence of menstrual flow are due to the accumulation of blood and old menstrual secretions (hematocolpos) above the intact hymen. This condition is caused by a failure of the cells of the lower part of the vaginal plate and the wall of the urogenital sinus to degenerate (see p. 241). Surgical incision of the hymen, followed by dilation, cures the condition.

12. This man has a cyst of the appendix of the right testis; this is a remnant of the paramesonephric duct. Since such a cyst may grow larger, may become infected, and may cause the patient some concern, it should be removed surgically.

13. This child is suffering from female pseudohermaphroditism, that is, the child is a female, as shown by the presence of the female sex chromatin. However, the presence of large amounts of androgens resulted in the hypertrophy of the clitoris so that it resembles a penis, and hypertrophy and partial fusion of the labia majora so that they resemble a scrotum. In this child the vaginal orifice is represented by the dimple in between the labia majora. The upper part of the vagina and the uterus, the uterine tubes, and the ovaries are normal. The cause of the excessive production of androgens by the adrenal cortex is fully discussed on page 244.

14. A full chromosome examination of a somatic cell in this case would have revealed a count of 46 with a sex chromosome pattern of XY. Palpation of both inguinal canals revealed the presence of a firm ovoid structure present posterior to the superficial inguinal ring on both sides. Surgical removal of these structures followed by histological examination showed the presence of testicular tissue with no evidence of spermatogenesis. The diagnosis is testicular feminization syndrome. It is believed that although the testes in such cases are rudimentary, they are capable of producing both androgens

and estrogens. Unfortunately, the target organs are incapable of responding to the androgens. The estrogens are responsible for the development of the normal female secondary sexual characteristics. Since these individuals are psychologically oriented as females they should be raised as females even though they are male pseudohermaphrodites. Both testes should be removed surgically, as in this case, since they are prone to malignant change. Estrogen therapy should then be given to maintain the female sexual characteristics.

CHAPTER 17

1. This child is suffering from hemophilia. If a hemophiliac marries a normal woman, his sons will be normal and cannot pass on the disease. If a female carrier marries a normal man, as in this case, half her sons will have hemophilia and half will be normal. The daughters will not suffer from the disease, but half the daughters will carry the trait. The disease is carried on the X chromosome and is handed down from unaffected carrier females to sons. If a hemophiliac son marries a normal woman, all the daughters will be unaffected carriers of the disease, and his sons will be normal and cannot pass on the disease. Hemophilia exists in all degrees of severity. This case appears to be moderately severe, since extensive bruising occurred without obvious cause. This child would be ill advised to play competitive games at school. There are many reported cases in which the disease appears to become less serious with age. However, in many of these cases, it is probable that the patient has learned to avoid traumatizing circumstances.

2. The detection of the presence of Rh antibodies in the mother's serum is important since they will cross the placental barrier and destroy the fetal Rh-positive red cells.

A knowledge of the presence of antibodies will enable the obstetrician and pediatrician to initiate the appropriate treatment, such as premature delivery or exchange transfusion at the time of delivery. The determination of the husband's Rh genotype provides the obstetrician with helpful information in predicting the outcome of subsequent pregnancies. An Rh-negative woman who has in the past been transfused with Rh-positive blood, is likely to have already formed anti-Rh antibodies. She is likely to have increased her susceptibility to stimulation by an Rh-positive fetus, should she become pregnant.

3. This patient has sickle cell anemia. Examination of a sample of blood prepared with sodium metabisulfite showed the presence of numerous sickled erythrocytes. The jaundice can be explained on the basis of the excessive destruction of the abnormal erythrocytes taking place, with the consequent liberation of bile pigments into the bloodstream. The weakness and breathlessness could also be accounted for by the severe degree of anemia. The acute abdominal pains and the skin ulceration resulted from thrombosis and stagnation of the blood in the capillaries, which are associated with the sickling phenomenon. The enlarged liver was due to overactivity of the reticuloendothelial system, whose cells are loaded with blood pigments and iron in this disease.

4. The diagnosis is cystic hygroma. The swelling in this disease results from the presence of a large number of small cysts filled with clear lymph and lined by endothelium. The cysts may be independent of one another or may communicate freely. The condition is due to a failure of the primitive endothelial-lined lymph sacs to join with the lymphatic system (see p. 260). Because of the likelihood that the swelling will continue to increase in size, the danger of sudden enlargement due to hemorrhage,

and the possibility of infection, a cystic hygroma should be excised.

5. This patient has idiopathic hereditary lymphedema (Milroy's disease). The condition is both congenital and familial. The lymph vessels in the area involved, most commonly the legs, are found to be aplastic or hypoplastic. It is believed that the formation of the peripheral lymphatic system has been abnormal and that there is a failure in its proper connection with the central lymphatic vessels. The condition usually becomes progressively worse with age. However, frequent elevation of the affected part, together with elastic support, should be advised in order to keep the edema to a minimum.

CHAPTER 18

1. The pituitary gland develops from two sources: (a) a small ectodermal diverticulum, Rathke's pouch, which grows superiorly from the roof of the stomodeum, and (b) a small ectodermal downgrowth, which grows inferiorly from the floor of the diencephalon. A craniopharyngioma is a form of cystic epidermoid tumor that is thought to arise from remnants of Rathke's pouch. Such remnants sometimes become incorporated in the mesenchymal tissue which later forms the body of the sphenoid bone.

2. The following congenital anomalies may produce masses in the tongue: (a) lingual thyroid, (b) thyroglossal cyst, (c) lymphangioma, (d) hemangioma, and (e) neurofibroma. The absence of a thyroid gland in the normal position in the neck, together with the position of the mass beneath the foramen cecum, makes the diagnosis of a lingual thyroid certain. A thyroglossal cyst may be located within the tongue, but the thyroid gland would be felt in its normal position. Surgical ex-

cision of the lingual thyroid is the treatment of choice in this case, since the mass is large and is causing the patient discomfort. To avoid hypothyroidism, the excised mass of thyroid tissue should be transplanted into the soft tissues of the neck. If autotransplantation fails, the patient will have to receive thyroid hormone continuously for life.

3. This child is a cretin and has all the symptoms and signs of hypothyroidism. The treatment in such a case is the oral administration of thyroid hormone, which must be given as a single dose daily for the rest of the patient's life. The sooner the diagnosis is made, the sooner the treatment can be started and the better the prognosis. Delay may result in irreversible brain damage.

4. This patient has a thyroglossal cyst. It has developed as the result of a persistence of a small amount of epithelium that continues to secrete mucus within a segment of the thyroglossal duct. A cyst may develop at any point along the thyroglossal tract. Such a cyst is prone to infection, and for this reason it should be removed surgically. To avoid recurrence of the condition, it is important that all remnants of the thyroglossal duct be removed along with the cyst.

5. The parathyroid glands are developed from the entodermal lining of the pharynx. The inferior parathyroid glands arise from the lining of the third pharyngeal pouch on each side and are closely related to the developing thymus gland (see p. 267). As the thymic diverticulum on each side grows down the neck, it pulls the inferior parathyroid with it, so that usually it finally comes to rest on the posterior surface of the lateral lobe of the thyroid gland near its lower pole; it separates off completely from the thymus. If the parathyroid glands should remain attached to the thymus, they may be pulled down into the lower

part of the neck or thoracic cavity. The superior parathyroid glands are developed from the fourth pharyngeal pouch on each side and take up their final position on the posterior aspect of the lateral lobes of the thyroid gland, at about the level of the isthmus. They are much more constant in position than the inferior glands.

The variable position of the inferior parathyroid glands caused the surgeon some concern. The glands are supplied by the inferior thyroid arteries, and these should be carefully followed during the surgical operation until the inferior parathyroid glands are identified.

CHAPTER 19

1. This patient has spina bifida occulta involving the fifth lumbar vertebra. The condition is a result of failure of the embryonic mesenchyme to grow in between the neural tube and the surface ectoderm and form the vertebral arch; the vertebral canal remains open posteriorly. The defect has therefore existed since before birth and could not be seen or felt on physical examination because it was covered by the postvertebral muscles. The spinal cord and spinal nerve roots are usually normal. No treatment is required.
2. This child has a myelocele. In addition to the failure of the formation of the vertebral arches of the fourth and fifth lumbar vertebrae, the neural tube failed to close in this region. The oval raw area seen in this patient is the neural groove that has not united. The central canal is discharging clear cerebrospinal fluid onto the surface. The deformities of the knee joints and feet are due to the maldevelopment of the spinal cord in the lumbar region, with consequent interference with the innervation of certain muscle groups in the legs.
3. This child has hydrocephalus. A postmortem examination performed 1 year later showed that the aqueduct of Sylvius was not normally developed and consisted of a number of small tubules. This had resulted in the excessive accumulation of cerebrospinal fluid within the lateral and third ventricles of the brain. The distension of the ventricles, with the consequent enlargement of the brain and increased intracranial pressure, forced apart the bones of the cranial vault so that the head became greatly enlarged. The downward pressure on the orbital plates of the frontal bone caused the eyes to look downward. The optic atrophy was probably caused by the stretching of the optic nerve. The increased muscle tone of the lower limbs was almost certainly due to destruction of the corticospinal tracts by the expanding lateral ventricles. Although in some cases the head ceases to enlarge spontaneously, in the majority the hydrocephalus is progressive and death ultimately occurs. Surgical treatment of hydrocephalus may be attempted (see p. 299).
4. This child has cranioschisis between the frontal and nasal bones. A cephalic meningocele is associated with this defect. The fluctuation apparent on palpation is due to the presence of cerebrospinal fluid within the subarachnoid space, which could be returned to the intracranial cavity by exerting gentle pressure on the swelling. The pulse is due to transmission of the pulse wave from the cerebral arteries through the cerebrospinal fluid.

CHAPTER 20

1. Peripheral nerves show considerable variation in their arrangement, and this is commonly found in the brachial plexus. There may be variations in the formation of (a) the roots of the plexus, (b) the trunks of the plexus, and (c) the cords and branches. Moreover, there may be variations in the relation of the plexus to the axillary artery.

Embryologically, the contributions from the spinal nerves may be determined by the position of the limb bud in relation to the spinal cord. A postfixed plexus is one in which T2 gives a major contribution to the plexus, whereas that from C4 is deficient or absent. In the same manner a prefixed plexus is one in which C4 gives a major contribution to the plexus, whereas that from T2 is lacking or absent.

2. This is an example of a variation of the arrangement of the peripheral nerves found in the brachial plexus. In this case it is possible that, during the formation of the plexus in the embryo, the nerve axons destined for the median nerve from the lateral cord accompanied the musculocutaneous nerve for a short distance and finally left as a branch of the musculocutaneous nerve to join the median nerve. This variation is relatively common.

3. This boy has neurofibromatosis. The presence of brown pigmented patches and pigmented fibromas of the skin is characteristic of the disease. Because it is often associated with multiple neurofibromas occurring in the spinal and cranial nerves and in parts of the central and autonomic nervous systems, it is advisable to perform a careful neurological examination in these cases. This condition is inherited as an autosomal dominant trait.

CHAPTER 21

1. This child has a congenital medial strabismus (squint) of the right eye. The condition is due to an imbalance of the extraocular muscles. Although strabismus can be caused by abnormalities of the central nervous system, in many cases the condition is due to a simple congenital muscle imbalance, and about half the cases are familial. The condition never cures itself spontaneously and all cases should be referred to an ophthalmologist for treatment

as soon as possible. In this case the deviating right eye, which was not being used for seeing, failed to develop good central vision, and the child actually suppressed the image. Covering the normal undeviated eye immediately revealed the impaired vision in the deviating eye.

2. The rubella virus is a potent teratogenic agent (see p. 420). The virus is transmitted to the fetus via the placenta, and the effects on the fetus are usually multiple. If the mother is infected with rubella between the fourth and seventh weeks of pregnancy, a time when the lens is actively developing, congenital cataract may appear in the child. In a similar manner the organ of Corti of the ear may undergo viral destruction. The most common heart anomalies caused by rubella are pulmonary stenosis, patent ductus arteriosus, and ventricular septal defects. Remember that a child born of a mother who has been infected by rubella will have the virus within its tissues for many months after birth. This fact will cause you to delay surgical removal of the cataract for at least 2 years (Scheie and Albert—see Chap. 21 references).

3. This child has a small coloboma of the iris of the left eye. The condition is due to a failure of closure of the optic fissure. The anomaly may be minimal, as in this case, or may extensively involve the uveal tissue, with defects in the ciliary body and retina.

4. This child has congenital atresia of the external auditory meatus; the defect involves the inner end of the cartilaginous part of the meatus. Associated with this condition is a small auricular appendage containing a core of cartilage.

CHAPTER 22

1. This child is suffering from icthyosis simplex. The disease is often familial and has a genetic background.

2. This boy has a dermoid cyst, which has resulted from the burying by skin fusion of ectodermal cells along the line of closure, between the maxillary process and the frontonasal process, on the right side. Because a dermoid cyst will gradually increase in size, may become infected, and is cosmetically unpleasant, it should be excised.

3. The diagnosis is congenital alopecia.

4. This child has congenital hypertrichosis involving the limbs. It can be treated easily by using proprietary depilatory agents.

5. This woman has an additional nipple and areola (polythelia) on the right side. The nipple in such cases is very small, and there is no evidence of the presence of underlying breast tissue. It should be noted that the site of the additional nipple in this case is along a line corresponding to the position of the milk ridge. The darkening of the nipple and areola, which occurred at the time of puberty, was produced by the influence of the female sex hormones on the melanocytes in the epidermis; the normally placed nipples and areolae also darkened at this time. Polythelia is a common anomaly and should not be confused with pigmented moles.

6. Congenital retracted or inverted nipple is due to a failure in the development of the nipple during the later embryological stages. The ectodermal thickening which forms the nipple does not become raised, due to an absence of proliferation of the underlying mesenchyme. The condition is bilateral in about one-quarter of the cases. Congenital inverted nipple must not be confused with a nipple that has become recently retracted from an underlying scirrhous carcinoma. The expectant mother should be encouraged to draw the nipple out, using traction with the fingers, during the remaining months of the pregnancy. If the nipple fails to protrude with this treatment, breast-feeding is out of the question.

7. This woman has an accessory breast on the left side (polymastia). Following parturition the accessory breast will become swollen and painful. Later the breast will shrink in size and give no further discomfort.

8. This woman has micromastia on the right side. It is common to find some degree of asymmetry between the two breasts, particularly in women with very large breasts. In this case the plastic surgeon decided to augment the size of the right breast by the implantation of a foam-like plastic material into the retromammary tissues.

9. Mild enlargement and tingling sensations in both breasts is common in most boys at puberty. The condition usually regresses within a few months. It is believed to be due to the secretion of estrogens as well as androgens by the testes at the time of puberty. Gynecomastia rarely persists for more than 2 years. This should be fully explained to this boy and his parents. If the enlargement of the left breast persists, or the breast further increases in size and is emotionally upsetting to the patient, some form of plastic operation should be undertaken to reduce the size of the breast.

10. This child is a complete albino. The disease is inherited by a single recessive gene, which is not sex-linked. In this condition there is a genetic absence of the enzyme tyrosinase in the melanocytes. It is unusual to find complete albinism in man. In the commoner incomplete form the hair is yellow or light brown and the irides are light blue or pink.

CHAPTER 23

1. This child has congenital torticollis. Most cases of congenital torticollis are believed

to result from excessive stretching of the sternocleidomastoid muscle during a difficult delivery. The tender swelling noted by the mother was due to the presence of blood clot, which had followed hemorrhage into the damaged muscle. Later the blood clot had become invaded by fibrous tissue, which contracted down and shortened the muscle, thus producing the deformity. This was followed by a secondary shortening of the fasciae and other muscles on that side of the neck. If congenital torticollis is left untreated, the deformity worsens as the neck elongates, and there is a gradual atrophy of the face on the affected side, the cervical vertebrae often becoming wedge-shaped. In a mild case the shortened muscle should be gently stretched and exercised daily as soon as the diagnosis is made. In this 6-year-old child, operative division of the affected sternocleidomastoid and other shortened muscles and fasciae is the treatment of choice.

2. This child has arthrogryphosis multiplex. This is a relatively rare disorder of unknown etiology, although some authorities believe that a contributing factor may be severe loss of mobility of the limb joints while the fetus is in utero. The joint capsules and ligaments are thickened and inelastic, and the muscles acting on the joints are atrophied. In many cases there is evidence of degeneration of the nerve cells in the anterior horns of the spinal cord. Associated with this disease it is quite common to find other congenital anomalies such as cleft palate, hypoplasia of the mandible, and absent sacrum.

3. This child has the typical signs of achondroplasia (see p. 377). The condition is inherited as a mendelian dominant trait and is the commonest cause of dwarfism.

4. This little girl has osteogenesis imperfecta. The disease is fully discussed on page 377. This case is moderately severe, since the child already has multiple fractures and is greatly deformed. Some of the fractures probably occurred before birth. The prognosis in such a case is poor. There is no specific treatment. When holding these children, great care must be exercised to avoid further fractures. The correct treatment of all fractures must be instituted when they occur, and osteotomy may be carried out where bones have united in bad positions.

5. This girl and her mother have craniocleidodysostosis. This condition is caused by the inheritance of an autosomal dominant gene resulting in the incomplete formation or absence of the clavicles. The membrane bones of the skull are also involved, causing the fontanelles to remain wide open. No treatment is necessary, since the excessive mobility of the shoulders is not a hindrance. However, in some cases the sternal or acromial ends of the clavicle may develop and exert pressure on the brachial plexus. In these cases, the offending bony fragments should be removed.

6. This man has diaphyseal aclasis. In this condition the bony tumor on each leg consists of spongy bone covered by compact bone. It is surmounted by a cap of hyaline cartilage from which continuous growth in size takes place. The exostoses are usually bilateral, as in this case. They originate from the metaphyseal region of bones. The treatment is to remove exostoses that are causing trouble by pressure on neighboring structures such as muscles, tendons, or nerves.

7. This child has Klippel-Feil syndrome, in which the cervical vertebrae are reduced in number, and those that are present are deformed and often fused into one bony mass. It is often associated with Sprengel's shoulder (high position of the scapula), torticollis, and spina bifida. The condi-

tion is deforming and causes some disability, but no treatment is necessary.

8. This girl has a congenital scoliosis due to a hemivertebra at the T5 level with compensatory curves above and below this defect. Apart from the congenital scoliosis, she has congenital fusion of the fifth and sixth ribs on the left side. A hemivertebra is caused by a failure in development of one of the two ossification centers that appear in the centrum of the body of each vertebra. A hemivertebra in the thoracic region is often associated with aplasia or fusion of adjacent ribs. In this case the child has no symptoms and the compensatory curves are well balanced so that no special treatment is required.

9. This man has spondylolisthesis involving the fifth lumbar vertebra. During the year that he had experienced low back pain, the body of the fifth lumbar vertebra had slowly become dislocated in front of the sacrum. The embryological explanation for this condition is given on page 379.

10. This woman has a cervical rib on the right side of the neck, causing pressure on the lower trunk of the brachial plexus (C8 and T1). Pressure on the nerve trunk is responsible for the pain and paresthesia on the medial side of the right forearm and hand and the atrophy of the small muscles of the right hand. As the patient became tired toward the end of the day, the shoulder girdles dropped, increasing the tension on the nerve trunk as it passed over the cervical rib. Further depression of the shoulder caused occlusion of the subclavian artery as it passed over the cervical rib. A cervical rib occurs as the result of excessive development of the anterior tubercle of the transverse process of the seventh cervical vertebra. The different varieties are discussed on page 381. The treatment in this case is to remove the additional rib surgically.

11. This child has a funnel chest. Although the precise cause is unknown, it is believed by some authorities to be due to a congenitally short central tendon of the diaphragm. The diaphragm pulls exclusively upon the lower end of the sternum, which gradually becomes depressed. If the depression of the sternum is so severe as to cause embarrassment to the patient or is interfering with pulmonary function, some form of surgical correction should be attempted. In this case there were no symptoms, so that the parents were advised against surgical interference.

12. *Amelia* is the name given to the condition in which a child is born with one or more limbs absent. Thalidomide was widely used in Britain and Western Germany between 1960 and 1962. It has been found to be a potent teratogenic agent and may well have been responsible for amelia in this case. Needless to say, this drug has been withdrawn from clinical use.

13. This boy has a right-sided Sprengel's shoulder. The right scapula is unable to rotate because it is fixed to the vertebral column by a bar of bone. The scapula is normally formed high up in the neck, and during development it progressively descends to the posterior surface of the upper part of the thorax. Why the descent should be arrested in this disease is not fully understood. In this case the development of a bridge of bone anchoring the scapula to the vertebral column probably played a part in its arrest. However, many cases have been reported in which the descent of the scapula is arrested in the absence of a bony bridge.

14. Bilateral congenital absence of the radius is the diagnosis. Some form of surgical treatment is required to correct the deformity and improve the function of the hand.

15. This child has trigger thumb on the right side. The condition is due to a localized congenital narrowing of the fibrous flexor

sheath covering the flexor pollicis longus tendon. It is often accompanied by a localized thickening of the flexor pollicis longus tendon. When passive pressure is applied to the distal end of the thumb, the tendon is pulled through the narrowed portion of the sheath, and the thumb jerks into the extended position. Gentle passive exercises of the thumb by the mother at each bath time for 6 months often results in a spontaneous cure. If this fails, the flexor sheath should be incised at about 1 year of age.

16. This child has local gigantism affecting the little and ring fingers of the right hand (macrodactyly). The most likely cause for this condition in this case is neurofibromatosis involving the digital branches of the ulnar nerve. Occasionally, a hemangioma may be responsible for local enlargement of a digit.

17. This girl has a congenital dislocation of the right hip joint.

18. This baby has bilateral congenital talipes equinovarus—talipes (clubfoot), equino (plantar-flexed at the ankle joint), varus (adducted and inverted at the talonavicular joint). The treatment is repeated manipulation and splinting in the over-corrected position. The functional result in children treated early is extremely good.

CHAPTER 24

1. Labor or parturition is the series of processes by which the baby, the fetal membranes, and the placenta are expelled from the genital tract of the mother. The attitude of the fetus, transverse lie, and the presenting part are terms that are defined on page 395.

2. In a primigravida the fundus of the uterus reaches the level of the xiphoid process at approximately the ninth month of gestation.

3. Seven days are added to the date of onset of the last menstrual period; i.e., November 10 + 7 = November 17. Three months are then subtracted; i.e., November 17 − 3 months = August 17 of the following year. This is the expected date of delivery.

4. The theoretical causes for the onset of labor in a normal person are fully discussed on page 396.

5. The process of labor is divided into three stages. The first stage, or stage of dilatation, begins with the onset of regular, forceful uterine contractions and ends with complete dilatation of the cervix. The second stage, or stage of expulsion, begins with the complete dilatation of the cervix and ends with the complete delivery of the baby. The third, or placental, stage begins immediately following the delivery of the baby and ends with the expulsion of the placenta and fetal membranes.

6. The signs and symptoms of labor are: (a) Painful, rhythmic uterine contractions. During each contraction the uterus feels hard on palpation. (b) The appearance at the vaginal orifice of the blood-stained cervical plug of mucus. (c) The cervix begins to dilate.

7. In a primigravida the second stage of labor normally lasts about 50 minutes. In the multigravida the second stage is usually of considerably shorter duration, since the maternal soft tissues offer less resistance.

8. The bloody show is the presence of the blood-stained plug of cervical mucus which appears at the vaginal orifice at the onset of labor. As the liquor amnii and the fetal membranes are forced down into the cervical canal, the cervix slowly dilates. The pulling away of the membranes from the uterine wall in the region of the internal os of the cervix is responsible for the bleeding.

9. Placental separation takes place at the spongy layer of the decidua basalis.

10. The *afterbirth* is the term sometimes used for the expelled placenta and fetal membranes after they have left the birth canal.

11. The lochia is the name given to the discharge from the genital tract of the mother that occurs during the first 6 to 8 weeks of the puerperium. It is first bright red and consists of blood and decidual remains; later it becomes brown, then yellow, then finally stops.

12. Following separation and expulsion of the placenta and fetal membranes from the uterine cavity, the walls become lined with endometrium within 2 to 3 weeks after delivery.

CHAPTER 25

1. The cheese-like material is called *vernix caseosa*. This material is a mixture of the epitrichium (see p. 343) and the secretions of the sebaceous glands. The fine hairs seen on the shoulders and back are the remains of the first hairs to appear on the skin surface and are known as *lanugo hairs*. In the majority of children these are cast off just before birth or very soon afterward.

2. The neonatal period is the first 4-week period after birth.

3. It is now generally accepted that rhythmic respiratory movements do not take place in the mature fetus in utero unless it is subjected to partial asphyxia or is stimulated physically.

4. The normal average respiratory rate in the newborn is approximately 40 per minute and is regular. This is a considerably higher rate than in the normal adult, which is approximately 16 times per minute and is regular. In the newborn the ribs are nearly horizontal in position, and very little movement of the thoracic cage takes place. Respiration is mainly brought about by the diaphragm, and this is accompanied by reciprocal movement of the muscles of the anterior abdominal wall.

5. The lungs are not fully expanded when a child takes his first breath. Some degree of atelectasis may be present for several days after birth. Adequate amounts of surfactant must be present in the lungs at birth to overcome the surface-tension forces within the alveoli so that effective ventilation can be established. Surfactant is thought to be produced by the cells lining the alveoli.

6. In the newborn the peripheral circulation is initially slow. In a normal child this cyanosis disappears within a few hours and the skin becomes pink. The child should be covered by a blanket and kept in a warm room.

7. If the umbilical cord is not tied immediately at birth, the blood flow through the umbilical arteries and the umbilical vein may continue for several minutes after delivery, although at a rapidly decreasing rate (see p. 405). When the application of a ligature is delayed, the fetal blood is expressed from the placenta by the contracting uterus and returned to the fetus, thus increasing the blood volume within the fetus by as much as 100 ml. It should be remembered, however, that at birth the baby has a very high red cell count, which was necessary during intra-uterine life but is not necessary after birth. Allowing the infant to have extra blood from the placenta at birth is unnecessary since the excess of cells is broken down soon afterward and the baby is more likely to be jaundiced from the additional bilirubin produced. Delay is also liable to cause exposure and chilling of the baby. It is now generally agreed that there is no advantage in delaying the tying of the umbilical cord beyond a minute after delivery.

8. The pulse rate is rapid, with an average of 130 beats per minute.

9. There is a wide variation in the normal total leukocyte count in the newborn; values of 10,000 to 35,000 per cubic millimeter are considered normal. On the third or fourth day the count drops rapidly. The majority of cells are neutrophils. After the third week the lymphocytes predominate, and this predominance persists until the fourth year.

10. Icterus neonatorum (physiological jaundice) is very common. In nearly half of all healthy babies, the bilirubin content of the blood is raised sufficiently to cause a mild degree of jaundice. The condition is due to the immaturity of the liver enzymes, causing a temporary impairment of the excretion of bilirubin by the liver and an increased destruction of erythrocytes at this time. It is more likely to occur in premature babies because of the greater immaturity of the liver.

11. Almost immediately after birth the body temperature falls by as much as 3 degrees. Increased general metabolic activity and improved vasomotor control of the peripheral blood vessels result in the temperature rising and becoming stabilized within 8 hours.

12. The first stools are referred to as *meconium*. Meconium is dark green in color, sticky, and odorless. It consists of a mixture of digestive secretions, bile pigments, desquamated cells, and lanugo and vernix caseosa swallowed with the amniotic fluid; 3 or 4 days later the stools become greenish-yellow, and after the fifth day the yellow milk stools appear.

13. A baby commonly empties his bladder immediately after birth. However, quite often, the emptying of the bladder may be delayed for as long as 24 hours.

14. During the first 3 to 5 days, the child loses up to 10 percent of his birth weight by loss of fluid from the body and a relatively low fluid intake.

15. A newborn baby normally keeps his fists clenched for about 2 months after birth.

16. It is normal for a newborn baby to exhibit a positive Babinski response, i.e., the toes are extended when the lateral plantar surface is stroked.

17. A newborn baby can hear at birth and responds to loud noises. The sensitivity of hearing improves after a few days as the result of aeration of the middle ear and the draining away of amniotic fluid. A baby does not shed tears until the end of the third or fourth week, when the lacrimal glands start to function.

18. The caput succedaneum is a diffuse swelling of the scalp found at birth and is caused by edema that has formed as a result of pressure of the scalp against the dilated cervix during the early stages of labor. It usually disappears in 2 days.

19. *Witch's milk* is the layman's term for the milky fluid which can sometimes be expressed from the nipples of newborn children of both sexes. It is due to the stimulation of the mammary glands in the child by the mother's estrogen, which has entered the fetal circulation across the placenta. The secretion ceases shortly after birth.

20. Yes. This fact is compensated for to some extent by the acquisition of passive immunity from the mother by the passage of antibodies across the placenta before birth.

CHAPTER 26

1. It has been estimated that about 2 percent of all newborn infants have defects that are either lethal at birth or will cause death or disability if left untreated.

2. Hydrocephalus may be recognized by virtue of the fact that the head remains above the pelvic brim, and on abdominal

examination the enlarged head may be felt on palpation to be softer than normal and more globular. Anencephaly and esophageal atresia may be suspected in cases of hydramnios. The transudation of cerebrospinal fluid from the exposed choroid plexuses will cause hydramnios in cases of anencephaly, and the failure of the fetus to swallow the amniotic fluid in cases of esophageal atresia will also produce hydramnios. Multiple deformities may be expected when the rare condition of oligohydramnios occurs. Adhesions of the membranes to the face, talipes equinovarus, and the presence of skin dimples over bony points due to pressure exerted on the fetus by the uterus are a few examples.

3. (a) Hydrocephalus is often associated with spina bifida, talipes, and cleft palate. (b) Mongolism tends to be associated with congenital heart disease and duodenal atresia. (c) Agenesis of the kidneys is often associated with lung abnormalities.

4. Clinical signs and congenital anomalies are discussed on page 413 and also under the different sections dealing with congenital anomalies.

5. According to the 1966 worldwide survey reported by the World Health Organization, the incidence of certain congenital anomalies varies greatly in different parts of the world; for example, the incidence of neural tube defects was 0.6 per 1,000 in Calcutta, India, and 10.2 per 1,000 in Belfast, Northern Ireland. Other examples are given on page 415.

6. The etiological factors responsible for many forms of congenital anomalies are described on pages 416 to 423.

7. The incidence of Down's syndrome in Western countries is estimated to be about 1 in 600 births. In complete mongolism, the eyes are small and the palpebral fissures slant downward at the medial ends. The epicanthal folds are prominent on either side. The skull is small and brachycephalic, with a flattened occipital region. The mouth is small and the tongue protrudes and is fissured. The hands are short and broad, and a deep transverse crease is seen across the palms. Mongoloids are mentally defective. An examination of the chromosome structure reveals trisomy 21, which confirms the diagnosis.

8. Some important syndromes are: Down's syndrome (trisomy 21), cri du chat syndrome (partial deletion of the short arm of one of the chromosome 5 pair), Klinefelter's syndrome (47 chromosomes, with a sex chromosomal constitution of XXY), Turner's syndrome (45 chromosomes, with a sex chromosomal constitution of XO).

9. Expectant mothers should be warned of the danger of taking drugs other than a mild purgative. They should always consult their obstetrician before taking any drug. Rubella is a potent teratogenic agent. If an expectant mother should come into contact with a person who has German measles, she should contact her obstetrician at once.

10. The terrible disappointment and concern expressed by the father and mother of a congenitally deformed child is not difficult to understand. The obstetrician, pediatrician, and nursing staff should comfort and give assurance to the couple. Having recovered from the initial shock the parents should be given positive advice as to the day-to-day management of the child. They should be told of the modern surgical and remedial treatment that is now available, and the future program of medical treatment should be carefully outlined to them. Every effort must be made by all medical personnel and the family to prepare the child so that he can live an independent existence. This may

require the help of speech therapists, physiotherapists, and occupational therapists and the use of artificial limbs and other appliances. For children who are severely mentally handicapped, the help of local residential training centers may be required.

The risk of a second child with a congenital anomaly is high in only a few cases. Nevertheless, the advice to parents must be based on a very careful medical history, the nature of the anomaly in the first child, and counseling from an expert geneticist.

Index